Non-Coding RNAs and Extracellular Vesicles in Cancer Crosstalk: Diagnostic and Therapeutic Implications

Non-Coding RNAs and Extracellular Vesicles in Cancer Crosstalk: Diagnostic and Therapeutic Implications

Guest Editors

Simona Taverna
Giuseppe Cammarata

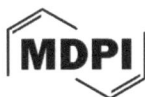

Basel • Beijing • Wuhan • Barcelona • Belgrade • Novi Sad • Cluj • Manchester

Guest Editors

Simona Taverna
Institute of Translational
Pharmacology
National Research Council
Palermo
Italy

Giuseppe Cammarata
Institute of Translational
Pharmacology
National Research Council
Palermo
Italy

Editorial Office
MDPI AG
Grosspeteranlage 5
4052 Basel, Switzerland

This is a reprint of the Special Issue, published open access by the journal *Cancers* (ISSN 2072-6694), freely accessible at: https://www.mdpi.com/journal/cancers/special_issues/FLD3RHO0KX.

For citation purposes, cite each article independently as indicated on the article page online and as indicated below:

Lastname, A.A.; Lastname, B.B. Article Title. *Journal Name* **Year**, *Volume Number*, Page Range.

ISBN 978-3-7258-4309-1 (Hbk)
ISBN 978-3-7258-4310-7 (PDF)
https://doi.org/10.3390/books978-3-7258-4310-7

© 2025 by the authors. Articles in this book are Open Access and distributed under the Creative Commons Attribution (CC BY) license. The book as a whole is distributed by MDPI under the terms and conditions of the Creative Commons Attribution-NonCommercial-NoDerivs (CC BY-NC-ND) license (https://creativecommons.org/licenses/by-nc-nd/4.0/).

Contents

Valentina Bollati, Paola Monti, Davide Biganzoli, Giuseppe Marano, Chiara Favero, Simona Iodice, et al.
Environmental and Lifestyle Cancer Risk Factors: Shaping Extracellular Vesicle OncomiRs and Paving the Path to Cancer Development
Reprinted from: *Cancers* 2023, 15, 4317, https://doi.org/10.3390/cancers15174317 1

Anna Paola Carreca, Rosaria Tinnirello, Vitale Miceli, Antonio Galvano, Valerio Gristina, Lorena Incorvaia, et al.
Extracellular Vesicles in Lung Cancer: Implementation in Diagnosis and Therapeutic Perspectives
Reprinted from: *Cancers* 2024, 16, 1967, https://doi.org/10.3390/cancers16111967 19

Giuseppa Augello, Alessandra Cusimano, Melchiorre Cervello and Antonella Cusimano
Extracellular Vesicle-Related Non-Coding RNAs in Hepatocellular Carcinoma: An Overview
Reprinted from: *Cancers* 2024, 16, 1415, https://doi.org/10.3390/cancers16071415 40

Edoardo Garbo, Benedetta Del Rio, Giorgia Ferrari, Massimiliano Cani, Valerio Maria Napoli, Valentina Bertaglia, et al.
Exploring the Potential of Non-Coding RNAs as Liquid Biopsy Biomarkers for Lung Cancer Screening: A Literature Review
Reprinted from: *Cancers* 2023, 15, 4774, https://doi.org/10.3390/cancers15194774 62

Giuseppe Fabio Parisi, Maria Papale, Giulia Pecora, Novella Rotolo, Sara Manti, Giovanna Russo and Salvatore Leonardi
Cystic Fibrosis and Cancer: Unraveling the Complex Role of CFTR Gene in Cancer Susceptibility
Reprinted from: *Cancers* 2023, 15, 4244, https://doi.org/10.3390/cancers15174244 82

Simona Taverna, Anna Masucci and Giuseppe Cammarata
PIWI-RNAs Small Noncoding RNAs with Smart Functions: Potential Theranostic Applications in Cancer
Reprinted from: *Cancers* 2023, 15, 3912, https://doi.org/10.3390/cancers15153912 99

Ya-Ting Chuang, Jen-Yang Tang, Jun-Ping Shiau, Ching-Yu Yen, Fang-Rong Chang, Kun-Han Yang, et al.
Modulating Effects of Cancer-Derived Exosomal miRNAs and Exosomal Processing by Natural Products
Reprinted from: *Cancers* 2023, 15, 318, https://doi.org/10.3390/cancers15010318 118

Giusy Daniela Albano, Rosalia Gagliardo, Angela Marina Montalbano and Mirella Profita
Non-Coding RNAs in Airway Diseases: A Brief Overview of Recent Data
Reprinted from: *Cancers* 2023, 15, 54, https://doi.org/10.3390/cancers15010054 143

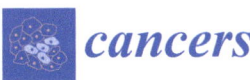

Article

Environmental and Lifestyle Cancer Risk Factors: Shaping Extracellular Vesicle OncomiRs and Paving the Path to Cancer Development

Valentina Bollati [1,2,*], Paola Monti [1], Davide Biganzoli [3], Giuseppe Marano [4], Chiara Favero [1], Simona Iodice [1], Luca Ferrari [1,2], Laura Dioni [1], Francesca Bianchi [5,6], Angela Cecilia Pesatori [1,2] and Elia Mario Biganzoli [4,*]

[1] Epiget Lab, Department of Clinical Sciences and Community Health, University of Milan, 20133 Milan, Italy; paola.monti@unimi.it (P.M.); chiara.favero@unimi.it (C.F.); simona.iodice@unimi.it (S.I.); luca.ferrari@unimi.it (L.F.); laura.dioni@unimi.it (L.D.); angela.pesatori@unimi.it (A.C.P.)
[2] Occupational Health Unit, Fondazione IRCCS Ca' Granda Ospedale Maggiore Policlinico, 20122 Milan, Italy
[3] Center of Functional Genomics and Rare Diseases, Buzzi Children's Hospital, 20154 Milan, Italy; davide.biganzoli@asst-fbf-sacco.it
[4] Unit of Medical Statistics, Bioinformatics and Epidemiology, Department of Biomedical and Clinical Sciences (DIBIC), University of Milan, 20133 Milan, Italy; giuseppe.marano@unimi.it
[5] Dipartimento di Scienze Biomediche per la Salute, University of Milan, 20133 Milan, Italy; francesca.bianchi@unimi.it
[6] U. O. Laboratorio Morfologia Umana Applicata, IRCCS Policlinico San Donato, 20097 Milan, Italy
* Correspondence: valentina.bollati@unimi.it (V.B.); elia.biganzoli@unimi.it (E.M.B.); Tel.: +39-02-503220127 (V.B.); +39-02-50319886 (E.M.B.)

Simple Summary: In this study, we aim to shed light on a fascinating new aspect of cellular communication involving extracellular vesicles (EVs) and their cargo of microRNAs (EV-miRNAs). These EVs were once thought of as cellular waste but are now known to play a crucial role in transferring vital information between cells. We investigated how EV-miRNAs respond to various environmental and lifestyle factors and how this might be linked to the development and progression of cancer. By analyzing the associations between these factors and specific miRNAs related to common cancers (oncomiRs), we aim to better understand the complex regulatory networks of miRNAs in response to exogenous influences. The findings could revolutionize our understanding of cancer development and have important implications for future exposome studies in the research community.

Abstract: Intercellular communication has been transformed by the discovery of extracellular vesicles (EVs) and their cargo, including microRNAs (miRNAs), which play crucial roles in intercellular signaling. These EVs were previously disregarded as cellular debris but are now recognized as vital mediators of biological information transfer between cells. Furthermore, they respond not only to internal stimuli but also to environmental and lifestyle factors. Identifying EV-borne oncomiRs, a subset of miRNAs implicated in cancer development, could revolutionize our understanding of how environmental and lifestyle exposures contribute to oncogenesis. To investigate this, we studied the plasma levels of EV-borne oncomiRs in a population of 673 women and 238 men with a body mass index > 25 kg/m^2 (SPHERE population). The top fifty oncomiRs associated with the three most common cancers in women (breast, colorectal, and lung carcinomas) and men (lung, prostate, and colorectal carcinomas) were selected from the OncomiR database. Only oncomiRs expressed in more than 20% of the population were considered for statistical analysis. Using a Multivariate Adaptive Regression Splines (MARS) model, we explored the interactions between environmental/lifestyle exposures and EV oncomiRs to develop optimized predictor combinations for each EV oncomiR. This innovative approach allowed us to better understand miRNA regulation in response to multiple environmental and lifestyle influences. By uncovering non-linear relationships among variables, we gained valuable insights into the complexity of miRNA regulatory networks. Ultimately, this research paves the way for comprehensive exposome studies in the future.

Keywords: oncomiR; exposome; lifestyle factors; environmental exposures; SPHERE population; MARS models

1. Introduction

Environmental and lifestyle factors exert a profound influence on chronic diseases, particularly in the context of cancer development and related clinical outcomes [1,2]. These factors encompass diverse elements [3,4], ranging from exposure to environmental carcinogens and dietary habits [5] to physical activity levels [6], adiposity [7], smoking, alcohol consumption [8], and socioeconomic status [9]. The intricate interplay between these factors and cancer etiology underscores the necessity for a comprehensive approach to cancer prevention and management. By addressing the environmental and lifestyle determinants of cancer, we can implement targeted interventions and promote healthier behaviors [10], aiming to reduce non-intrinsic cancer risks and enhance clinical outcomes in a personalized way.

Individuals with pre-existing hypersusceptibility conditions, such as those associated with adiposity (excessive body fat), might experience an amplified influence from the exposome, i.e., an accumulation of lifelong environmental exposures [11,12]. Adiposity-related conditions, like being overweight/obesity and metabolic syndrome, foster a hormonally dysregulated and pro-inflammatory environment both at systemic and tissue levels. This inflamed host environment can synergize with external exposures, augmenting the vulnerability to cancer development and progression [11,13].

Extracellular vesicles (EVs), encompassing exosomes and microvesicles, are small membrane-bound structures released by various cell types [14]. Once considered cellular debris, EVs are now recognized as sophisticated carriers of cellular cargo, including proteins, lipids, and nucleic acids [15]. Owing to their ability to traverse biological barriers, EVs serve as conduits for intercellular communication and facilitate information exchanges between cells, even across distant locations within the body [14]. These distinctive attributes render EVs versatile entities with significant roles in diverse physiological processes and disease contexts, including cancer [16,17].

MicroRNAs (miRNAs) are pivotal regulators of gene expression among the myriad of molecules transported by EVs. MiRNAs, short non-coding RNA molecules, play a critical role in post-transcriptional gene regulation by targeting messenger RNAs (mRNAs) for degradation or translational inhibition [18]. Within this group, oncomiRs, a subset of miRNAs, have garnered attention for their involvement in cancer-related processes, including tumor initiation, growth, metastasis, and therapy resistance [19,20].

Understanding the mechanisms driving the selective packaging of oncomiRs into EVs and their subsequent release into the extracellular space has become central in cancer research. EVs enriched with oncomiRs can engage in cell-to-cell communication, delivering functional oncomiRs to recipient cells—ranging from neighboring cancer cells to fibroblasts, adipocytes, and immune cells. This transfer reshapes the gene expression profiles and behavior of recipient cells, contributing to the ability of cancer cells to shape both local and distant microenvironments. EVs containing miRNAs thus dynamically orchestrate multidirectional communication, serving as the hubs of the intercellular network, ultimately transforming the microenvironment in a pro-tumoral manner. This intriguing phenomenon fuels interest in cancer biology as it may hold substantial implications for innovative diagnostics and therapeutic strategies.

The SPHERE project [21], with its unique attributes, has enabled the investigation of EVs and their miRNA content's role in mediating the impact of air particulate matter (PM) on cardiovascular health. The SPHERE study offers comprehensive insights into the microRNA content of EVs within a population of over 2000 individuals characterized by a body mass index (BMI) exceeding 25 and a well-defined exposome.

In this paper, we delve into the captivating domain of EVs and oncomiRs, probing the oncomiRs associated with specific cancer types based on their dependency on major exposome factors in the SPHERE screening subpopulation of 911 non-oncological subjects with assessed miRNome.

Given the complexity of analyzing these data, it is essential to consider the application of inductive inference methods rooted in machine learning, extending multivariate analysis and regression approaches. In this context, adopting automated methods for variable selection and their preferably non-linear/non-additive effects on EV-contained miRNA expression is pivotal. Within the realm of multiple regression models, the Multivariate Adaptive Regression Splines (MARS) methodology appears promising, given its ability to automatically identify non-linear effects and interactions (effect modifiers) among predictors.

2. Materials and Methods

2.1. Study Design and Participants

We recruited 911 subjects who were overweight/obese from the Center for Obesity and Work at IRCCS Fondazione Ca'Granda—Ospedale Maggiore Policlinico, Milan, Italy, between September 2010 and March 2015 (recruitment of the subset reported in the present paper ended on January 2013). This was the screening subset of the cross-sectional study, SPHERE (Susceptibility to Particle Health Effects, miRNAs, and Exosomes), funded by the European Research Council (ERC); it focused on investigating the interplay between particle health effects, miRNAs, and EVs [21,22]. Briefly, the eligibility criteria included being over 18 years old, having a BMI ≥ 25 kg/m^2, residing in the Lombardy region (Italy), and providing informed consent and blood/urine samples. Exclusions were recent (i.e., in the last 5 years) cancer, heart disease, stroke, or other chronic conditions. This study followed the Helsinki Declaration principles and received ethics committee approval from the Fondazione IRCCS Ca'Granda Ospedale Maggiore Policlinico di Milano (approval number 1425). The participation rate was 92%.

2.2. Isolation and Purification of EVs and miRNA-EVs from Plasma

EV preparation and miRNA analysis have been described elsewhere [22]. Briefly, blood was collected in EDTA tubes in the morning and transported to the EPIGET Lab (University of Milan) within 2 h. Blood was centrifuged at $1200 \times g$ for 15 min at room temperature to obtain plasma, followed by additional centrifugation steps (1000, 2000, and $3000 \times g$ for 15 min at 4 °C) to remove debris. Plasma was ultracentrifuged (Beckman Coulter Optima-MAX-XP, Brea, CA, USA) at $110,000 \times g$ for 75 min at 4 °C to obtain an EV-rich pellet, which was resuspended in filtered PBS. MiRNAs were isolated from frozen EV pellets using the miRNeasy Kit and RNeasy CleanUp Kit (Qiagen, Germantown, MD, USA) and stored at -80 °C.

2.3. miRNA Analysis

For reverse transcription (RT), Megaplex™ RT Primers (Pool A v2.1 and Pool B v3.0) and the TaqMan® Micro RNA Reverse Transcriptase Kit (Life Technologies, Foster City, CA, USA) were used. Two reactions were performed to cover 754 target miRNAs, including 16 replicates of 4 internal controls (ath-miR159a, RNU48, RNU44, and U6). Each reaction consisted of 0.75 µL of Megaplex RT Primers (Pool A or Pool B), 0.15 µL of dNTPs, 0.75 µL of $10 \times$ RT Buffer, 0.90 µL of MgCl2, 0.1 µL of RNase Inhibitor, 1.5 µL of MultiScribe™ Reverse Transcriptase, and 3.3 µL of miRNAs. After incubation on ice for 5 min, the mixture underwent a thermal protocol in a C1000 Thermal Cycler (Biorad, Hercules, CA, USA) with specific temperature cycles. The resulting cDNA samples were stored at -20 °C until further use. For preamplification, each cDNA requiring preamplification was loaded onto a 96-well plate and combined with TaqMan® PreAmp Master Mix, nuclease-free water, and Megaplex™ PreAmp Primers. The preamplification reaction involved specific thermal conditions and the preamplified samples were stored at 4 °C until analysis with the OpenArray® System. The preamplified cDNA was diluted and mixed with TaqMan OpenArray® Real-Time PCR Master Mix. The reaction mix was aliquoted into the wells of a 384-well OpenArray® plate using the MicroLab STAR Let instrument (Hamilton Robotics, Birmingham, UK). The plate was then loaded into a TaqMan™ OpenArray® Human miRNA Panel using the QuantStudio™ AccuFill System Robot (Life Technologies, Foster City, CA, USA). Finally, the mixture was analyzed with the QuantStudio™ 12K Flex Real-Time PCR System and the OpenArray® Platform (QS12KFlex) following the manufacturer's instructions.

In total, 545 miRNAs were included in the analysis after the exclusion of non-amplified miRNAs. The application of the global mean was identified as the optimal normalization method; miRNA expression levels were quantified using relative quantification, represented as $2^{-\Delta Ct}$. Leveraging the OncomiR database [23], we extracted the top 50 oncomiRs for each of the 3 most prevalent cancers in both women (breast, colorectal, and lung carcinomas) and men (lung, prostate, and colorectal carcinomas) [24]. Notably, this selection process was underpinned by stringent criteria, including a significance threshold of a p-value < 0.0001 and a false discovery rate (FDR) < 0.0001. OncomiRs expressed at detectable levels in more than 20% of our populations were considered for statistical analysis. This threshold was chosen after looking at the distributions of the miRNA measures allowing for the best compromise between the number of selected miRNAs and their detection prevalence in the population, thereby ensuring that our findings possess broader applicability.

2.4. Statistical Analysis

The data consisted of 911 records, including information about 75 EV oncomiR expressions and exposome factors. The latter consisted of numerical variables: age, BMI, residence PM10 exposure (annual average), C-reactive protein (CRP), homocysteine, coffee consumption (cup/week), alcohol consumption (glass/week), number of previous pregnancies; and categorical variables: education (primary school or less, secondary school, high school, university or more), occupation (employee, unemployed, retired, housewife), residence traffic exposure (mild, moderate, high), lifestyle (sedentary, active, sportive), smoking habit (never, former smoker, current smoker), passive smoker (no, yes), menopausal status (no, yes), use of antidepressants (no, yes), use of oral contraceptives (no, yes).

The strategy of analysis sketched in the following section was applied separately for female and male data. In the first step, multivariate relationships among miRNA expressions and exposure variables were investigated via a multivariate analysis approach using Factor Analysis of Mixed Data (FAMD) methods [25,26]. In this context, exposure variables were considered active variables and miRNA expressions were considered supplementary (or passive) variables. According to FAMD methods, the following strategy of analysis was adopted: (1) the number of relevant principal axes that summarize the active variables was chosen by evaluating the indices of the explained inertia; (2) the relationships among the exposure variables and principal axes were evaluated by a plot of squared correlation coefficients; (3) finally, the relationships among the miRNA expressions and exposure variables were evaluated by the plotting the orthogonal projections of the former ones onto the principal axes (passive projections plot).

The "ggstatsplot" package [27] was used to perform Spearman correlation analysis on miRNA expression and "ggplot2" was used to visualize the results by generating a heatmap.

Multivariate Adaptive Regression Spline (MARS) models [28] were fitted to explore non-linear and non-additive relationships between single miRNA expressions and exposure variables. According to MARS methods, a regression model is built by performing two automatic selection steps. In the former one, called the forward step, additive and interaction effects, also including the non-linear effects of numerical variables, are included in the model according to the reduction of a sum-of-squares residual error. Non-linear effects are represented using linear splines called "hinge functions". In the latter step, called the backward step, the aim is to improve the generalizability of the model determined at the end of the previous step. To such an end, the optimal number of variables is selected using the Generalized Cross-Validation (GCV) statistic and the model is then pruned according to this choice. It is worth noting that the forward step can be customized. First, by specifying the "degree" option, one can choose the maximum order of interactions: degree = 1 means no interactions (in other terms, only additive effects can be included in the model), degree = 2 means order one interaction and so on. Second, in an analogous fashion, it is possible to avoid the specification of the non-linear effects of numerical variables (linearity constraints).

In the current study, miRNA expressions were considered dependent variables and exposure factors were considered candidate predictors. For each EV oncomiR, several models were fitted according to the order of interactions (degree = 1 and degree = 2) and the presence/absence of the constraints on non-linear effects. According to the bias vs. variance trade-off, it is important to acknowledge that linear relationships between response variables and predictors may oversimplify the complexity of real-world relationships; but, they do so with a gain in interpretability. Therefore, in exploratory analyses, we decided to evaluate models with hinge functions along with models with linear effects because the former could be unstable and too complex to be interpreted, despite reducing the bias.

For each of the fitted models, the goodness of fit was evaluated using R^2 and generalized R^2 coefficients. The importance of each predictor (i.e., exposure variables) was evaluated by the nsubset [29]. All of the analyses were performed using the R software release 4.2.3 [30], with the packages FactoMineR [31] and Earth [32], and the Knime Analytic Platform release 4.7.0 [33].

3. Results

3.1. Characteristics of the Study Population

For a total of 911 subjects, 238 males and 673 females were included in this study. A description of the study participants is reported in Table 1.

Table 1. Description of the study population.

		Males (N = 238)	Females (N = 673)
Age	years, mean ± SD	50.9 ± 13.3	51.6 ± 13.4
BMI	kg/m^2, mean ± SD	33.9 ± 4.7	33.6 ± 5.7
Education	Primary school or less	21 (8.8%)	85 (12.6%)
	Secondary school	61 (25.6%)	178 (26.4%)
	High school	117 (49.2%)	315 (46.8%)
	University or more	39 (16.4%)	95 (14.1%)
Occupation	Employee	166 (69.8%)	375 (55.7%)
	Unemployed	15 (6.3%)	55 (8.2%)
	Retired	57 (23.95%)	160 (23.8%)
	Housewife	-	83 (12.3%)
Residence traffic exposure	Mild	53 (22.2%)	148 (22.0%)
	Moderate	117 (49.2%)	329 (48.9%)
	Heavy	68 (28.6%)	196 (29.1%)
PM10 annual average	from the ARPA monitoring station µg/m^3, mean ± SD	43.0 ± 4.4	42.7 ± 4.7
Physical activity	Sedentary	148 (62.2%)	433 (64.4%)
	Active	66 (27.7%)	206 (30.6%)
	Sportive	24 (10.1%)	34 (5.0%)
Antidepressants	Yes	15 (6.3%)	100 (14.9%)
	No	223 (93.7%)	573 (85.1%)

Table 1. *Cont.*

		Males (N = 238)	Females (N = 673)
Smoking	Never Ex Current	88 (37.0%) 108 (45.4%) 42 (17.6%)	377 (56.0%) 198 (29.4%) 98 (14.5%)
Passive smoke exposure	Yes No	110 (46.2%) 128 (53.8%)	293 (43.5%) 380 (56.5%)
Alcohol	weekly consumption, median [Q1, Q3]	2 [0; 7]	0 [0; 2]
Coffee	weekly consumption, median [Q1, Q3]	9 [5; 20]	7 [3; 16]
C-reactive protein	mg/L, median [Q1, Q3]	0.22 [0.11; 0.45]	0.31 [0.14; 0.6]
Homocysteine	µmol/L, median [Q1, Q3]	12 [10.2; 14.2]	9.8 [8.3; 12.1]
Birth control pill	Yes No	-	26 (3.9%) 647 (96.1%)
Number of previous pregnancies	median [Q1, Q3]	-	2 [1; 3]
Menopause	Yes No	-	355 (55.1%) 287 (44.9%)

Briefly, the study participants had mean ages of 50.9 ± 13.3 years and 51.6 ± 13.4 years in males and females, respectively. The mean BMIs were equal to 33.9 ± 4.7 kg/m^2 (males) and 33.6 ± 5.7 kg/m^2 (females). Study subjects were, for a large percentage, employed (males 69.8%; females 55.7%), sedentary (males 62.2%; females 64.4%), and non-current smokers (males 82.4%; females 85.5%). The association between the different continuous predictors was assessed by Spearman's rank correlation coefficients and is reported in Figure 1A (females) and Figure 1B (males) together with scatter plots with smoothing trend lines for continuous predictors.

Concerning females, no major monotonic associations were observed; although, moderate ($r > 0.1$) correlations involved age with homocysteine, age and number of pregnancies, BMI and CRP, BMI and number of pregnancies, and CRP and alcohol consumption (Figure 1A). Similarly, in males, moderate positive correlations involved age with the PM10 annual average and alcohol consumption, BMI and CRP, BMI and alcohol consumption, CRP and homocysteine, alcohol and homocysteine, coffee consumption, and alcohol consumption(Figure 1B).

Concerning the FAMD, the plot showing the joint contributions of each variable is reported in Figure 2. In females, the first principal component, Dim1, is primarily related to age, menopausal status, and working status variables. Dim2 is predominantly related to BMI and PCR, with physical activity variables also contributing to a lesser extent. Lastly, the third principal component, Dim3, mainly comprises the PM10 annual average.

Conversely, for males, the first principal component, Dim1, is predominantly related to age and working status variables, with smoking also contributing significantly. Dim2 is mainly related to PCR and coffee consumption, where these variables show opposition in their influence, along with traffic and physical activity variables playing a secondary role. Finally, the third principal component, Dim3, is primarily composed of BMI.

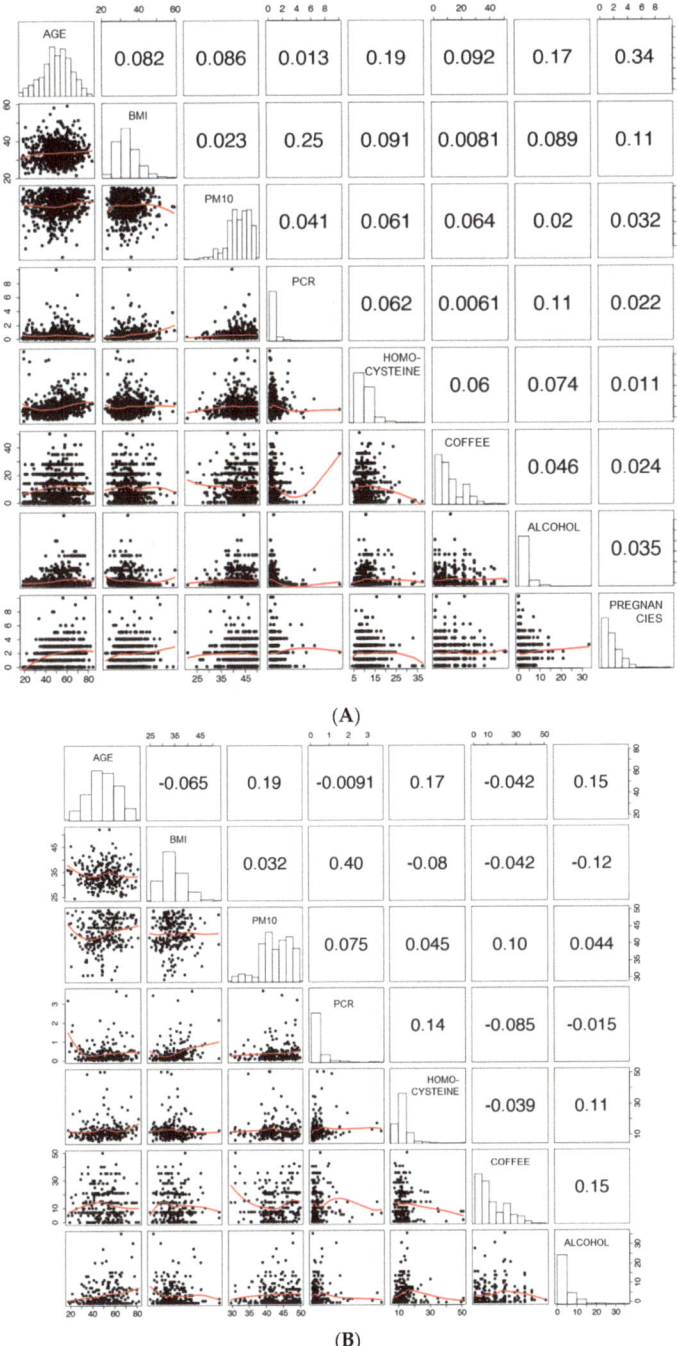

Figure 1. Correlation among numerical variables. (**Panel A**) Female data. (**Panel B**) Male data. On the lower panels, scatterplots for each variable pair are reported. The red curves were obtained by the non-parametric regression method (lowess smoother). On the upper panel are the reported Spearman correlation coefficients for each variable pair.

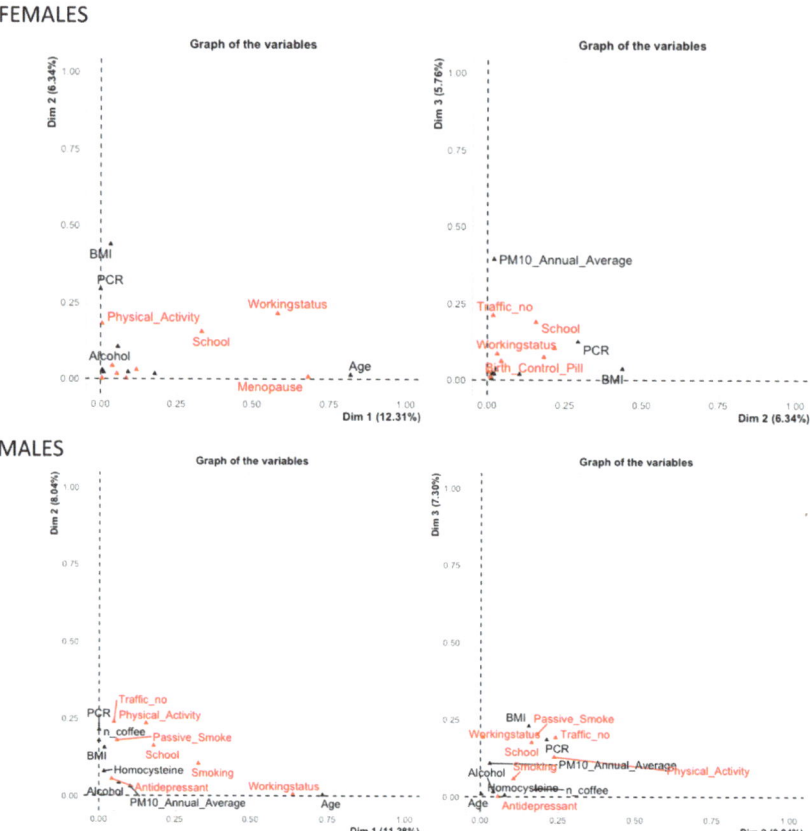

Figure 2. Multivariate analysis of miRNA expressions and exposure variables. Factor Analysis of Mixed Data (FAMD) was used to investigate the joint contributions of various variables in females and males. Continuous variables are reported in red and categorical variables are in black. Labels of variables with minor contributions were omitted.

3.2. miRNA Selection and Expression Levels in the Study Subjects

Supplementary Table S1 presents a comprehensive list of miRNAs identified from the OncomiR database that were ranked in the top 50 based on their association with specific cancer types. Table S1 includes the percentage of expression in females and males regarding the SPHERE study along with an indication of their recorded average up-regulation/downregulation in cancer tissues. Spearman's correlation coefficients were calculated and presented in a correlation matrix heatmap, based on the average correlation values for each column and row, and are displayed in Supplementary Figure S1 for females (Panel A) and males (Panel B).

In Figure 3A, the overlapping miRNAs across various cancer types are displayed. In Panel B, we present the miRNAs observed in female cancers, expressed in at least 20% of the women included in this study. Similarly, Panel C reports the equivalent selection of miRNAs for male cancers.

Additionally, Figures 4 and 5 report (in females and males, respectively) the relationships of the miRNA subsets for each cancer type as supplementary (or passive) variables and continuous predictors (active variables). Only major associations are reported because the small observed correlations between the sets of active and passive variables lead to most of the miRNA projections that tend to gather very close to the centroid of the axes.

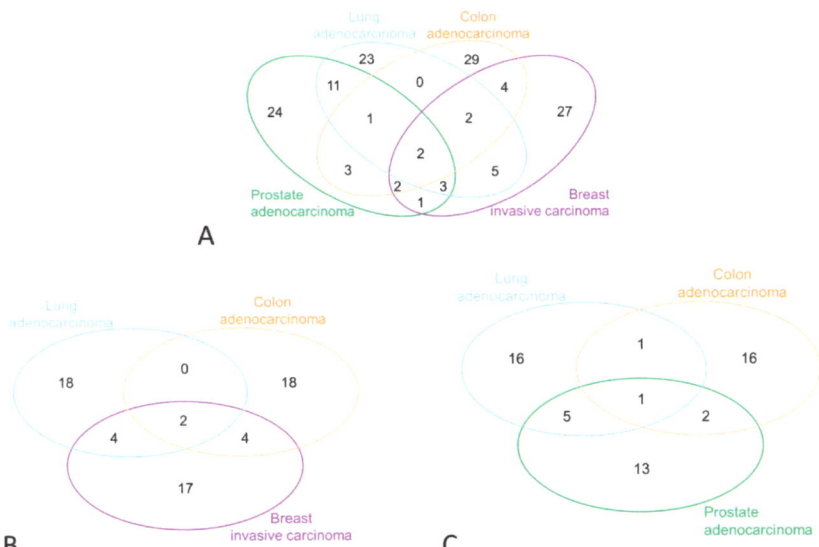

Figure 3. miRNA expression patterns in different cancer types. (**Panel A**) illustrates overlapping miRNAs across various cancer types (females AND males). (**Panel B**) displays miRNAs observed in female cancers, expressed in at least 20% of the women in this study. (**Panel C**) presents the equivalent selection of miRNAs for male cancers.

3.3. Multivariate Adaptive Regression Splines

The MARS algorithm was applied to explore the non-linear and non-additive relationships between miRNA expression and the selected risk factors in order to evaluate the importance of the explanatory variables we considered. Supplementary Table S2 reports the results of the models we applied in the female group of subjects while the models for the male group are reported in Supplementary Table S3. In addition, both of the above tables include additional results obtained by fitting models with continuous predictors constrained to linear effects. Finally, the goodness of fit of each model, evaluated using R2 and generalized R2 coefficients, is described in Supplementary Tables S4 (females) and S5 (males).

In females, as we considered MARS models with Degree 1 (i.e., MARS model using only additive terms to fit the data), the higher R-squared value for the model was observed for hsa-miR-136-5p, indicating that 25% of the variance in this miRNA expression could be explained by the selected risk factors (PM10, BMI, passive smoke, working status, and homocysteine). This association is coherent with the projections of continuous variables from the FAMD analysis of Figure 5 showing the major role of hsa-miR-136-5p as a passive variable. As we considered MARS models with Degree 2 (i.e., MARS model considering also interactions among predictors to fit the data), the higher R-squared value for the model was observed for hsa-miR-301a-3p, indicating that 29% of the variance in this miRNA expression could be explained by a complex combination of selected risk factors (age: alcohol, PM10 with antidepressants, PCR, working status and alcohol, antidepressants with education, PCR, homocysteine, birth control, number of pregnancies, consumption of coffee, PCR with smoking status and alcohol consumption, and alcohol consumption with physical activity).

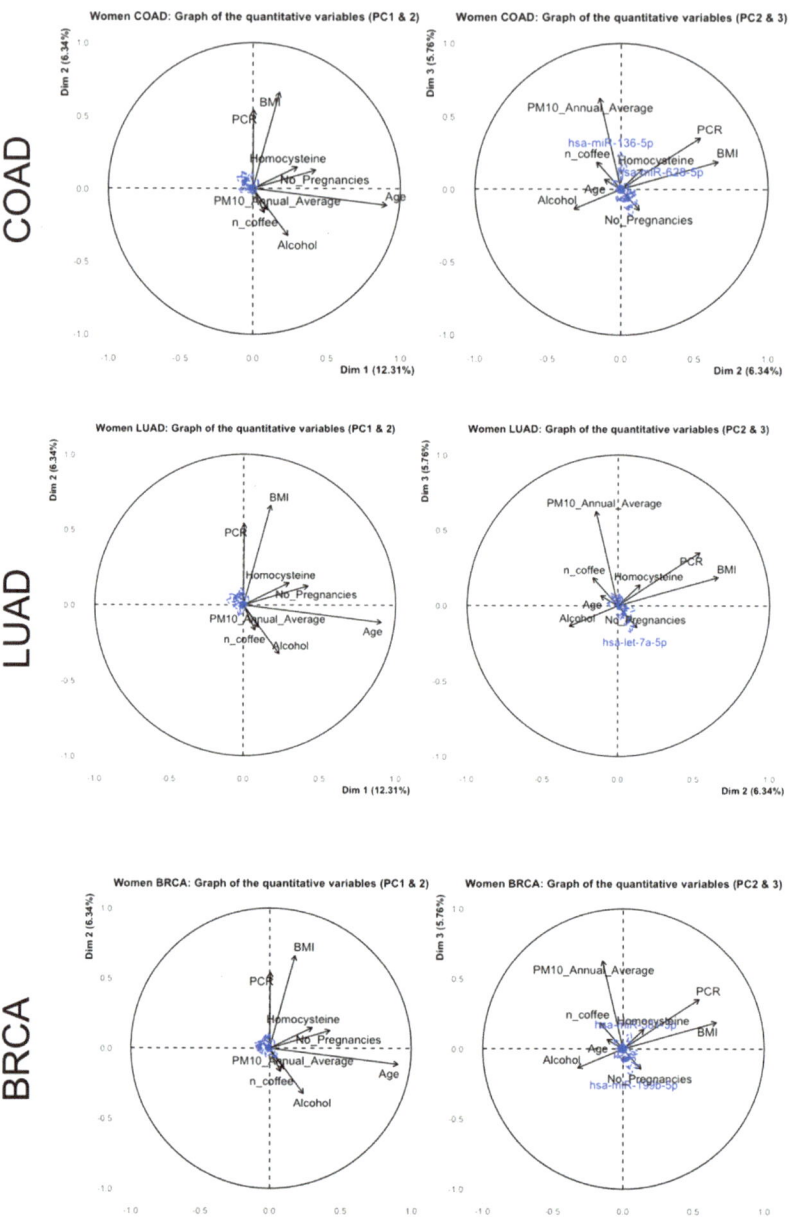

Figure 4. Relationships of miRNA subsets for each cancer type in females (Colon cancer—COAD, Lung cancer—LOAD, Breast cancer—BRCA). The miRNA subsets are presented as supplementary (passive) variables while continuous predictors are represented as active variables.

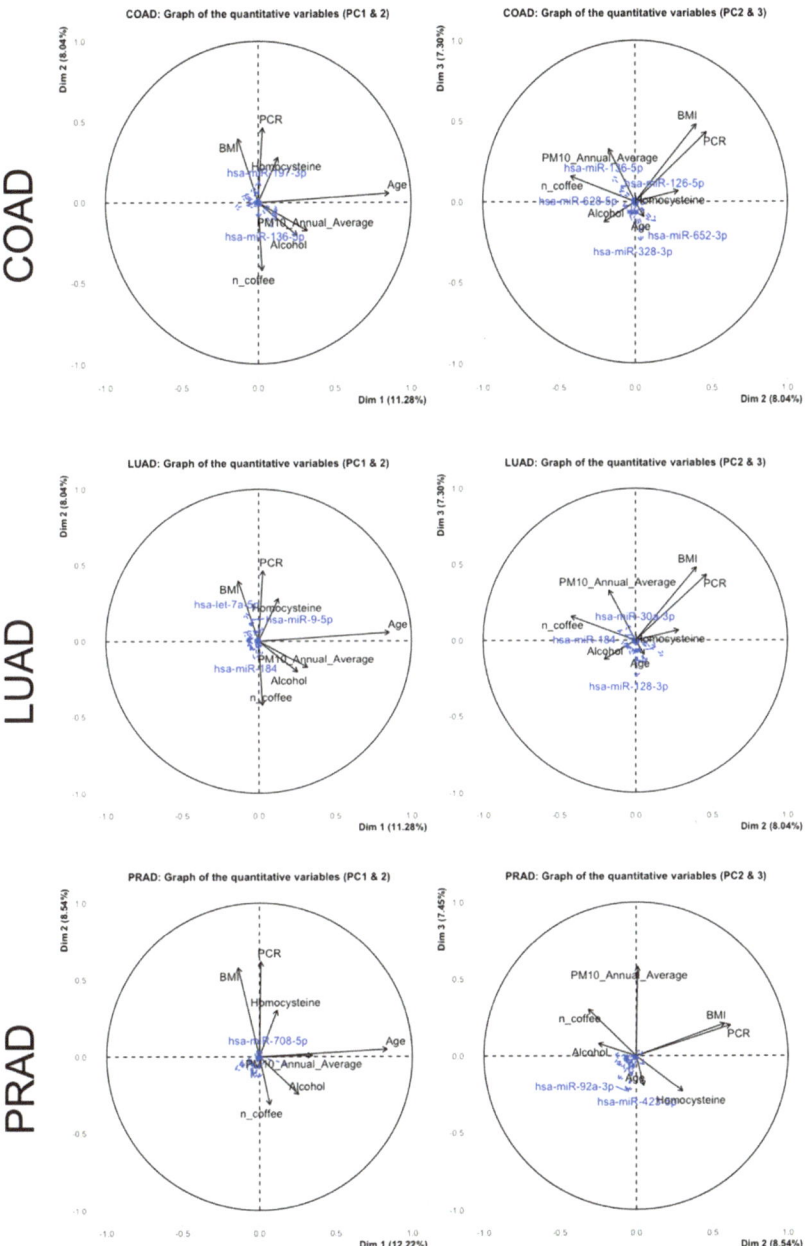

Figure 5. Relationships of miRNA subsets for each cancer type in males (COAD, LOAD, PRAD). The miRNA subsets are presented as supplementary (passive) variables while continuous predictors are represented as active variables.

As we considered MARS models with Degree 1 and hinges, in males, the higher R-squared value for the model was observed for hsa-miR-136-5p, indicating that 37% of the variance in this miRNA expression could be explained by the selected risk factors (PM10 annual average, age, and alcohol). As we considered MARS models with Degree 2, the higher R-squared value for the model was observed for hsa-miR-338-5p, indicating that 61% of the variance in this miRNA expression could be explained by a complex combination of selected risk factors (AgexCoffee; BMIxCoffee, PM10xCoffee; EducationxHomocysteine; PCRxCoffee; HomocysteinexCoffee; SmokingxCoffee; Physical ActivityxCoffee; Working statusxCoffee; and AlcoholxCoffee).

Intriguingly, the PM10 annual average emerged as the top-ranked variable in terms of its importance for numerous miRNAs, both in females (Supplementary Table S2) and males (Supplementary Table S3).

Given the complexity of the results, we here provide detailed descriptions for the associations involving predictors with a top-ranking priority (i.e., 1st). Individual raw outputs are reported in the Supplementary File "Material S1" M1.

Age was identified as a robust predictor of miRNA expression in females with hsa-miR-324-3p, hsa-miR-671-3p, hsa-miR-7-1-3p, and hsa-miR-9-5p, for which the predictor showed maximum importance. In males, age was similarly found to be a key predictor, correlating with hsa-miR-574-3p, hsa-miR-125a-5p, and hsa-miR-126-3p. Notably, a distinctive link between age and hsa-miR-125a-5p was observed exclusively in males; meanwhile, in females, age ranked as the second most important factor influencing miR-125a-5p expression.

Furthermore, BMI showed notable associations with miRNA expression, specifically hsa-miR-378a-3p and hsa-miR-708-5p in females and hsa-miR-9-5p, hsa-miR-103a-3p, and hsa-miR-140-5p in males. Interestingly, hsa-miR-378a-3p displayed a remarkable association with BMI, ranking fourth among the associated predictors for males.

Regarding biochemical parameters, CRP emerged as the top factor associated with the modulation of hsa-miR-338-5p in both females and males. In addition, homocysteine exhibited significant associations with hsa-miR-590-5p, ranking as the primary predictor in females and the secondary predictor in males.

The consumption of coffee demonstrated a significant correlation with miRNA expression in both females (hsa-miR-144-5p, hsa-miR-130b-3p, and hsa-miR-7-1-3p) and males (hsa-miR-139-3p, hsa-miR-378a-3p, and hsa-miR-148a-3p).

Lastly, hsa-miR-26b-3p exhibited a strong association with physical activity in females (as related to BRCA) but was not included in the male oncomiRNA list we selected a priori; thus, it was not further investigated.

4. Discussion

The present study investigated the association between selected oncomiRNAs and various factors, including age, BMI, biochemical parameters, and coffee consumption, shedding light on potential regulatory mechanisms and their relevance in the context of exposome research. Moreover, we investigated the gender-specific patterns observed in the associations, emphasizing the importance of considering this variable in miRNA-related research. Our objective is to enhance the comprehension of the complex association dependence of miRNAs with diverse factors. This highlights the importance of developing multivariable methodological approaches for overcoming the analysis of one exposure at a time, as is conventionally performed in exposome research. Emphasizing the relevance of considering non-linear relationships among variables, we seek to advance the understanding of miRNA regulation in response to multiple environmental influences. By exploring the broader context of miRNA regulation, our findings could offer valuable insights into the complexity of molecular interactions and pave the way for more comprehensive and robust exposome studies in the future.

In our investigation, age emerged as a robust and influential predictor of miRNA expression in both female and male subjects. Specifically, we observed major associations between age and the expression levels of miR-324-3p, miR-671-3p, miR-7-1-3p, and miR-9-5p in females and miR-574-3p, miR-125a-5p, and miR-126-3p in males.

An intriguing finding in our study was the gender-specific association of age with miR-125a-5p. Age significantly influenced miR-125a-5p expression in both females and males, providing robust evidence for the role of this association in two independent sets of subjects. In males, however, age was the single selected predictor of miR-125a-5p while a more complex pattern of modulation was observed in females. Namely, the hinge model showed the role of PM10, age, BMI, and PCR ranked by importance; the same variables (plus coffee consumption) were observed in Degree 2 models with interactions. Under linear constraint age, PM10, menopause, and BMI were showing their ranked importance. Considering linear interactions, the selected models showed the major role of being retired and post-menopause. The difference between linear and hinge models could be related to underlying non-linear and non-additive dependence relations on the considered continuous variables possibly surrogated by the associated categorical factors of menopause and working status.

These results suggest that age plays a central role in shaping miRNA expression profiles in both genders. Furthermore, the gender-specific associations underscore the importance of considering sex as a biological variable in miRNA-related studies as it may uncover unique regulatory patterns and provide insights into gender-specific molecular mechanisms associated with age-related processes.

Additionally, miR-125a-5p has been extensively studied in the context of cancer [34,35]. It acts as a tumor suppressor in various cancers by targeting oncogenes or genes involved in cell proliferation, invasion, and metastasis [36,37]. Its down-regulation in cancer cells can contribute to tumor progression [38,39]. Our findings confirm the age-dependent down-regulation in the expression of miR-125a-5p, which has been previously reported in mouse models [40].

We further observed significant associations between BMI and miRNA expression, with gender-specific patterns present. In females, miR-378a-3p and miR-708-5p showed an association with BMI; meanwhile, in males, miR-9-5p, miR-103a-3p, and miR-140-5p were found to be associated. These results suggest distinct miRNA regulatory patterns in relation to BMI in females and males, reflecting potential gender-specific molecular mechanisms linked to adiposity and metabolic processes. The SPHERE population consisted of individuals with high BMIs and previous studies have emphasized the significant role of BMI in modulating EV-miRNA expression [21]. Specifically, miR-378a has been implicated in adipogenesis and obesity [41–44] while miR-708-5p was found to be up-regulated in individuals with obesity and metabolic syndrome [45].

In the context of obesity, miR-9-5p has been frequently reported as dysregulated in adipose tissue and serum, pointing to its potential involvement in the pathogenesis of obesity [46]. It is known to influence adipocyte differentiation by targeting key genes in adipogenesis [47]. Moreover, miR-9-5p has been associated with the regulation of inflammatory processes [48,49]; given that obesity is characterized by chronic low-grade inflammation in adipose tissue [50], the dysregulation of miR-9-5p in obesity may contribute to adipose tissue inflammation and insulin resistance. Similarly, miR-103a-3p has been found to be down-regulated in blood samples of individuals with obesity [51,52] and its role in modulating insulin sensitivity is well-established [52]. Additionally, miR-140-5p has been reported to be up-regulated in the plasma of obese or diabetic patients and its levels can be influenced by treatment with metformin or bariatric surgery, indicating a potential correlation with insulin sensitivity [52,53]. Moreover, miR-140-5p overexpression has been positively correlated with BMI and waist-to-hip ratio [53].

In our investigation of biochemical parameters, we identified CRP as the most influential factor regulating miR-338-5p expression in both females and males. Furthermore, homocysteine showed significant associations with miR-590-5p, ranking as the primary predictor in females and the secondary predictor in males. To the best of our knowledge, no previous studies have reported an association between CRP and miR-338-5p. However, a recent paper demonstrated that overexpressed miR-338-5p effectively suppressed IL-6 expression at both the mRNA and protein levels, both in vitro and in vivo, and vice versa [54]. Additionally, luciferase reporter assays confirmed that miR-338-5p directly regulated IL-6 expression by binding to its mRNA 3′ untranslated region [55]. Given that IL-6 is a known inducer of hepatic C-reactive protein (CRP) synthesis, this discovery suggests a potential link between miR-338-5p and CRP [54]. These findings shed light on a novel regulatory mechanism that may have implications for our understanding of the interplay between miRNAs and inflammatory pathways and could provide insights into the molecular basis of miR-338-5p modulation by CRP.

MiR-590-5p plays a crucial role in cellular homeostasis, including cancer, with recent evidence showing its dual function as both an oncogene and a tumor suppressor, depending on the specific cancer context [56]. Although the link between miR-590-5p and homocysteine is not clear, miR-590-5p has been implicated in processes related to vascular endothelial function [57] and inflammation [58], which are pathways closely connected to homocysteine metabolism. However, it is important to note that the relationship between miR-590-5p and homocysteine is likely to be influenced by various factors related to the cellular context, including other molecular interactions. More comprehensive studies are needed to elucidate the specific mechanisms underlying this potential link and its functional consequences in health and disease.

The significant correlation we found between coffee consumption and miRNA expression in both females and males is a fascinating finding. Coffee contains numerous bioactive compounds, such as caffeine and polyphenols, which have been shown to exert protective effects against cancer by acting as antioxidants and modulating various cellular pathways [59]. Numerous epidemiological studies have explored the association between coffee consumption and cancer risk, revealing intriguing findings. Overall, the evidence suggests that moderate coffee consumption is associated with a potentially reduced risk of certain cancers. Some studies have shown an inverse relationship between coffee consumption and the risk of developing cancers, such as liver, colorectal, and endometrial cancer [60]. Moreover, coffee consumption has been linked to a lower risk of certain types of hormone-related cancers, like estrogen-receptor-negative breast cancer [61]. In the literature, we have not found any possible associations between coffee consumption and the expression of the microRNAs we identified (miR-144-5p, miR-130b-3p, miR-7-1-3p, miR-139-3p, miR-378a-3p, and miR-148a-3p). This field of study is still in its very early stages and further research is required to assess the effect of these dietary compounds.

The intriguing link between miR-26b-3p and physical activity sheds light on the complex regulatory network of microRNAs in response to both exercise and everyday physical behaviors. It emphasizes miR-26b-3p's potential role as a significant player in processes related to physical activity. Notably, in this context, "physical activity" encompasses habitual behaviors beyond structured exercise. However, to fully comprehend the functional significance and implications of miR-26b-3p in relation to physical activity, further comprehensive studies are warranted.

One of the major advantages of a machine learning method like MARS is its ability to automatically select relevant variables from a large set of predictors and their interactions, also considering non-linear relationships under their hinge function representation. This provides an additional level of information with respect to multivariate projection techniques like FAMD and simple univariable linear regression. Whereas the MARS method can capture non-linear and non-additive relationships, the resulting models are still relatively interpretable, providing relevant exploratory information for setting biological hypotheses and building refined models with optimal control of the bias vs. variance tradeoff and enhanced predictive capability. Therefore, we are aware of the limitations as well as the advantages of the applied MARS method; more sophisticated modeling, rather than multivariable regression, is requested by the integrative analysis of multi-omics data in order to infer about regulatory/causal networks. This is outside of the scope of the present paper but lays the ground for future developments of our analyses of the SPHERE data.

5. Conclusions

This study not only enhances our understanding of miRNA regulation in response to multiple environmental and lifestyle influences but also underscores the critical role of methodology in unraveling the complexities of cancer risk factors. By uncovering non-linear relationships among variables, we gain valuable insights into the complexity of miRNA regulatory networks. Furthermore, our adoption of the MARS methodology, with its inherent capacity to automatically identify non-linear and non-additive effects (interactions) among predictors, exemplifies the power of computational techniques in elucidating the interplay between multifaceted variables. This innovation approach not only advances our comprehension of EV oncomiR network regulation but also serves as a model for future studies seeking to decipher complex molecular systems. As we move forward, we envisage a horizon of comprehensive exposome studies that will further define the dynamic relationships between our environment, our genetic makeup, and the complex landscape of cancer development.

Supplementary Materials: The following supporting information can be downloaded at: https://www.mdpi.com/article/10.3390/cancers15174317/s1.

Author Contributions: Conceptualization, V.B. and E.M.B.; methodology, L.D. and P.M.; formal analysis, D.B. and G.M.; investigation, L.F. and F.B.; resources, V.B.; data curation, C.F. and S.I.; writing—original draft preparation, V.B. and E.M.B.; writing—review and editing, L.F., F.B. and A.C.P. All authors have read and agreed to the published version of the manuscript.

Funding: This study was supported by the EU Programme "Ideas", European Research Council (ERC-2011-StG 282,413 to VB).

Institutional Review Board Statement: This study was conducted according to the guidelines of the Declaration of Helsinki and approved by the Ethics Committee of Fondazione IRCCS Cà Granda Ospedale Maggiore Policlinico (approval number 1425).

Informed Consent Statement: Informed consent was obtained from all subjects involved in this study.

Data Availability Statement: The data presented in this study are available on request from the corresponding author.

Acknowledgments: We acknowledge Luisella Vigna and the Occupational Medicine Medical Residents for their help in examining and recruiting study subjects. We are grateful to the nurses of the "Medicina del Lavoro" Unit, Fondazione IRCCS Ca' Granda Ospedale Maggiore Policlinico, Enrico Radice, Raquel Cacace and Barbara Marinelli for database development and preparation. We acknowledge Sai Spandana Adivishnu for her help with the data preparation for the analysis. We extend our heartfelt gratitude to the HEBE consortium for their invaluable contribution to fostering the rich cultural background that laid the foundation for the development of the scientific discussion leading to this paper.

Conflicts of Interest: The authors declare no conflict of interest.

References

1. Zhang, Y.-B.; Pan, X.-F.; Chen, J.; Cao, A.; Zhang, Y.-G.; Xia, L.; Wang, J.; Li, H.; Liu, G.; Pan, A. Combined lifestyle factors, incident cancer, and cancer mortality: A systematic review and meta-analysis of prospective cohort studies. *Br. J. Cancer* **2020**, *122*, 1085–1093. [CrossRef] [PubMed]
2. Vineis, P.; Wild, C.P. Global cancer patterns: Causes and prevention. *Lancet* **2014**, *383*, 549–557. [CrossRef]
3. Anand, P.; Kunnumakara, A.B.; Sundaram, C.; Harikumar, K.B.; Tharakan, S.T.; Lai, O.S.; Sung, B.; Aggarwal, B.B. Cancer is a Preventable Disease that Requires Major Lifestyle Changes. *Pharm. Res.* **2008**, *25*, 2097–2116. [CrossRef]
4. Irigaray, P.; Newby, J.; Clapp, R.; Hardell, L.; Howard, V.; Montagnier, L.; Epstein, S.; Belpomme, D. Lifestyle-related factors and environmental agents causing cancer: An overview. *Biomed. Pharmacother.* **2007**, *61*, 640–658. [CrossRef] [PubMed]
5. Steck, S.E.; Murphy, E.A. Dietary patterns and cancer risk. *Nat. Rev. Cancer* **2020**, *20*, 125–138. [CrossRef] [PubMed]
6. Friedenreich, C.M.; Ryder-Burbidge, C.; McNeil, J. Physical activity, obesity and sedentary behavior in cancer etiology: Epidemiologic evidence and biologic mechanisms. *Mol. Oncol.* **2021**, *15*, 790–800. [CrossRef] [PubMed]

7. Biganzoli, E.; Desmedt, C.; Fornili, M.; de Azambuja, E.; Cornez, N.; Ries, F.; Closon-Dejardin, M.-T.; Kerger, J.; Focan, C.; Di Leo, A.; et al. Recurrence dynamics of breast cancer according to baseline body mass index. *Eur. J. Cancer* 2017, *87*, 10–20. [CrossRef] [PubMed]
8. GBD 2019 Cancer Risk Factors Collaborators. The global burden of cancer attributable to risk factors, 2010–2019: A systematic analysis for the Global Burden of Disease Study 2019. *Lancet* 2022, *400*, 563–591. [CrossRef]
9. Ward, E.; Jemal, A.; Cokkinides, V.; Singh, G.K.; Cardinez, C.; Ghafoor, A.; Thun, M. Cancer Disparities by Race/Ethnicity and Socioeconomic Status. *CA A Cancer J. Clin.* 2004, *54*, 78–93. [CrossRef]
10. Martin-Moreno, J.M.; Ruiz-Segovia, N.; Diaz-Rubio, E. Behavioural and structural interventions in cancer prevention: Towards the 2030 SDG horizon. *Mol. Oncol.* 2021, *15*, 801–808. [CrossRef] [PubMed]
11. Catalán, V.; Avilés-Olmos, I.; Rodríguez, A.; Becerril, S.; Fernández-Formoso, J.A.; Kiortsis, D.; Portincasa, P.; Gómez-Ambrosi, J.; Frühbeck, G. Time to Consider the "Exposome Hypothesis" in the Development of the Obesity Pandemic. *Nutrients* 2022, *14*, 1597. [CrossRef]
12. Nguyen, H.-L.; Geukens, T.; Maetens, M.; Aparicio, S.; Bassez, A.; Borg, A.; Brock, J.; Broeks, A.; Caldas, C.; Cardoso, F.; et al. Obesity-associated changes in molecular biology of primary breast cancer. *Nat. Commun.* 2023, *14*, 4418. [CrossRef]
13. Deng, T.; Lyon, C.J.; Bergin, S.; Caligiuri, M.A.; Hsueh, W.A. Obesity, Inflammation, and Cancer. *Annu. Rev. Pathol. Mech. Dis.* 2016, *11*, 421–449. [CrossRef] [PubMed]
14. Colombo, M.; Raposo, G.; Théry, C. Biogenesis, secretion, and intercellular interactions of exosomes and other extracellular vesicles. *Annu. Rev. Cell Dev. Biol.* 2014, *30*, 255–289. [CrossRef] [PubMed]
15. Margolis, L.; Sadovsky, Y. The biology of extracellular vesicles: The known unknowns. *PLoS Biol.* 2019, *17*, e3000363. [CrossRef]
16. van Niel, G.; Carter, D.R.F.; Clayton, A.; Lambert, D.W.; Raposo, G.; Vader, P. Challenges and directions in studying cell-cell communication by extracellular vesicles. *Nat. Rev. Mol. Cell Biol.* 2022, *23*, 369–382. [CrossRef]
17. Yokoi, A.; Ochiya, T. Exosomes and extracellular vesicles: Rethinking the essential values in cancer biology. *Semin. Cancer Biol.* 2021, *74*, 79–91. [CrossRef]
18. O'Brien, J.; Hayder, H.; Zayed, Y.; Peng, C. Overview of MicroRNA Biogenesis, Mechanisms of Actions, and Circulation. *Front. Endocrinol.* 2018, *9*, 402. [CrossRef]
19. Svoronos, A.A.; Engelman, D.M.; Slack, F.J. OncomiR or Tumor Suppressor? The Duplicity of MicroRNAs in Cancer. *Cancer Res.* 2016, *76*, 3666–3670. [CrossRef] [PubMed]
20. Otmani, K.; Rouas, R.; Lewalle, P. OncomiRs as noncoding RNAs having functions in cancer: Their role in immune suppression and clinical implications. *Front. Immunol.* 2022, *13*, 913951. [CrossRef]
21. Bollati, V.; Iodice, S.; Favero, C.; Angelici, L.; Albetti, B.; Cacace, R.; Cantone, L.; Carugno, M.; Cavalleri, T.; De Giorgio, B.; et al. Susceptibility to particle health effects, miRNA and exosomes: Rationale and study protocol of the SPHERE study. *BMC Public Health* 2014, *14*, 1137. [CrossRef]
22. Pergoli, L.; Cantone, L.; Favero, C.; Angelici, L.; Iodice, S.; Pinatel, E.; Hoxha, M.; Dioni, L.; Letizia, M.; Albetti, B.; et al. Extracellular vesicle-packaged miRNA release after short-term exposure to particulate matter is associated with increased coagulation. *Part. Fibre Toxicol.* 2017, *14*, 32. [CrossRef] [PubMed]
23. World Cancer Research Fund International. Worldwide Cancer Data. *Global Cancer Statistics for the Most Common Cancers in the World*. Available online: http://wcrf.orf/cancer-trends/worldwide-cancer-data (accessed on 1 January 2023).
24. Wong, N.; Chen, Y.; Chen, S.; Wang, X. OncomiR: An online resource for exploring pan-cancer microRNA dysregulation. *Bio-informatics* 2018, *34*, 713–715. [CrossRef]
25. Société Française de Statistique. *Journal de la Société Française de Statistique*; Société Française de Statistique: Paris, France, 1998.
26. Husson, F.; Le, S.; Pagès, J. *Exploratory Multivariate Analysis by Example Using R*, 2nd ed.; CRC Press: Boca Raton, FL, USA, 2017.
27. Kassambara, A. Ggcorrplot: Visualization of a Correlation Matrix using 'ggplot2'_. R Package Version 0.1.4, 2022. Available online: https://CRAN.R-project.org/package=ggcorrplot (accessed on 1 June 2023).
28. Hastie, T.; Tibshirani, R.; Friedman, J.H. *The Elements of Statistical Learning: Data Mining, Inference, and Prediction*, 2nd ed.; Springer: New York, NY, USA, 2009; p. xxii. 745p.
29. Milborrow, S. Notes on the Earth Package. 2017. Available online: http://www.milbo.org/doc/earth-notes.pdf (accessed on 1 June 2023).
30. R Core Team. *R: A Language and Environment for Statistical Computing*; R Foundation for Statistical Computing: Vienna, Austria, 2023; Available online: https://www.r-project.org/ (accessed on 1 June 2023).
31. Lê, S.; Josse, J.; Husson, F. FactoMineR: An R Package for Multivariate Analysis. *J. Stat. Softw.* 2008, *25*, 1–18. [CrossRef]
32. Milborrow, S. Derived from mda: Mars by T. Hastie and R. Tibshirani. 2023 Earth: Multivariate Adaptive Regression Splines. R Package Version 5.3.2. Available online: https://CRAN.R-project.org/package=earth (accessed on 1 June 2023).
33. Berthold, M.R.; Cebron, N.; Dill, F.; Gabriel, T.R.; Kötter, T.; Meinl, T.; Ohl, P.; Sieb, C.; Thiel, K.; Wiswedel, B. KNIME: The Konstanz Information Miner; Springer: Berlin/Heidelberg, Germany, 2008; pp. 319–326. [CrossRef]
34. Hsieh, T.-H.; Hsu, C.-Y.; Tsai, C.-F.; Long, C.-Y.; Chai, C.-Y.; Hou, M.-F.; Lee, J.-N.; Wu, D.-C.; Wang, S.-C.; Tsai, E.-M. miR-125a-5p is a prognostic biomarker that targets HDAC4 to suppress breast tumorigenesis. *Oncotarget* 2015, *6*, 494–509. [CrossRef]

35. Bhattacharjya, S.; Nath, S.; Ghose, J.; Maiti, G.P.; Biswas, N.; Bandyopadhyay, S.; Panda, C.K.; Bhattacharyya, N.P.; Roychoudhury, S. miR-125b promotes cell death by targeting spindle assembly checkpoint gene MAD1 and modulating mitotic progression. *Cell Death Differ.* **2013**, *20*, 430–442. [CrossRef]
36. Jiang, L.; Huang, Q.; Chang, J.; Wang, E.; Qiu, X. MicroRNA HSA-miR-125a-5p induces apoptosis by activating p53 in lung cancer cells. *Exp. Lung Res.* **2011**, *37*, 387–398. [CrossRef] [PubMed]
37. Zhang, Y.; Zhang, D.; Lv, J.; Wang, S.; Zhang, Q. MiR-125a-5p suppresses bladder cancer progression through targeting FUT4. *BioMedicine* **2018**, *108*, 1039–1047. [CrossRef]
38. Yang, X.; Qiu, J.; Kang, H.; Wang, Y.; Qian, J. miR-125a-5p suppresses colorectal cancer progression by targeting VEGFA. *Cancer Manag. Res.* **2018**, *10*, 5839–5853. [CrossRef]
39. Makwana, K.; Patel, S.A.; Velingkaar, N.; Ebron, J.S.; Shukla, G.C.; Kondratov, R.V. Aging and calorie restriction regulate the expression of miR-125a-5p and its target genes Stat3, Casp2 and Stard13. *Aging* **2017**, *9*, 1825–1843. [CrossRef]
40. Huang, N.; Wang, J.; Xie, W.; Lyu, Q.; Wu, J.; He, J.; Qiu, W.; Xu, N.; Zhang, Y. MiR-378a-3p enhances adipogenesis by targeting mitogen-activated protein kinase 1. *Biochem. Biophys. Res. Commun.* **2015**, *457*, 37–42. [CrossRef]
41. Gerin, I.; Bommer, G.T.; McCoin, C.S.; Sousa, K.M.; Krishnan, V.; MacDougald, O.A.; Warren, J.S.; Oka, S.-I.; Zablocki, D.; Sadoshima, J.; et al. Roles for miRNA-378/378* in adipocyte gene expression and lipogenesis. *Am. J. Physiol. Metab.* **2010**, *299*, E198–E206. [CrossRef]
42. Eichner, L.J.; Perry, M.-C.; Dufour, C.R.; Bertos, N.; Park, M.; St-Pierre, J.; Giguère, V. miR-378* Mediates Metabolic Shift in Breast Cancer Cells via the PGC-1β/ERRγ Transcriptional Pathway. *Cell Metab.* **2010**, *12*, 352–361. [CrossRef] [PubMed]
43. Pan, D.; Mao, C.; Quattrochi, B.; Friedline, R.H.; Zhu, L.J.; Jung, D.Y.; Kim, J.K.; Lewis, B.; Wang, Y.-X. MicroRNA-378 controls classical brown fat expansion to counteract obesity. *Nat. Commun.* **2014**, *5*, 4725. [CrossRef] [PubMed]
44. Mir, F.A.; Mall, R.; Iskandarani, A.; Ullah, E.; Samra, T.A.; Cyprian, F.; Parray, A.; Alkasem, M.; Abdalhakam, I.; Farooq, F.; et al. Characteristic MicroRNAs Linked to Dysregulated Metabolic Pathways in Qatari Adult Subjects with Obesity and Metabolic Syndrome. *Front. Endocrinol.* **2022**, *13*, 937089. [CrossRef] [PubMed]
45. Wang, L.; Shang, C.; Pan, H.; Yang, H.; Zhu, H.; Gong, F. MicroRNA Expression Profiles in the Subcutaneous Adipose Tissues of Morbidly Obese Chinese Women. *Obes. Facts* **2021**, *14*, 78–92. [CrossRef]
46. Zhang, H.-G.; Wang, X.-B.; Zhao, H.; Zhou, C.-N. MicroRNA-9-5p promotes osteoporosis development through inhibiting osteogenesis and promoting adipogenesis via targeting Wnt3a. *Eur. Rev. Med. Pharmacol. Sci.* **2019**, *23*, 456–463. [CrossRef]
47. Su, H.; Liang, Z.; Weng, S.; Sun, C.; Huang, J.; Zhang, T.; Wang, X.; Wu, S.; Zhang, Z.; Zhang, Y.; et al. miR-9-5p regulates immunometabolic and epigenetic pathways in β-glucan-trained immunity via IDH3α. *J. Clin. Investig.* **2021**, *6*, 144260. [CrossRef]
48. Bazzoni, F.; Rossato, M.; Fabbri, M.; Gaudiosi, D.; Mirolo, M.; Mori, L.; Tamassia, N.; Mantovani, A.; Cassatella, M.A.; Locati, M. Induction and regulatory function of miR-9 in human monocytes and neutrophils exposed to proinflammatory signals. *Proc. Natl. Acad. Sci. USA* **2009**, *106*, 5282–5287. [CrossRef]
49. Mraz, M.; Haluzik, M. The role of adipose tissue immune cells in obesity and low-grade inflammation. *J. Endocrinol.* **2014**, *222*, R113–R127. [CrossRef]
50. Villard, A.; Marchand, L.; Thivolet, C.; Rome, S. Diagnostic Value of Cell-free Circulating Micrornas for Obesity and Type 2 Diabetes: A Meta-analysis. *J. Mol. Biomarkers Diagn.* **2015**, *6*, 6. [CrossRef] [PubMed]
51. Assmann, T.S.; Riezu-Boj, J.I.; Milagro, F.I.; Martínez, J.A. Circulating adiposity-related microRNAs as predictors of the response to a low-fat diet in subjects with obesity. *J. Cell Mol. Med.* **2020**, *24*, 2956–2967. [CrossRef]
52. Trajkovski, M.; Hausser, J.; Soutschek, J.; Bhat, B.; Akin, A.; Zavolan, M.; Heim, M.H.; Stoffel, M. MicroRNAs 103 and 107 regulate insulin sensitivity. *Nature* **2011**, *474*, 649–653. [CrossRef] [PubMed]
53. Li, X.; Ye, Y.; Wang, B.; Zhao, S. miR-140-5p Aggravates Insulin Resistance via Directly Targeting GYS1 and PPP1CC in Insulin-Resistant HepG2 Cells. *Diabetes Metab. Syndr. Obesity Targets Ther.* **2021**, *14*, 2515–2524. [CrossRef] [PubMed]
54. Bermudez, E.A.; Rifai, N.; Buring, J.; Manson, J.E.; Ridker, P.M. Interrelationships Among Circulating Interleukin-6, C-Reactive Protein, and Traditional Cardiovascular Risk Factors in Women. *Arter. Thromb. Vasc. Biol.* **2002**, *22*, 1668–1673. [CrossRef]
55. Zhang, Y.; Zhang, Z.; Wei, R.; Miao, X.; Sun, S.; Liang, G.; Chu, C.; Zhao, L.; Zhu, X.; Guo, Q.; et al. IL (Interleukin)-6 Contributes to Deep Vein Thrombosis and Is Negatively Regulated by miR-338-5p. *Arter. Thromb. Vasc. Biol.* **2020**, *40*, 323–334. [CrossRef]
56. Barwal, T.S.; Singh, N.; Sharma, U.; Bazala, S.; Rani, M.; Behera, A.; Kumawat, R.K.; Kumar, P.; Uttam, V.; Khandelwal, A.; et al. miR-590–5p: A double-edged sword in the oncogenesis process. *Cancer Treat. Res. Commun.* **2022**, *32*, 100593. [CrossRef] [PubMed]
57. Zhou, Q.; Zhu, Y.; Wei, X.; Zhou, J.; Chang, L.; Sui, H.; Han, Y.; Piao, D.; Sha, R.; Bai, Y. MiR-590-5p inhibits colorectal cancer angiogenesis and metastasis by regulating nuclear factor 90/vascular endothelial growth factor A axis. *Cell Death Dis.* **2016**, *7*, e2413. [CrossRef] [PubMed]
58. Yu, M.; Luo, Y.; Cong, Z.; Mu, Y.; Qiu, Y.; Zhong, M. MicroRNA-590-5p Inhibits Intestinal Inflammation by Targeting YAP. *J. Crohn's Colitis* **2018**, *12*, 993–1004. [CrossRef]
59. Molnar, R.; Szabo, L.; Tomesz, A.; Deutsch, A.; Darago, R.; Raposa, B.L.; Ghodratollah, N.; Varjas, T.; Nemeth, B.; Orsos, Z.; et al. The Chemopreventive Effects of Polyphenols and Coffee, Based upon a DMBA Mouse Model with microRNA and mTOR Gene Expression Biomarkers. *Cells* **2022**, *11*, 1300. [CrossRef]

60. Wang, A.; Wang, S.; Zhu, C.; Huang, H.; Wu, L.; Wan, X.; Yang, X.; Zhang, H.; Miao, R.; He, L.; et al. Coffee and cancer risk: A meta-analysis of prospective observational studies. *Sci. Rep.* **2016**, *6*, srep33711. [CrossRef] [PubMed]
61. Li, J.; Seibold, P.; Chang-Claude, J.; Flesch-Janys, D.; Liu, J.; Czene, K.; Humphreys, K.; Hall, P. Coffee consumption modifies risk of estrogen-receptor negative breast cancer. *Breast Cancer Res. BCR* **2011**, *13*, R49. [CrossRef] [PubMed]

Disclaimer/Publisher's Note: The statements, opinions and data contained in all publications are solely those of the individual author(s) and contributor(s) and not of MDPI and/or the editor(s). MDPI and/or the editor(s) disclaim responsibility for any injury to people or property resulting from any ideas, methods, instructions or products referred to in the content.

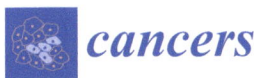

Review

Extracellular Vesicles in Lung Cancer: Implementation in Diagnosis and Therapeutic Perspectives

Anna Paola Carreca [1,*,†], Rosaria Tinnirello [2,†], Vitale Miceli [2], Antonio Galvano [3], Valerio Gristina [3], Lorena Incorvaia [3], Mariangela Pampalone [1], Simona Taverna [4] and Gioacchin Iannolo [2,*]

- [1] Ri.MED Foundation, 90127 Palermo, Italy; mpampalone@fondazionerimed.com
- [2] Department of Research, IRCCS ISMETT (Istituto Mediterraneo per i Trapianti e Terapie ad Alta Specializzazione), Via E. Tricomi 5, 90127 Palermo, Italy; rtinnirello@ismett.edu (R.T.); vmiceli@ismett.edu (V.M.)
- [3] Department of Precision Medicine in Medical, Surgical and Critical Care, University of Palermo, 90133 Palermo, Italy; antonio.galvano@unipa.it (A.G.); valerio.gristina@unipa.it (V.G.); lorena.incorvaia@unipa.it (L.I.)
- [4] Institute of Translational Pharmacology (IFT), National Research Council (CNR), 90146 Palermo, Italy; simona.taverna@cnr.it
- * Correspondence: apcarreca@fondazionerimed.com (A.P.C.); giannolo@ismett.edu (G.I.)
- † These authors contributed equally to this work.

Simple Summary: Cell–cell communication mechanisms are gathering growing scientific interest, particularly in the context of cancer cells and the tumor microenvironment. Extracellular vesicles are gaining increased interest due to their relevance in tumor molecular characterization, classification, diagnosis, prognosis evaluation, and response to treatment. Many advances have been made in the clinical and therapeutic fields, exploiting increasingly precise biomolecular engineering strategies. This review aims to focus on the role of extracellular vesicles (EVs) as diagnostic and therapeutic tools in lung cancer.

Abstract: Lung cancer represents the leading cause of cancer-related mortality worldwide, with around 1.8 million deaths in 2020. For this reason, there is an enormous interest in finding early diagnostic tools and novel therapeutic approaches, one of which is extracellular vesicles (EVs). EVs are nanoscale membranous particles that can carry proteins, lipids, and nucleic acids (DNA and RNA), mediating various biological processes, especially in cell–cell communication. As such, they represent an interesting biomarker for diagnostic analysis that can be performed easily by liquid biopsy. Moreover, their growing dataset shows promising results as drug delivery cargo. The aim of our work is to summarize the recent advances in and possible implications of EVs for early diagnosis and innovative therapies for lung cancer.

Keywords: lung cancer; NSCLC; SCLC; EVs; BALF; liquid biopsy; personalized medicine; organ failure

1. Introduction

Cancer is the leading cause of mortality globally [1], and a massive effort is being focused on finding novel therapeutic approaches and standardizing methods that can contribute to early neoplastic detection. Non-invasive techniques that do not involve radiation analysis represent a crucial goal. Among different tumors, the principal cause of death is lung cancer [1]. Lung cancer can be classified into two main histological subtypes: Small-Cell Lung Carcinoma (SCLC) and Non-Small Cell Lung Carcinoma (NSCLC), with a higher prevalence of NSCLC (about 80–85%) [2]. In the last decade, the high level of mortality due to lung cancer has prompted the onset of many multicenter studies seeking to improve early tumor detection by consolidated analysis (imaging by X-ray, PET, and PET/CT) and blood tests correlation. The 2004 COSMOS study (Continuous Observation of Smoking Subject) (ClinicalTrials.gov ID NCT01248806) enrolled more than 5000 asymptomatic smoker volunteers from the population because of their higher risk of developing lung cancer. Subjects were followed for 5 years with blood tests, spirometry, and annual low-dose spiral CT radiological examinations for nodules, alongside an evaluation of the correlation between COPD and lung cancer. Furthermore, many more studies comprising thousands of healthy patients have evaluated circulating biomarkers and radiomic analyses. For example, the CLEARLY study (Circulating and Imaging Biomarkers to Improve Lung Cancer EARLY Detection) (ClinicalTrials.gov ID NCT04323579), which started in 2018, is a multifactorial "bio-radiomic" protocol designed to detect early lung cancer in association with circulating biomarkers and radiomic data. Prognostic radiomic profiles for early detection have been correlated with molecular and cellular biomarkers such as microRNAs (miRNAs), proteins, circulating tumor cells (CTCs), and extracellular vesicles (EVs). EVs are involved in various processes, such as cell proliferation, differentiation, and the inflammatory response.

During the last ten years, circulating EVs have gained growing attention not only as biomarkers, but also for their ability to mediate cell–cell regulation and be manipulated for therapeutic purposes [3]. EV components have been implicated in many biological processes, and among them, a clear involvement in cancer invasion and metastasis has been observed [4]. Particularly noteworthy are the modulatory effects of EVs released from tumors and non-tumor cells such as mesenchymal stromal cells (MSCs) [5,6]. Many studies have been carried out to evaluate the effects and compositions of different EVs in tumor progression. The presence of regulatory messenger RNA (mRNA), which can modulate cancer cell proliferation, has been found within EVs [7]. Additionally, EV analysis has revealed the presence of controller proteins from neighboring cells [8], such as from the tumoral counterpart. Released EVs shuttle molecules involved in cell adhesion, migration, aggressiveness, and resistance to chemotherapeutic treatments [9]. The most remarkable molecules carried by EVs are miRNAs, which modulate multiple processes (growth, differentiation, apoptosis, migration, and drug/radioresistance) by their interaction with non-coding RNAs (ncRNAs), such as mRNAs, long non-coding RNAs (lncRNAs), and circular RNAs (circRNAs) [10]. Through these interactions, a single miRNA strand can control multiple genes, inhibiting their translation. This uniqueness gives relevance both to regulation processes and diagnosis and therapy. Engineering EVs with specific ncRNAs represents a promising outcome of the last few years, whereas the identification of an miRNA-specific signature from onset tumors still represents a challenging target. This review focuses on the role of EVs in diagnosis as components of liquid biopsy and in therapies for lung cancer, exploiting their use as theranostic agents. Despite many groups in the past describing the relationship between EVs and lung cancer, we hope that our work can help to suggest future diagnostic and therapeutic directions, improving their applications in fighting lung cancer [11–13].

2. Extracellular Vesicles

Extracellular vesicles (EVs) represent a crucial functional component of intercellular communication, acting as important mediators in both physiological and pathological processes in different organs and pathologies [14,15]. The classification of EVs reveals a complex landscape characterized by several factors. EVs were originally isolated from blood cells and showed significant variability in terms of their cellular origin, molecular content, size, and therapeutic efficacy [16,17]. Their classification based on size categorizes EVs into apoptotic bodies (1–5 µm), microvesicles (0.1–1 µm), and exosomes (30–150 nm) [18]. However, alternative classifications have been proposed, introducing considerations such as tissue of origin (e.g., prostasomes and oncosomes) and functional parameters [19]. EV proteins constitute a key aspect of their classification, reflecting both the cellular origin and the contents of the originating compartments. Exosomes (Exo) are generated by the endocytic pathway through the interaction between the endocytic vesicles and the endosomal sorting complex required for transport (ESCRT) system, and afterwards, they are released by the fusion of multivesicular bodies (MVBs) with the plasma membrane [20]. ESCRTs are involved in Exo production regulation also through the autophagy system. Autophagy-related genes (*Atg*) represent key factors for Exo release and their expression has been found to be deregulated in cancer cells, promoting proliferation and metastasis [21]. The complex network between autophagy and Exo trafficking includes many regulatory proteins and was recently revised by Zubkova and coworkers [22]. Conversely, microvesicles (MV) and apoptotic bodies arise directly from the plasma membrane [22]. In particular, MVs derive from membrane budding, whereas apoptotic bodies form from the blebbing of cells that undergo apoptosis. Cancer cells promote EV release to induce cancer development, proliferation, and metastasis. Among the EVs derived from cancer cells are oncosomes, which differ by size and composition from other EVs (Figure 1, Table 1).

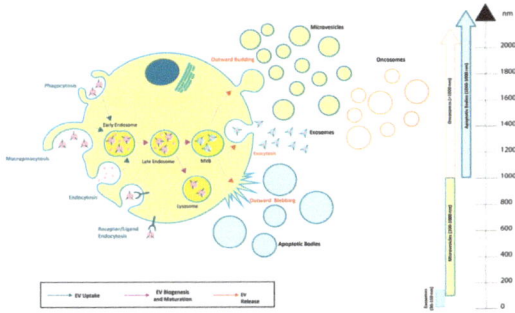

Figure 1. Overview of extracellular vesicle subtypes and their uptake, biogenesis, and release. They are classified into different sub-classes and are generated through the endosomal pathway, released as exosomes (30–150 nm), microvesicles (0.1–1 μm), apoptotic bodies (1–5 μm), and oncosomes (>1 μm).

Table 1. EV classification.

	Characteristics of Extracellular Vesicles (EVs) Subtypes			
EV Subtypes	**Origin**	**Markers**	**Cargo**	**Reference**
Exosomes	MVBs fuse with plasma membrane	CD63, CD81, CD9, HSP60, HSP70, Alix, TSG101	Genomic DNA, mRNA, miRNA, circRNA, lncRNA, MHC class I and II	[23–25]
Microvesicles	Outward budding of plasma membrane	Anneximin A1, Integrins, CD62, CD40 ligand	mRNA, miRNA, circRNA, lncRNA, Lipids, Adesion proteins	[26–28]
Oncosomes	Exclusively shed by cancer cells;Outward budding of plasma membrane	CAV-1, Keratin 18, ARF6, GAPDH	Genomic DNA, mRNA, miRNA, circRNA, lncRNA, MHC calss I and II	[29–32]
Apoptotic bodies	Outward blebbing from cells in apoptosis	Caspase 3, Annexin V, CD63, CD81	miRNA, mRNA, Fragmented DNA, Histones	[33–35]

Integral membrane proteins, specifically tetraspanins like CD9, CD63, and CD81, stand out as important markers. Furthermore, EVs may contain membrane and cytoskeletal proteins, lysosomal enzymes, cytokines, chemokines, antigen presentation-related proteins (MHC class I and II complexes), and nucleic acids such as DNA, mRNAs, and miRNAs, all of which contribute significantly to EV classification [23,36]. The existence of DNA in EVs demonstrated in the past decade adds an intriguing dimension to their molecular composition. DNA in EVs, different in type (single- or double-stranded, mitochondrial) and form (fragment or chromatin-bound), may aid in discriminating EVs based on their cell of origin [37,38]. However, due to a lack of sufficient biomarkers and an overlap in size range, it is difficult to discriminate between the various types of vesicles.

EVs function as messengers and can be involved in key physiological conditions such as coagulation, pregnancy, metabolism, immunity, and apoptosis [39–43]. Under pathological or stress conditions induced by various stimuli, EVs show dynamic responses by altering both their quantity and molecular composition [44–48]. These altered vesicles hold promise as prospective biomarkers for various diseases, serving as reservoirs for potentially dangerous molecules. The pivotal role of EVs extends to their involvement in neurodegenerative diseases [47], blood disorders [49], metabolic processes [50], and cancer progression [51], where they act as intercellular communicators between cells and distant organs. EVs carry functional biomolecules, such as mRNA, proteins, miRNA, and metabolites, and can deliver them to cells across short and long distances, using the blood as a transport medium. The growing interest in EVs as disease biomarkers is reflected in their detectability across various body fluids.

The innate targeting capacity of EVs has shown considerable potential in cancer therapy [52–54], where, to mitigate challenges such as rapid clearance, low uptake rates, and off-target effects, researchers have explored EV engineering strategies that involve the modification of the EV surface and internal cargos [55]. Recent studies have demonstrated that EV surface cargos significantly influence their uptake, providing a basis for engineering strategies. The surface markers, including integrins, CD63, and tetraspanin 8 [56,57], contribute to EV tropism and are susceptible to engineering to improve their uptake efficiency [58]. EVs' potential in cancer therapy extends to artificial targeting strategies, where specific surface molecules are designed to bind to molecules expressed on the surface of the desired recipient cells. This approach includes receptor–ligand interactions, enzymatic modifications, and antigen–antibody combinations [55]. In particular, engineered EVs with ankyrin repeat proteins expressed on the surface of the cell membrane exhibited specific binding to HER2-positive breast cancer cells, showing the potential of the receptor–ligand interaction strategy [59]. Antibody-mediated strategies involve engineering EV surfaces with anti-CD3 and anti-EGFR antibodies, leading to the T-cell-mediated elimination of EGFR-positive cancer cells [60]. Enzymatic strategies using hyaluronidase on the EV surface aim to increase EV uptake by degrading the tumor extracellular matrix, improving permeability for both tumor-specific CD8 T cells and drugs in the tumor microenvironment [61].

Upon uptake, the EV cargo modulates the activity of recipient cells [62,63], and, in this context, EVs secreted by MSCs (MSC-EVs) are a promising therapeutic component of the MSC secretome. Most preclinical studies involving MSC-EV therapy are based on vesicles produced by MSCs [3,64,65]. Moreover, to potentiate the functional activity of MSC-EVs, the strategy of priming/preconditioning their cells of origin was explored by using chemicals, cytokines, and growth factors, as well as specific culture conditions [3,64,66–69]. For instance, human MSC-EVs produced after stimulation with dimethyloxaloylglycine further stimulated angiogenesis through the Akt/mTOR pathway to enhance bone healing [70]. Tumor necrosis factor-alpha (TNF-α) was able to prime MSCs and improve the bone regenerative properties of MSC-derived EVs, as evidenced by the increased proliferation and osteogenic differentiation of osteoblastic cells in vitro [71]. Furthermore, several studies explored the effects of inflammatory priming on MSC-EVs, revealing distinct EV functions compared to other priming conditions. For instance, it was recently demonstrated that EVs derived from IFN-γ-primed MSCs have improved immunomodulatory properties compared to the 3D culture priming of MSC-EVs, which instead showed enhanced angiogenic properties [66]. In this scenario, the yield, size, and surface marker composition of MSC-derived EVs exhibited substantial variations with various priming treatments, and it is intriguing to understand how the EV content and their beneficial properties can be modulated. These studies will no doubt lay the foundation for potential advancements in MSC-EV therapeutics.

3. EVs in Diagnosis

While lung cancer represents, in most cases, a very inoperable disease with a low response to radiation therapy or chemotherapy and a low survival rate (with <17% for NSCLC and <7% for SCLC), the most important factor contributing to an increase in survival rate is early diagnosis and the selection of specific targeted therapeutic procedures.

The identification of tumor characteristics based on molecular markers plays a key role in treatment effectiveness. Recently, a minimally invasive approach known as liquid biopsy was introduced, which involves sampling a small portion of body fluids to search for circulating tumor cells (CTCs), circulating proteins, and nucleic acids [72]. In this scenario, EVs, and particularly Exo, contain mediators influencing tumor progression as components of carcinogenesis that can help to identify and classify tumor onset and prevent its diffusion.

Several methods can be used to isolate EVs, such as differential ultracentrifugation, size exclusion chromatography, gradient centrifugation, the co-precipitation method, and microfluidic devices [73]. Yet, this represents a major challenge for EV application, since the development of high-throughput methodologies to allow for the rapid isolation of EVs from many samples would enhance their use in diagnosis [74].

EVs are known to participate in intercellular communication, immune responses, metabolism, and tumor progression, as they are capable of horizontally transmitting a wide range of biomolecules to target cells, making them important biomarkers for diagnosis, as well as promising molecular carriers for targeted therapies. The information they carry can influence the behavior of target cells in multiple ways. In particular, they can act as indicators, transferring membrane proteins and receptors to target cells, or even altering their phenotype through the horizontal transfer of genetic information. It has been demonstrated that EVs can deliver not only proteins or lipids, but also miRNAs, other ncRNAs, and mRNAs [75]. The analysis of EV miRNA levels in lung cancer patients showed a significant difference compared to control samples, suggesting that circulating EV miRNAs might represent a useful screening tool [76]. Compared to other circulating biomarkers such as cell-free DNA (cfDNA) and CTC, EVs have the advantage of being more abundant and more stable, given their lipid layer, which also protects the transported cargo. These characteristics are very important in order to establish sensitive and easily repeatable protocols for the early diagnosis of disease. Their role is central in certain pathological phenomena; for instance, it is now widely demonstrated that a tumor cell can release more than 20,000 of these vesicles in 48 h [77], with a role in conditioning the tumor microenvironment (TME). The TME includes several components such as the extracellular matrix (ECM), endothelial cells, cancer-associated fibroblasts (CAFs), and a strong immune component such as tumor-associated macrophages (TAMs), natural killer cells (NK), and T and B lymphocytes. Sanchez and coworkers examined the involvement of EVs and their miRNA cargo in the TME, demonstrating how they stimulate the formation of the neointima by activating macrophages within the TME, thus generating a niche for inflammation [78]. The analysis of EVs can represent a low-impact source for lung cancer characterization; notably, it has been demonstrated that EVs derived from bronchoalveolar lavage fluid (BALF) liquid biopsy can be used proficiently for epidermal growth factor receptor (EGFR) genotyping and the evaluation of EGFR mutations [79]. This method, together with the digital droplet PCR (ddPCR) and next-generation sequencing (NGS) techniques, can allow for the stratification of patients for TKI treatment without invasive methods such as tissue biopsy [79]. In this way, it is possible to quantify (copies/mL) and identify, if present, variants relating to the mutated EGFR, perhaps due to targetable resistance mechanisms involved in resistance to cancer therapy [80]. In this regard, a prospective phase 2 study was carried out to promote EGFR genotyping for subsequent therapeutic interventions through the analysis of EV-BALF liquid biopsy obtained from advanced NSCLC patients [81]. The study, for the first time, established that this platform represents a valid tool for immediate genotyping and allows for rapid results for therapeutic initiation in advanced NSCLC patients [81]. Moving forward, genotyping the miRNA content in EVs has been widely investigated. A recent study evaluated, with low-dose computed tomography (LDCT), the presence of indeterminate pulmonary nodules (IPNs) in association with circulating EV miRNAs [82]. The NGS analysis demonstrated a specific miRNA signature associated with the patient's prognostic survival [82]. Similarly, another study described an miRNA signature (hsa-miR-106b-3p, hsa-miR-125a-5p, hsa-miR-3615, and hsa-miR-450b-5p) from plasma-circulating EVs with the identification of early-stage lung cancer [83]. An analogous result was obtained with the RT-PCR analysis of six miRNAs (miR-7, miR-21, miR-126, Let-7a, miR-17, and miR-19) in EV-BALF. Despite the limited number of patients, the study suggested a correlation between the expression of the analyzed miRNAs and early-stage lung cancer [84]. High-throughput transcriptomic analyses allowed for the identification of circular RNAs (circRNAs), resulting from the back-splicing of pre-mRNA, among numerous RNA strands. Although first described in the early 1970s, circRNAs were, until very recently, regarded as byproducts of splicing without any important biological function. The main function of circRNAs is the inhibition of miRNAs. They act as miRNA sponges, establishing a complex and precise system in the interaction with RNA-binding proteins and in the regulation of gene expression [85]. Recently, circRNAs were found to be enriched and stable in cancer EVs, suggesting their potential use as cancer biomarkers or therapeutic targets. It has been supposed that EVs could represent a mechanism for the release of circRNAs [86,87].

Cancer patients show circRNA expression levels in the ratio of 2:1 vs healthy controls [88]. A valid example of the role of EVs in prognosis is given by the Hongya et al. study on circVMP1, which was found to be correlated with the progression of NSCLC and resistance to cisplatin therapy [89].

Indeed, there is much evidence for circRNAs being involved in promoting tumor migration, NSCLC development, resistance to therapies, and tumorigenesis, with different pathways of molecular interaction. Through the miR377-5p/NOVA2 axis, circ_007288 promotes the development of NSCLC [90], while circ_0000376 stimulates tumorigenesis and promotes drug resistance by positively modulating the action of KPNA4 and sponging miR1298-5p [91].

Circ_0020123 is particularly interesting for the multiple interaction pathways in which it is involved in lung cancer and appears to be capable of promoting cell proliferation and migration on tumor growth in vivo, acting on the THBS2/miR590-5p axis [92] and favoring cisplatin resistance in NSCLC cells by targeting miR-14-3p [93].

In the study conducted by Wei et al., circ_0020123 acts as a competitive endogenous RNA (ceRNA) to interact with miR-1283, thus promoting the expression levels of PDZD8, a cytoskeletal regulatory protein involved in tumor migration and proliferation [94], also involved in the LARP1/miR-330-5p tumor axis mechanism with the homonymous CircRNA (circ_PDZD8) [95] or suppressing tumor growth either if not expressed [96] or through sponging miR-1299, regulating HMGB3 [97]. Many studies on circRNA in lung cancer have demonstrated a repressive role in the disease. The relevance of circRNAs and their RNA splice variants for tumor progression and therapy response has been demonstrated in preclinical models [98]. Given the plethora of pathways in which circRNAs are involved, the use of a specific database is fundamental to shed light on the many possible pathways, and this is one of the objectives with which CircInteractome was born [99].

Recent studies have explored the role of circRNAs derived from the lung and carried by EVs [100], and most of them are focused on their expression and role in lung cancer [101] (Table 2).

In a pioneering work in this field, Zhu and coworkers identified the presence of circHIPK3 in lung cancer released EVs [102]. This circRNA has been proposed as a novel EV-derived biomarker for lung cancer, whose action is connected with miR-637 reduction and acts as a tumor suppressor on cellular migration, invasion, and proliferation in NSLC [102].

Moreover, it was reported that the circRNAs contained in EVs act as novel genetic information molecules, mediating the interactions between cancer cells and other cells of the TME and regulating key steps in cancer progression [10,103,104]. Nowadays, the use of EV-circRNAs as biomarkers for cancer diagnosis and prognosis shows various limitations for sample sizes and a lack of standardized evaluation systems, so further analysis will support their specific application as early diagnostic markers.

On the other side, engineering strategies for EV-circRNAs could solve the limitations due to the size of circRNAs for efficient packaging and delivery systems, overcoming pharmacodynamics, pharmacokinetics, and safety considerations [105].

Table 2. circRNA effects on lung cancer.

CircRNA #	Function	Pathway	Reference
Circ_0012673	Promote cell proliferation	Sponge miR-22; upregulate ErbB3	[106]
Circ_0067934	Promote cell proliferation, migration, and invasion	Modulate markers of epithelial-to-mesenchymal transition (EMT)	[107]
Circ_007288	Promote cell proliferation	Sponge miR-377-5p/NOVA2	[90]
Circ_0000376	To induce resistance to cisplatin and promote tumorigenesis	Sponge miR-1298-5p/KPNA4	[91]
Circ_PDZD8	Promote cell proliferation	Sponge miR330-5p/LARP1	[95]
Circ_0072309	To promote tumor progression and invasion	Sponge miR607/FTO	[108]
Circ_ATAD1	Enhance cancer progression	Sponge miR-191-5p	[109]
Circ_0092887	Induce resistance to taxane	Sponge miR490-5p/UBE2T	[110]
Circ_0007385	Promote cell proliferation, migration, tumourigenesis, and invasion	Sponge miR-181	[111]
Circ_0013958	Promote cell proliferation and invasion and prevent apoptosis	Sponge miR-134/cyclin D1	[112]
Circ_0020123	Inhibit proliferation and invasion	Sponge miR1299/HMGB3	[97]
Circ_008305	Inhibit tumor metastasis	Sponge miR-429/miR-200b-3p/PTK2	[113]
Circ_CRIM1	Inhibit tumor metastasis and invasion	Sponge miR-93 and miR-182;	[114]
Circ_RNF13	Inhibit tumor proliferation and metastasis	Sponge miR-93-5p	[115]
CircSH3PXD2A	Inhibit tumor chemoresistance	miR-375-3p/YAP1	[116]

In addition to nucleic acid evaluation, recent progress in EV analysis has been implemented by looking at the protein content by proteomic profiling. Lung cancer EVs contain several tumor-associated proteins, such as EGFR, KRAS, inducer of extracellular matrix metalloproteinase, claudins, and RAB family proteins. In NSCLC, other proteins have been found such as exo markers like CD91, CD317, and EGFR. CD151, CD171, and tetraspanin 8 represent very reliable markers for lung cancer characterization and identification. Furthermore, METTL1 and the HIST family of proteins have been found to be overexpressed mostly in tumor samples [117]. Many studies are focusing on identifying the protein profiles of EVs from different stages and histologies of lung cancer, which is very important as a potential diagnostic tool [118,119]. A good example is given by Hoshino et al., who were able to characterize the complete proteomic profile of EVs from the plasma of 16 different cancer types and identified the proteins up- or down-regulated in cancer-associated EVs. Notably, the study revealed that cancer-derived proteins were not potential tumor tissue biomarkers and that approximately 50% of them arose from distant organs. Tumor-specific proteins were detected only in plasma, supporting the systemic nature of cancer and strengthening the potential use of EVs as liquid biopsy markers for early cancer diagnosis [117]. It has been reported that NSCLC-EVs shuttle specific proteins capable of inducing metastasis. Taverna et al. demonstrated that Amphiregulin, a ligand of EGFR contained in NSCLC-EVs, could induce metastasis, activating the EGFR pathway in pre-osteoclasts with an enhanced activity of proteolytic enzymes, leading to bone metastasis formation [120]. NSCLC EVs show an increased expression of *FAM3C*, a gene encoding for interleukin-like EMT inducer (ILEI). This results in an enhanced detection of FAM3C from lung tumor patients vs healthy subjects [121]. Furthermore, Du and coworkers identified that SCLC tumor-cell-derived EVs expressing PD-L1 play an important role in EVs and immune system crosstalk, suggesting a potential use of EV PD-L1 in the design of anticancer strategies [122]. From a prognostic point of view, the expression proteins of the A549 cell line (NSCLC) were analyzed before and after cisplatin treatment [123] by mass spectrometry (LC–MS/MS analysis). The results define a protein profile enriched for cholesterol metabolism pathway activation, indicating the role of EVs in lipogenesis activation and cell proliferation after chemotherapeutic treatment [123]. Nonetheless, a uniform consensus on protein markers from EVs is still missing for the restricted human sample datasets to drive interpretations of data analyses. To date, various resources have deposited the contents of EVs, especially regarding miRNAs, which can be consulted online: EVpedia [124,125] and Exocarta [126]. While the observation of new diagnostic information is strongly promoted, ctDNA represents an interesting target for liquid biopsy investigations in lung cancer detection [127]. However, the study of EVs and their protein cargo or CTCs has not yet entered clinical practice, and their application is limited to research studies (Table 3).

Table 3. Diagnostic application of EVs from different body fluids in lung cancer.

Disease	Body Fluid Samples Source	Description	Reference
Lung Cancer	BALF	LC-MS analysis of proteome profile. DNMT3B protein complex as potential therapeutic target.	[128]
Early-Stage Lung Adenocarcinoma	BALF	Quantitative analysis of miRNAs with diagnostic value. miR-126 and Let-7a possible diagnostic biomarkers: higher levels in lung adenocarcinoma than in control subjects.	[84]
Early-Stage Lung Adenocarcinoma/Invasive Stage Lung Adenocarcinoma	Plasma	A signature drawn up with four miRNAs (hsa-miR-106b-3p, hsa-miR-125a-5p, hsa-miR-3615, and hsa-miR-450b-5p) for early diagnosis.	[83]
Advanced-Stage Lung Adenocarcinoma	BALF	Next-Generation Sequencing (NGS) of EV DNA content to identify genetic alterations, suitable for a clinical approach.	[129]
(Advanced) NSCLC	BALF	EGFR mutation analysis on BALF EVs as method more accurate, specific and rapid than cfDNA evaluation.	[79]
(Advanced) NSCLC	Plasma and BALF	BALF EV DNA analysis as alternative diagnostic method in accordance with tissue biopsy and greater efficiency for detecting the p.T790 M mutation in the patients resistant to EGFR-TKIs.	[130]
(Advanced) NSCLC	BALF	A phase 2 study on BALF EV as platform for EGFR genotyping and rapid therapeutic intervention.	[81]
Adenocarcinoma, Squamous Cell Carcinoma, NSCLC	Bronchial Washing	Detection of *EGFR* mutation and evaluation of its prognostic value.	[131]
Early-Stage Malignant Pleural Mesothelioma (MPM) vs Benign Conditions and Metastatic Adenocarcinomas	Pleural Effusions	Characterization of surface marker or proteins differentially expressed as diagnostic markers.	[132]
Indeterminate Pulmonary Nodules (IPNs)	Plasma	CircEV-miR profile as a molecular model to distinguish the benign and malignant IPNs. miR-30c-5p, miR-30e-5p, miR-500a-3p, miR-125a-5p, and miR-99a-5p: five miRNAs differentially expressed and associated to an overall survival.	[82] Chinese Clinical Trials: ChiCTR1800019877

4. EVs in Lung Cancer Therapy

Until a few years ago, the most common lung cancer treatment was chemotherapy. Recent progress in oncology has prompted the use of immune-checkpoint monoclonal antibody blockades in association with chemotherapeutic treatment [133] or as a single agent, depending on PD-1 IHC expression. On the other hand, next-generation sequencing technologies allow for the identification of the most recurrent mutations in lung cancers, providing a unique tool for evaluating oncogene addiction and the role of targeted therapy. Some of the identified mutations include epidermal growth factor receptor (EGFR), where mutations occur in 15% of NSCLC adenocarcinoma cases [134]. This allows for the targeting of these tumors by specific tyrosine kinase inhibitors (TKIs) and/or monoclonal antibodies, as recommended by current guidelines [135]. Different TKIs have been employed in several clinical trials, which have demonstrated a positive effect on progression-free survival (PFS) and fewer side effects compared to standard chemotherapy (platinum) [136]. Unfortunately, many patients have shown resistance to the specific EGFR inhibitor treatment. To overcome this problem, TKI treatment can be associated with anti-EGFR monoclonal antibodies (cetuximab, necitumumab, and panitumumab), as supported by numerous clinical trials reviewed by Ciardiello and colleagues [137]. Another therapeutic target identified in lung cancers is anaplastic lymphoma kinase (ALK), whose translocation with the EML4 gene affects 5% of NSCLC patients [138]. Specific TKI inhibitors have been identified: crizotinib, second-generation ceritinib and alectinib, and the new-generation lorlatinib, recently preferred for resistance mutations [139]. Interestingly, crizotinib has also been employed as a treatment for NSCLC patients positive for ROS-1 chromosomal rearrangements with clinical signs similar to ALK mutations [140,141]. Similar to NSCLC cancers, some mutations have been identified in mainly SCLC patients. In particular, these alterations concern the suppressor genes TP53 and RB1 [142]. Despite their identification, SCLC tumors do not show targetable mutations, and recently, researchers have been focusing their attention on RB1 as a potential therapy target, as demonstrated by in vivo studies [143,144]. Innovative therapeutic approaches have been studied in the last few years, revealing that EVs play a relevant role in physiological and pathological conditions, such as cancer and cardiovascular and neurodegenerative diseases. Over the last ten years, EV research has focused on their potential application as therapeutic agents. As already underlined, EVs can carry molecules, particularly non-coding RNAs, influencing cancer growth, progression, metastasis, or drug resistance [145]. Therefore, non-coding RNA has gained importance as a therapeutic tool and has been employed in several clinical studies (Table 4). Among the ncRNAs, a pivotal role is played by miRNA, which can be easily carried and delivered by EVs or other vectors. Specifically, miR34 has been widely studied in different tumors. Recently two different phase I multicenter trials were conducted to study by dose escalation the safety, pharmacokinetics, and pharmacodynamics of an miR-34 mimic (MRX34), administered by liposomal injection in patients with melanoma (NCT02862145) and other selected solid tumors: primary liver cancer SCLC, NSCLC, lymphoma, melanoma, multiple myeloma, and renal cell carcinoma (NCT01829971). The melanoma trial was withdrawn due to high toxicity, and the other study on solid tumors showed stable disease (SD) in 6 out of 47 patients [146]. This study represented the first miRNA-based clinical trial on cancer [147]. The capacity of miR-34 to inhibit tumor growth has been demonstrated by various studies, and the ability of EVs to carry this miRNA and inhibit tumor growth in a paracrine way has been assessed [148]. EVs can be considered a peculiar vector for anti-cancer delivery systems due to their natural and advantageous properties, such as their high biocompatibility and limited systemic toxicity. Specific nanocarrier-targeted action can be improved by engineering and functionalizing their surface, for example, by inducing the expression of specific proteins on the EV membrane or through the loading of miRNA, which can be inserted exogenously on isolated EVs (electroporation, sonication, and RNA cholesterol conjugation), or indirectly by genetic modification of the donor cells before EV isolation (RNA transfection, RNA encoding plasmid transfection, and virus transfection) [145]. For example, EVs isolated from mesenchymal stem cells have been demonstrated to transfer miRNA efficiently in different kinds of tumors. This observation has raised the possibility of engineering cells such as MSCs for miR-34 delivery to inhibit tumor growth by EV release [149]. Notable for their ability to migrate towards inflammation or tumoral regions, MSCs have the peculiar characteristic of being able to be genetically modified, and when employed for this purpose, they act as living delivery vectors [150,151]. It was observed recently that engineered bone marrow MSCs (BMSCs) can deliver miR-193a, reducing the cisplatin resistance of NSCLCs by targeting leucine-rich repeat-containing protein 1 (LRRC1) [152]. In the same way, BMSC-derived EVs carrying miR-126-3p suppressed the viability, migration, and invasion of NSCLC cells by targeting protein tyrosine phosphatase non-receptor type 9 (PTPN9) [153]. Similarly, another group showed that engineered BMSCs with miR-598 inhibited cell proliferation, migration, and invasion in NSCLC. They demonstrated that miR-598-loaded EVs acted in lung cells by down-regulating Derlin-1, the zinc finger E-box-binding homeobox 2 (ZEB2), and also Thrombospondin-2 (THBS2), in this way inhibiting growth and metastasis [154]. The same effect was obtained with exosomal miR-338-3p through the inhibition of MAPK signaling, reducing the cell adhesion molecule L1-like protein (CHL1) activity and the subsequent down-regulation of NSCLC proliferation and apoptosis [155]. Engineered exosomes loaded with miR-449a selectively inhibit the growth of homologous NSCLC [156]. Among them, Zhou and colleagues focused their attention on miR-449-a, which affects the migration and invasion of human NSCLC cells. They isolated exosomes from A549 cells and engineered them (miR-449a exo) to allow for the transfer of this miRNA, thereby demonstrating its anti-tumor activity both in in vitro and in vivo models [156]. Similarly, another group used MDA-MB-231 breast cancer cells as a source of engineered lung-targeted exosomes with miRNA-126, which reduced proliferation and migration through the PTEN/PI3K/AKT pathway in A549 cells and an in vivo lung metastasis mouse model [157].

Besides their application as miRNA carriers, EVs have been used for tumor RNA interference (RNAi) therapy through siRNA targeted against specific oncogenes. For example, KRAS, whose mutations account for 90% of pancreatic cancers and 20–25% of lung adenocarcinomas, represents an area of great interest for tumor-targeted gene therapy. Recently, lipid nanoparticles carrying KRAS siRNAs reduced its expression in several lung cancer cell lines, including human (A549 and H441) and mouse (CMT-167 and Lacun3) cells, and proliferation was observed through colony-forming assays [158].

During the last few years, various approaches have been studied and pursued to employ EVs as therapeutic applications or targets in lung cancer. It is well known that the EVs released by tumor cells can promote the spread and diffusion of the tumor and also counteract the immune response by inhibiting CD-positive T cells with anti-tumor functions [159] or favoring immune escape, attenuating cytotoxic CD8+ T cells through the expression of PD-L1, considered as a target for monoclonal therapy in NSCLC patients [160]. Because of these characteristics, EVs have been considered as target therapeutic strategies. Some pharmacological agents act on EV trafficking or lipid membrane metabolism and are extremely important for membrane fluidity and, as a consequence, for EV shedding/release. For example, GW4869 inhibits the membrane-neutral sphingomyelinase (nSMase) and exosome/EV biogenesis; it has been tested in PC9 lung adenocarcinoma cells, counteracting the antagonistic effects of gefitinib and cisplatin, which are widely used for NSCLC patient treatment [161].

Among the numerous molecular partners involved in membrane trafficking is Rab27A, a protein expressed in numerous cell types, including A549, which could regulate EV release. One research group demonstrated that specific shRNA against Rab27A carries a lower release of EVs and a reduction in tumor growth in an in vitro model of human lung adenocarcinoma cells [162].

Considering the impact of EVs on immune escape, over the years, clinical trials have been undertaken to apply them as a cancer vaccine [163–167] The EVs released by tumor cells proficiently trigger anti-tumor immunity; for example, in a study focused on EVs in vitro isolated from 3LL lung tumor cells, the activation of dendritic cells and T cells after being subjected to heat stress was induced through EV inflammatory chemokine contents [163]. Similarly, dendritic cells release vesicles (termed dexosomes) that have been demonstrated to prime T cells and present antigens to T CD8+ and CD4+ cells [168,169]. These cells and their secretome are of great scientific interest; indeed, dendritic cells were tested as autologous vaccinations in a clinical trial involving NSCLC patients, providing interesting immunologic responses [164]. A phase I clinical trial demonstrated the tolerance of engineering dexosomes with MAGE antigens in NSCLC patients' MAGE+ [167]. These dexosomes were also used in a phase II trial on NSCLC patients, resulting in the stabilization of 32% of the recruited patients [166].

In a similar way to miRNA delivery, researchers are attempting to use EVs for drug/chemotherapy delivery. EVs loaded with paclitaxel were administered to a metastatic mouse model of NSCLC [170]. In particular, this research group demonstrated that exosomes efficiently vehicle the paclitaxel [171] and subsequently improved the formulation of these exosomes, demonstrating that this new delivery system exerts a higher ability to reach cancer cells with a better therapeutic effect [170]. Recently, exosomes isolated from M1 macrophages were evaluated as a drug vehicle for cisplatin, both in in vitro (Lewis lung cancer cells) and in vivo mouse models. The study demonstrated that the exosomes from M1 macrophages as chemotherapy carriers improved the anti-lung cancer effect of cisplatin and induced tumor cell death; specifically, in vitro experiments demonstrated the involvement of apoptosis through Bax and Caspase-3 [172]. In another in vitro study with two NSCLC cell lines (H1299 and A549), researchers used exosomes loaded with gold nanoparticles conjugated with doxorubicin, obtaining a greater particle uptake by target cells and drug release and more specific cytotoxicity with fewer side effects [173].

Table 4. Therapeutic in vitro and in vivo application of EVs in lung cancers.

Target/Study Models	Subject	Description	Reference
(Advanced) NSCLC	Vaccination trial with tumor antigen-loaded dendritic cell-derived exosomes	Maintenance immunotherapy in 47 patients with dexosomes to improve their PFS.	NCT01159288
Solid tumors: primary liver cancer, SCLC, lymphoma, melanoma, multiple myeloma, renal cell carcinoma, NSCLC	Multicenter phase I study of MRX34, microRNA miR-RX34 liposomal injection	Phase I, open-label, multicenter, dose escalation study to investigate the safety, pharmacokinetics, and pharmacodynamics of the micro ribonucleic acid (microRNA) MRX34 in patients with unresectable primary liver cancer or advanced or metastatic cancer with or without liver involvement or hematologic malignancies.	NCT01829971 [147]
(Advanced) NSCLC	Phase I study of dexosome immunotherapy	Phase I study to evaluate safety and efficacy of autologous dexosomes loaded with tumor antigens (MAGE-A3, -A4, -A10, and MAGE-3DPO4), administered in 4 doses. Measurement of the immunologic responses and monitoring the clinical outcomes in 13 patients at different stages.	[167]
H1299 and A549 (NSCLC)	Nanosomes carrying doxorubicin anticancer activity against human lung cancer cells	In vitro analysis of gold nanoparticles (GNPs) loaded with doxorubicin to evaluate the release kinetics and the cytotoxic activity.	[173]
Mice injected with B16F10 cells to produce lung metastasis	EVs melanoma gold conjugated nanoparticle targeting lung tumors	The study provided an application system where exosomes isolated from cancer cells incorporated gold nanoparticles were tested in a mouse model to improve targeting system in metastatic foci.	[174]
In vitro: murine carcinoma cell line'(3LL-M27); in vivo: mouse model with pulmonary metastases	Paclitaxel-loaded EVs against cancer cells	In vitro and in vivo study aims to introduce a new formulation for Paclitaxel distribution through exosomes (PTX-exo, fom RAW 264.7 cell line), providing high stability in tumor environment and a better effectiveness in vivo murine model.	[171]
In vitro: A549 and H1299 (NSCLC); In vivo: mouse model with lung cancer xenograft	Celastrol EVs formulation against lung cancer	Study focused on the effect of the natural compound celastrol loaded into exosomes, a new delivery system improved efficacy and reduced dose toxicity.	[175]
In vitro: A549 and H1299 (NSCLC); In vivo: nude mice with xenograft	Anthocyanidins EVs against multiple cancer types	The study aimed to obtain a nano-formulation of the natural derived compound, anthos, with exosomes. Exosomes enhanced the anti-proliferative and anti-inflammatory activity of anthos (vs the free compound) and the therapeutic affect toward lung cancer.	[176]
Nude mice with lung tumor xenografts	Milk-derived exosomes for oral delivery of paclitaxel	A study on chemotherapeutic paclitaxel delivery through exosomes in a formulation for oral administration, which exhibited greater therapeutic efficacy and lower systemic toxicity.	[177]

5. Conclusions and Remarks

The potential applications of EVs in therapeutic and diagnostic approaches are far from being fully achieved. Over the last decade, the EV cancer field has experienced significant advancements that have fundamentally changed our understanding of intercellular communication and cancer biology.

However, a deeper knowledge of EV's role in lung cancer is crucial in order to define biomarkers for prognosis and diagnosis, as well as to develop new therapeutic strategies for such deadly tumors [1]. So, to transfer this knowledge from bench to bedside, other studies need to be conducted to clarify and confirm the potential role of EVs in lung cancer and beyond. Tumor heterogeneity, in particular looking at EGFR mutations, is currently under investigation to further correlate cellular modifications with therapeutic response [81].

Their utility as delivery vehicles for various drugs, proteins, and nucleic acids has been evaluated by many laboratories. Their lipid composition contributes to their stability in body fluids and provides, at the same time, valid support for their cellular delivery by cell membrane fusion [178]. Moreover, the immunological properties of MSC offer a unique tool for EV secretion, combining their specific transfer ability aptitude (drugs, nucleic acids, and proteins) with immunomodulatory pharmacological effects [179] or new therapeutic approaches in numerous diseases, including lung cancer (Table 4). Despite MSCs' natural tropism against tumors, which can represent a valid site-specific EV throughput tool, dendritic cell-derived exosomes can support the targeted tumor delivery of EVs and represent a promising example of vaccination due to their immunostimulatory capability (NCT01159288). On the other hand, from a diagnostic point of view and given the important role for cancer biology, the use of circulating EVs has gained a growing interest primarily for their availability. Conversely, one of the main challenges is represented from EVs' origin, because their release is not exclusively related to the disease but can arise from any tissue. A wider analysis of EVs' composition can support fast stratification and early detection. In this regard, a substantial analysis of EV circRNA signatures can identify lung-cancer-regulated miRNA [100,102]. Furthermore, a proteomic analysis of EV content offers the opportunity to acquire more information about EV biology and identify new biomarkers, contributing to early diagnosis and the design of valid treatments [180] (Figure 2). There are many difficulties and limitations, but the multi-omics approach has a very bright future and will undoubtedly provide much more information on these nano-sized biological entities. Despite numerous studies on experimental models and various pathologies, there are still many points that can be improved, for example, identifying cellular sources safe for immunogenicity and sources that can guarantee significant quantities, as well as trying to introduce standardized procedures to improve the workflow throughput. We hope that groundbreaking tests on the diagnostic and prognostic meaning of EV evaluation can draw new routine procedures for dissecting tumor heterogeneity and narrowing therapeutic intervention protocols.

Last, but not least, scientists must investigate EVs' structure deeply to maximize their engineering and applications as carrier systems (Figure 2). Another area to be further explored is related to their turnover. Studies have already focused on their release inhibition, and, considering the importance of the uptake step, it could be interesting to try to selectively reduce uptake mechanisms, although the pathways involved are numerous [181,182].

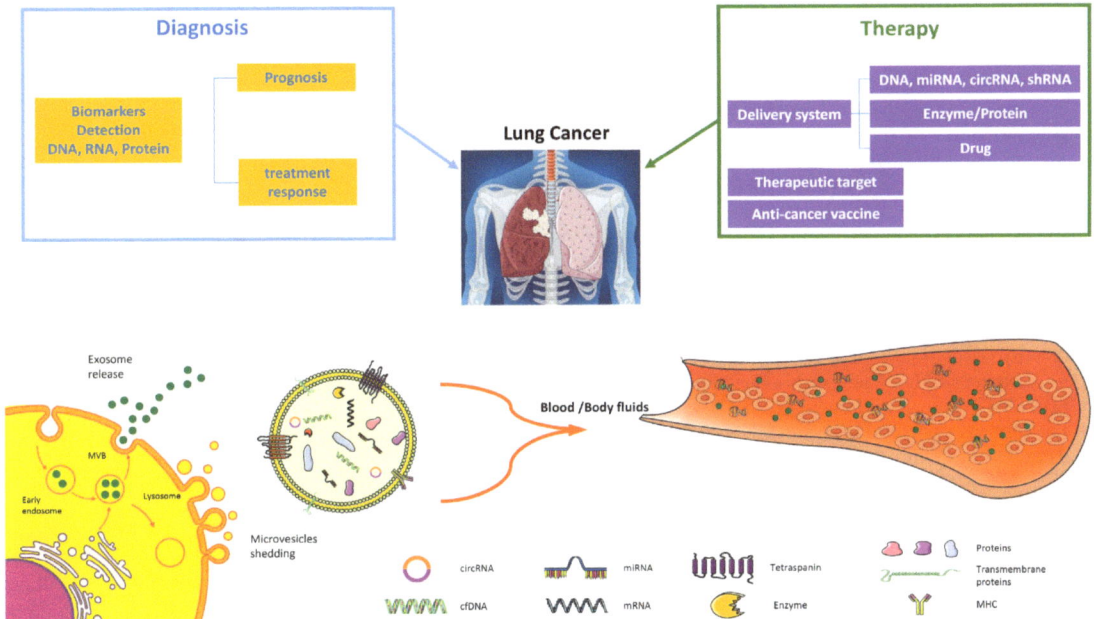

Figure 2. EVs in lung cancer diagnosis and therapy. EVs are important players in intercellular communication, released through the endosomal pathway by the plasma membrane as exosomes (30–150 nm), microvesicles (0.1–1 µm), and apoptotic bodies (1–5 µm). Tumor-derived EVs are good candidates for liquid biopsy since they contain many components such as tumor-derived DNA, mRNA, miRNAs, and proteins. Their analysis from plasma or body fluids (BALF) offers significant information about tumor diagnosis through biomarkers crucial for early detection or prognosis and treatment response. The potential application of EV in therapy comprises their application in targeted therapy through the delivery of specific miRNAs, drug delivery of chemotherapy agents, or their employment as anti-cancer vaccines.

Author Contributions: A.P.C. and G.I. conceived and designed the review. Data collection and interpretation were carried out by A.P.C., R.T., V.M., A.G., V.G., L.I., M.P., S.T. and G.I. All authors approved the final draft of the manuscript. All authors have read and agreed to the published version of the manuscript.

Funding: V.M. and G.I. work was supported by the Italian Ministry of Health, Ricerca Corrente.

Acknowledgments: The authors thank IRCCS ISMETT's Language Services Department for editing the manuscript.

Conflicts of Interest: The authors declare no conflicts of interest.

References

1. Sung, H.; Ferlay, J.; Siegel, R.L.; Laversanne, M.; Soerjomataram, I.; Jemal, A.; Bray, F. Global Cancer Statistics 2020: GLOBOCAN Estimates of Incidence and Mortality Worldwide for 36 Cancers in 185 Countries. *CA Cancer J. Clin.* **2021**, *71*, 209–249. [CrossRef]
2. Thai, A.A.; Solomon, B.J.; Sequist, L.V.; Gainor, J.F.; Heist, R.S. Lung cancer. *Lancet* **2021**, *398*, 535–554. [CrossRef]
3. Miceli, V.; Zito, G.; Bulati, M.; Gallo, A.; Busa, R.; Iannolo, G.; Conaldi, P.G. Different priming strategies improve distinct therapeutic capabilities of mesenchymal stromal/stem cells: Potential implications for their clinical use. *World J. Stem Cells* **2023**, *15*, 400–420. [CrossRef]
4. Grange, C.; Tapparo, M.; Collino, F.; Vitillo, L.; Damasco, C.; Deregibus, M.C.; Tetta, C.; Bussolati, B.; Camussi, G. Microvesicles released from human renal cancer stem cells stimulate angiogenesis and formation of lung premetastatic niche. *Cancer Res.* **2011**, *71*, 5346–5356. [CrossRef]

5. Zhang, C.; Qin, C.; Dewanjee, S.; Bhattacharya, H.; Chakraborty, P.; Jha, N.K.; Gangopadhyay, M.; Jha, S.K.; Liu, Q. Tumor-derived small extracellular vesicles in cancer invasion and metastasis: Molecular mechanisms, and clinical significance. *Mol. Cancer* **2024**, *23*, 18. [CrossRef]
6. Jothimani, G.; Pathak, S.; Dutta, S.; Duttaroy, A.K.; Banerjee, A. A Comprehensive Cancer-Associated MicroRNA Expression Profiling and Proteomic Analysis of Human Umbilical Cord Mesenchymal Stem Cell-Derived Exosomes. *Tissue Eng. Regen. Med.* **2022**, *19*, 1013–1031. [CrossRef]
7. Xiao, H.; Lasser, C.; Shelke, G.V.; Wang, J.; Radinger, M.; Lunavat, T.R.; Malmhall, C.; Lin, L.H.; Li, J.; Li, L.; et al. Mast cell exosomes promote lung adenocarcinoma cell proliferation—Role of KIT-stem cell factor signaling. *Cell Commun. Signal. CCS* **2014**, *12*, 64. [CrossRef]
8. Bhatta, B.; Luz, I.; Krueger, C.; Teo, F.X.; Lane, D.P.; Sabapathy, K.; Cooks, T. Cancer Cells Shuttle Extracellular Vesicles Containing Oncogenic Mutant p53 Proteins to the Tumor Microenvironment. *Cancers* **2021**, *13*, 2985. [CrossRef]
9. Di Giuseppe, F.; Carluccio, M.; Zuccarini, M.; Giuliani, P.; Ricci-Vitiani, L.; Pallini, R.; De Sanctis, P.; Di Pietro, R.; Ciccarelli, R.; Angelucci, S. Proteomic Characterization of Two Extracellular Vesicle Subtypes Isolated from Human Glioblastoma Stem Cell Secretome by Sequential Centrifugal Ultrafiltration. *Biomedicines* **2021**, *9*, 146. [CrossRef]
10. Cammarata, G.; de Miguel-Perez, D.; Russo, A.; Peleg, A.; Dolo, V.; Rolfo, C.; Taverna, S. Emerging noncoding RNAs contained in extracellular vesicles: Rising stars as biomarkers in lung cancer liquid biopsy. *Ther. Adv. Med. Oncol.* **2022**, *14*, 17588359221131229. [CrossRef]
11. Kato, T.; Vykoukal, J.V.; Fahrmann, J.F.; Hanash, S. Extracellular Vesicles in Lung Cancer: Prospects for Diagnostic and Therapeutic Applications. *Cancers* **2021**, *13*, 4604. [CrossRef]
12. Liu, Y.; Xia, Y.; Smollar, J.; Mao, W.; Wan, Y. The roles of small extracellular vesicles in lung cancer: Molecular pathology, mechanisms, diagnostics, and therapeutics. *Biochim. Biophys. Acta Rev. Cancer* **2021**, *1876*, 188539. [CrossRef]
13. Tine, M.; Biondini, D.; Damin, M.; Semenzato, U.; Bazzan, E.; Turato, G. Extracellular Vesicles in Lung Cancer: Bystanders or Main Characters? *Biology* **2023**, *12*, 246. [CrossRef]
14. Ginini, L.; Billan, S.; Fridman, E.; Gil, Z. Insight into Extracellular Vesicle-Cell Communication: From Cell Recognition to Intracellular Fate. *Cells* **2022**, *11*, 1375. [CrossRef]
15. Alberti, G.; Russo, E.; Corrao, S.; Anzalone, R.; Kruzliak, P.; Miceli, V.; Conaldi, P.G.; Di Gaudio, F.; La Rocca, G. Current Perspectives on Adult Mesenchymal Stromal Cell-Derived Extracellular Vesicles: Biological Features and Clinical Indications. *Biomedicines* **2022**, *10*, 2822. [CrossRef]
16. Russo, E.; Alberti, G.; Corrao, S.; Borlongan, C.V.; Miceli, V.; Conaldi, P.G.; Di Gaudio, F.; La Rocca, G. The Truth Is Out There: Biological Features and Clinical Indications of Extracellular Vesicles from Human Perinatal Stem Cells. *Cells* **2023**, *12*, 2347. [CrossRef]
17. Johnstone, R.M.; Adam, M.; Hammond, J.R.; Orr, L.; Turbide, C. Vesicle formation during reticulocyte maturation. Association of plasma membrane activities with released vesicles (exosomes). *J. Biol. Chem.* **1987**, *262*, 9412–9420. [CrossRef]
18. Di Bella, M.A. Overview and Update on Extracellular Vesicles: Considerations on Exosomes and Their Application in Modern Medicine. *Biology* **2022**, *11*, 804. [CrossRef]
19. Sailliet, N.; Ullah, M.; Dupuy, A.; Silva, A.K.A.; Gazeau, F.; Le Mai, H.; Brouard, S. Extracellular Vesicles in Transplantation. *Front. Immunol.* **2022**, *13*, 800018. [CrossRef]
20. Gurung, S.; Perocheau, D.; Touramanidou, L.; Baruteau, J. The exosome journey: From biogenesis to uptake and intracellular signalling. *Cell Commun. Signal. CCS* **2021**, *19*, 47. [CrossRef]
21. Guo, H.; Chitiprolu, M.; Roncevic, L.; Javalet, C.; Hemming, F.J.; Trung, M.T.; Meng, L.; Latreille, E.; Tanese de Souza, C.; McCulloch, D.; et al. Atg5 Disassociates the V(1)V(0)-ATPase to Promote Exosome Production and Tumor Metastasis Independent of Canonical Macroautophagy. *Dev. Cell* **2017**, *43*, 716–730.e717. [CrossRef]
22. Zubkova, E.; Kalinin, A.; Bolotskaya, A.; Beloglazova, I.; Menshikov, M. Autophagy-Dependent Secretion: Crosstalk between Autophagy and Exosome Biogenesis. *Curr. Issues Mol. Biol.* **2024**, *46*, 2209–2235. [CrossRef]
23. Thery, C.; Witwer, K.W.; Aikawa, E.; Alcaraz, M.J.; Anderson, J.D.; Andriantsitohaina, R.; Antoniou, A.; Arab, T.; Archer, F.; Atkin-Smith, G.K.; et al. Minimal information for studies of extracellular vesicles 2018 (MISEV2018): A position statement of the International Society for Extracellular Vesicles and update of the MISEV2014 guidelines. *J. Extracell. Vesicles* **2018**, *7*, 1535750. [CrossRef]
24. Wei, H.; Chen, Q.; Lin, L.; Sha, C.; Li, T.; Liu, Y.; Yin, X.; Xu, Y.; Chen, L.; Gao, W.; et al. Regulation of exosome production and cargo sorting. *Int. J. Biol. Sci.* **2021**, *17*, 163–177. [CrossRef]
25. Kalluri, R.; LeBleu, V.S. The biology, function, and biomedical applications of exosomes. *Science* **2020**, *367*, aau6977. [CrossRef]
26. Raposo, G.; Stahl, P.D. Extracellular vesicles—On the cusp of a new language in the biological sciences. *Extracell. Vesicles Circ. Nucl. Acids* **2023**, *4*, 240–254. [CrossRef]
27. Cable, J.; Witwer, K.W.; Coffey, R.J.; Milosavljevic, A.; von Lersner, A.K.; Jimenez, L.; Pucci, F.; Barr, M.M.; Dekker, N.; Barman, B.; et al. Exosomes, microvesicles, and other extracellular vesicles-a Keystone Symposia report. *Ann. N. Y. Acad. Sci.* **2023**, *1523*, 24–37. [CrossRef]
28. Turchinovich, A.; Drapkina, O.; Tonevitsky, A. Transcriptome of Extracellular Vesicles: State-of-the-Art. *Front. Immunol.* **2019**, *10*, 202. [CrossRef]

29. Clancy, J.W.; Sheehan, C.S.; Boomgarden, A.C.; D'Souza-Schorey, C. Recruitment of DNA to tumor-derived microvesicles. *Cell Rep.* **2022**, *38*, 110443. [CrossRef] [PubMed]
30. Schmidtmann, M.; D'Souza-Schorey, C. Extracellular Vesicles: Biological Packages That Modulate Tumor Cell Invasion. *Cancers* **2023**, *15*, 5617. [CrossRef] [PubMed]
31. Nicolini, A.; Ferrari, P.; Biava, P.M. Exosomes and Cell Communication: From Tumour-Derived Exosomes and Their Role in Tumour Progression to the Use of Exosomal Cargo for Cancer Treatment. *Cancers* **2021**, *13*, 822. [CrossRef]
32. Minciacchi, V.R.; Freeman, M.R.; Di Vizio, D. Extracellular vesicles in cancer: Exosomes, microvesicles and the emerging role of large oncosomes. *Semin. Cell Dev. Biol.* **2015**, *40*, 41–51. [CrossRef]
33. Crescitelli, R.; Lasser, C.; Szabo, T.G.; Kittel, A.; Eldh, M.; Dianzani, I.; Buzas, E.I.; Lotvall, J. Distinct RNA profiles in subpopulations of extracellular vesicles: Apoptotic bodies, microvesicles and exosomes. *J. Extracell. Vesicles* **2013**, *2*, 20677. [CrossRef]
34. Liu, D.; Kou, X.; Chen, C.; Liu, S.; Liu, Y.; Yu, W.; Yu, T.; Yang, R.; Wang, R.; Zhou, Y.; et al. Circulating apoptotic bodies maintain mesenchymal stem cell homeostasis and ameliorate osteopenia via transferring multiple cellular factors. *Cell Res.* **2018**, *28*, 918–933. [CrossRef]
35. Tang, H.; Luo, H.; Zhang, Z.; Yang, D. Mesenchymal Stem Cell-Derived Apoptotic Bodies: Biological Functions and Therapeutic Potential. *Cells* **2022**, *11*, 3879. [CrossRef]
36. Li, A.; Zhang, T.; Zheng, M.; Liu, Y.; Chen, Z. Exosomal proteins as potential markers of tumor diagnosis. *J. Hematol. Oncol.* **2017**, *10*, 175. [CrossRef]
37. Ghanam, J.; Chetty, V.K.; Barthel, L.; Reinhardt, D.; Hoyer, P.F.; Thakur, B.K. DNA in extracellular vesicles: From evolution to its current application in health and disease. *Cell Biosci.* **2022**, *12*, 37. [CrossRef]
38. Thakur, B.K.; Zhang, H.; Becker, A.; Matei, I.; Huang, Y.; Costa-Silva, B.; Zheng, Y.; Hoshino, A.; Brazier, H.; Xiang, J.; et al. Double-stranded DNA in exosomes: A novel biomarker in cancer detection. *Cell Res.* **2014**, *24*, 766–769. [CrossRef]
39. Huotari, J.; Helenius, A. Endosome maturation. *EMBO J.* **2011**, *30*, 3481–3500. [CrossRef]
40. Soekmadji, C.; Li, B.; Huang, Y.; Wang, H.; An, T.; Liu, C.; Pan, W.; Chen, J.; Cheung, L.; Falcon-Perez, J.M.; et al. The future of Extracellular Vesicles as Theranostics—An ISEV meeting report. *J. Extracell. Vesicles* **2020**, *9*, 1809766. [CrossRef]
41. Berckmans, R.J.; Nieuwland, R.; Boing, A.N.; Romijn, F.P.; Hack, C.E.; Sturk, A. Cell-derived microparticles circulate in healthy humans and support low grade thrombin generation. *Thromb. Haemost.* **2001**, *85*, 639–646.
42. Zhang, J.; Li, H.; Fan, B.; Xu, W.; Zhang, X. Extracellular vesicles in normal pregnancy and pregnancy-related diseases. *J. Cell. Mol. Med.* **2020**, *24*, 4377–4388. [CrossRef]
43. Akbar, N.; Azzimato, V.; Choudhury, R.P.; Aouadi, M. Extracellular vesicles in metabolic disease. *Diabetologia* **2019**, *62*, 2179–2187. [CrossRef]
44. Bewicke-Copley, F.; Mulcahy, L.A.; Jacobs, L.A.; Samuel, P.; Akbar, N.; Pink, R.C.; Carter, D.R.F. Extracellular vesicles released following heat stress induce bystander effect in unstressed populations. *J. Extracell. Vesicles* **2017**, *6*, 1340746. [CrossRef]
45. Chiaradia, E.; Tancini, B.; Emiliani, C.; Delo, F.; Pellegrino, R.M.; Tognoloni, A.; Urbanelli, L.; Buratta, S. Extracellular Vesicles under Oxidative Stress Conditions: Biological Properties and Physiological Roles. *Cells* **2021**, *10*, 1763. [CrossRef]
46. Sproviero, D.; Gagliardi, S.; Zucca, S.; Arigoni, M.; Giannini, M.; Garofalo, M.; Fantini, V.; Pansarasa, O.; Avenali, M.; Ramusino, M.C.; et al. Extracellular Vesicles Derived from Plasma of Patients with Neurodegenerative Disease Have Common Transcriptomic Profiling. *Front. Aging Neurosci.* **2022**, *14*, 785741. [CrossRef]
47. Thompson, A.G.; Gray, E.; Heman-Ackah, S.M.; Mager, I.; Talbot, K.; Andaloussi, S.E.; Wood, M.J.; Turner, M.R. Extracellular vesicles in neurodegenerative disease—Pathogenesis to biomarkers. *Nat. Rev. Neurol.* **2016**, *12*, 346–357. [CrossRef]
48. Martucci, G.; Arcadipane, A.; Tuzzolino, F.; Occhipinti, G.; Panarello, G.; Carcione, C.; Bonicolini, E.; Vitiello, C.; Lorusso, R.; Conaldi, P.G.; et al. Identification of a Circulating miRNA Signature to Stratify Acute Respiratory Distress Syndrome Patients. *J. Pers. Med.* **2020**, *11*, 15. [CrossRef]
49. Charla, E.; Mercer, J.; Maffia, P.; Nicklin, S.A. Extracellular vesicle signalling in atherosclerosis. *Cell Signal.* **2020**, *75*, 109751. [CrossRef] [PubMed]
50. Royo, F.; Moreno, L.; Mleczko, J.; Palomo, L.; Gonzalez, E.; Cabrera, D.; Cogolludo, A.; Vizcaino, F.P.; van-Liempd, S.; Falcon-Perez, J.M. Hepatocyte-secreted extracellular vesicles modify blood metabolome and endothelial function by an arginase-dependent mechanism. *Sci. Rep.* **2017**, *7*, 42798. [CrossRef] [PubMed]
51. Ren, W.; Hou, J.; Yang, C.; Wang, H.; Wu, S.; Wu, Y.; Zhao, X.; Lu, C. Extracellular vesicles secreted by hypoxia pre-challenged mesenchymal stem cells promote non-small cell lung cancer cell growth and mobility as well as macrophage M2 polarization via miR-21-5p delivery. *J. Exp. Clin. Cancer Res. CR* **2019**, *38*, 62. [CrossRef] [PubMed]
52. Jiang, S.; Chen, H.; He, K.; Wang, J. Human bone marrow mesenchymal stem cells-derived exosomes attenuated prostate cancer progression via the miR-99b-5p/IGF1R axis. *Bioengineered* **2022**, *13*, 2004–2016. [CrossRef] [PubMed]
53. Li, S.; Yan, G.; Yue, M.; Wang, L. Extracellular vesicles-derived microRNA-222 promotes immune escape via interacting with ATF3 to regulate AKT1 transcription in colorectal cancer. *BMC Cancer* **2021**, *21*, 349. [CrossRef] [PubMed]
54. Ono, M.; Kosaka, N.; Tominaga, N.; Yoshioka, Y.; Takeshita, F.; Takahashi, R.U.; Yoshida, M.; Tsuda, H.; Tamura, K.; Ochiya, T. Exosomes from bone marrow mesenchymal stem cells contain a microRNA that promotes dormancy in metastatic breast cancer cells. *Sci. Signal.* **2014**, *7*, ra63. [CrossRef] [PubMed]
55. Esmaeili, A.; Alini, M.; Baghaban Eslaminejad, M.; Hosseini, S. Engineering strategies for customizing extracellular vesicle uptake in a therapeutic context. *Stem Cell Res. Ther.* **2022**, *13*, 129. [CrossRef] [PubMed]

56. Rana, S.; Yue, S.; Stadel, D.; Zoller, M. Toward tailored exosomes: The exosomal tetraspanin web contributes to target cell selection. *Int. J. Biochem. Cell Biol.* **2012**, *44*, 1574–1584. [CrossRef] [PubMed]
57. Hoshino, A.; Costa-Silva, B.; Shen, T.L.; Rodrigues, G.; Hashimoto, A.; Tesic Mark, M.; Molina, H.; Kohsaka, S.; Di Giannatale, A.; Ceder, S.; et al. Tumour exosome integrins determine organotropic metastasis. *Nature* **2015**, *527*, 329–335. [CrossRef] [PubMed]
58. Williams, C.; Pazos, R.; Royo, F.; Gonzalez, E.; Roura-Ferrer, M.; Martinez, A.; Gamiz, J.; Reichardt, N.C.; Falcon-Perez, J.M. Assessing the role of surface glycans of extracellular vesicles on cellular uptake. *Sci. Rep.* **2019**, *9*, 11920. [CrossRef] [PubMed]
59. Limoni, S.K.; Moghadam, M.F.; Moazzeni, S.M.; Gomari, H.; Salimi, F. Engineered Exosomes for Targeted Transfer of siRNA to HER2 Positive Breast Cancer Cells. *Appl. Biochem. Biotechnol.* **2019**, *187*, 352–364. [CrossRef]
60. Cheng, Q.; Shi, X.; Han, M.; Smbatyan, G.; Lenz, H.J.; Zhang, Y. Reprogramming Exosomes as Nanoscale Controllers of Cellular Immunity. *J. Am. Chem. Soc.* **2018**, *140*, 16413–16417. [CrossRef]
61. Hong, Y.; Kim, Y.K.; Kim, G.B.; Nam, G.H.; Kim, S.A.; Park, Y.; Yang, Y.; Kim, I.S. Degradation of tumour stromal hyaluronan by small extracellular vesicle-PH20 stimulates CD103(+) dendritic cells and in combination with PD-L1 blockade boosts anti-tumour immunity. *J. Extracell. Vesicles* **2019**, *8*, 1670893. [CrossRef]
62. Lee, T.H.; Chennakrishnaiah, S.; Audemard, E.; Montermini, L.; Meehan, B.; Rak, J. Oncogenic ras-driven cancer cell vesiculation leads to emission of double-stranded DNA capable of interacting with target cells. *Biochem. Biophys. Res. Commun.* **2014**, *451*, 295–301. [CrossRef] [PubMed]
63. Valadi, H.; Ekstrom, K.; Bossios, A.; Sjostrand, M.; Lee, J.J.; Lotvall, J.O. Exosome-mediated transfer of mRNAs and microRNAs is a novel mechanism of genetic exchange between cells. *Nat. Cell Biol.* **2007**, *9*, 654–659. [CrossRef]
64. Miceli, V.; Bulati, M.; Iannolo, G.; Zito, G.; Gallo, A.; Conaldi, P.G. Therapeutic Properties of Mesenchymal Stromal/Stem Cells: The Need of Cell Priming for Cell-Free Therapies in Regenerative Medicine. *Int. J. Mol. Sci.* **2021**, *22*, 763. [CrossRef] [PubMed]
65. Miceli, V.; Bertani, A. Mesenchymal Stromal/Stem Cells and Their Products as a Therapeutic Tool to Advance Lung Transplantation. *Cells* **2022**, *11*, 826. [CrossRef]
66. Bulati, M.; Gallo, A.; Zito, G.; Busa, R.; Iannolo, G.; Cuscino, N.; Castelbuono, S.; Carcione, C.; Centi, C.; Martucci, G.; et al. 3D Culture and Interferon-gamma Priming Modulates Characteristics of Mesenchymal Stromal/Stem Cells by Modifying the Expression of Both Intracellular and Exosomal microRNAs. *Biology* **2023**, *12*, 1063. [CrossRef]
67. Bulati, M.; Miceli, V.; Gallo, A.; Amico, G.; Carcione, C.; Pampalone, M.; Conaldi, P.G. The Immunomodulatory Properties of the Human Amnion-Derived Mesenchymal Stromal/Stem Cells Are Induced by INF-gamma Produced by Activated Lymphomonocytes and Are Mediated by Cell-To-Cell Contact and Soluble Factors. *Front. Immunol.* **2020**, *11*, 54. [CrossRef] [PubMed]
68. Miceli, V.; Pampalone, M.; Vella, S.; Carreca, A.P.; Amico, G.; Conaldi, P.G. Comparison of Immunosuppressive and Angiogenic Properties of Human Amnion-Derived Mesenchymal Stem Cells between 2D and 3D Culture Systems. *Stem Cells Int.* **2019**, *2019*, 7486279. [CrossRef]
69. Miceli, V.; Chinnici, C.M.; Bulati, M.; Pampalone, M.; Amico, G.; Schmelzer, E.; Gerlach, J.C.; Conaldi, P.G. Comparative study of the production of soluble factors in human placenta-derived mesenchymal stromal/stem cells grown in adherent conditions or as aggregates in a catheter-like device. *Biochem. Biophys. Res. Commun.* **2020**, *522*, 171–176. [CrossRef]
70. Liang, B.; Liang, J.M.; Ding, J.N.; Xu, J.; Xu, J.G.; Chai, Y.M. Dimethyloxaloylglycine-stimulated human bone marrow mesenchymal stem cell-derived exosomes enhance bone regeneration through angiogenesis by targeting the AKT/mTOR pathway. *Stem Cell Res. Ther.* **2019**, *10*, 335. [CrossRef]
71. Lu, Z.; Chen, Y.; Dunstan, C.; Roohani-Esfahani, S.; Zreiqat, H. Priming Adipose Stem Cells with Tumor Necrosis Factor-Alpha Preconditioning Potentiates Their Exosome Efficacy for Bone Regeneration. *Tissue Eng. Part A* **2017**, *23*, 1212–1220. [CrossRef] [PubMed]
72. Casagrande, G.M.S.; Silva, M.O.; Reis, R.M.; Leal, L.F. Liquid Biopsy for Lung Cancer: Up-to-Date and Perspectives for Screening Programs. *Int. J. Mol. Sci.* **2023**, *24*, 2505. [CrossRef] [PubMed]
73. Shao, H.; Im, H.; Castro, C.M.; Breakefield, X.; Weissleder, R.; Lee, H. New Technologies for Analysis of Extracellular Vesicles. *Chem. Rev.* **2018**, *118*, 1917–1950. [CrossRef] [PubMed]
74. Cheng, L.; Hill, A.F. Therapeutically harnessing extracellular vesicles. *Nat. Rev. Drug Discov.* **2022**, *21*, 379–399. [CrossRef] [PubMed]
75. Albanese, M.; Chen, Y.A.; Huls, C.; Gartner, K.; Tagawa, T.; Mejias-Perez, E.; Keppler, O.T.; Gobel, C.; Zeidler, R.; Shein, M.; et al. MicroRNAs are minor constituents of extracellular vesicles that are rarely delivered to target cells. *PLoS Genet.* **2021**, *17*, e1009951. [CrossRef] [PubMed]
76. Rabinowits, G.; Gercel-Taylor, C.; Day, J.M.; Taylor, D.D.; Kloecker, G.H. Exosomal microRNA: A diagnostic marker for lung cancer. *Clin. Lung Cancer* **2009**, *10*, 42–46. [CrossRef] [PubMed]
77. Balaj, L.; Lessard, R.; Dai, L.; Cho, Y.J.; Pomeroy, S.L.; Breakefield, X.O.; Skog, J. Tumour microvesicles contain retrotransposon elements and amplified oncogene sequences. *Nat. Commun.* **2011**, *2*, 180. [CrossRef] [PubMed]
78. Sanchez, C.A.; Andahur, E.I.; Valenzuela, R.; Castellon, E.A.; Fulla, J.A.; Ramos, C.G.; Trivino, J.C. Exosomes from bulk and stem cells from human prostate cancer have a differential microRNA content that contributes cooperatively over local and pre-metastatic niche. *Oncotarget* **2016**, *7*, 3993–4008. [CrossRef] [PubMed]
79. Kim, I.A.; Hur, J.Y.; Kim, H.J.; Kim, W.S.; Lee, K.Y. Extracellular Vesicle-Based Bronchoalveolar Lavage Fluid Liquid Biopsy for EGFR Mutation Testing in Advanced Non-Squamous NSCLC. *Cancers* **2022**, *14*, 2744. [CrossRef]

80. Girard, N. Optimizing outcomes in EGFR mutation-positive NSCLC: Which tyrosine kinase inhibitor and when? *Future Oncol.* **2018**, *14*, 1117–1132. [CrossRef]
81. Kim, I.A.; Hur, J.Y.; Kim, H.J.; Kim, W.S.; Lee, K.Y. A prospective phase 2 study of expeditious EGFR genotyping and immediate therapeutic initiation through extracellular vesicles (EV)-based bronchoalveolar lavage fluid (BALF) liquid biopsy in advanced NSCLC patients. *Transl. Lung Cancer Res.* **2023**, *12*, 1425–1435. [CrossRef] [PubMed]
82. Zheng, D.; Zhu, Y.; Zhang, J.; Zhang, W.; Wang, H.; Chen, H.; Wu, C.; Ni, J.; Xu, X.; Nian, B.; et al. Identification and evaluation of circulating small extracellular vesicle microRNAs as diagnostic biomarkers for patients with indeterminate pulmonary nodules. *J. Nanobiotechnol.* **2022**, *20*, 172. [CrossRef] [PubMed]
83. Gao, S.; Guo, W.; Liu, T.; Liang, N.; Ma, Q.; Gao, Y.; Tan, F.; Xue, Q.; He, J. Plasma extracellular vesicle microRNA profiling and the identification of a diagnostic signature for stage I lung adenocarcinoma. *Cancer Sci.* **2022**, *113*, 648–659. [CrossRef] [PubMed]
84. Kim, J.E.; Eom, J.S.; Kim, W.Y.; Jo, E.J.; Mok, J.; Lee, K.; Kim, K.U.; Park, H.K.; Lee, M.K.; Kim, M.H. Diagnostic value of microRNAs derived from exosomes in bronchoalveolar lavage fluid of early-stage lung adenocarcinoma: A pilot study. *Thorac. Cancer* **2018**, *9*, 911–915. [CrossRef] [PubMed]
85. Chen, L.L. The expanding regulatory mechanisms and cellular functions of circular RNAs. *Nat. Rev. Mol. Cell Biol.* **2020**, *21*, 475–490. [CrossRef] [PubMed]
86. Lasda, E.; Parker, R. Circular RNAs Co-Precipitate with Extracellular Vesicles: A Possible Mechanism for circRNA Clearance. *PLoS ONE* **2016**, *11*, e0148407. [CrossRef] [PubMed]
87. Kim, K.M.; Abdelmohsen, K.; Mustapic, M.; Kapogiannis, D.; Gorospe, M. RNA in extracellular vesicles. *Wiley Interdiscip. Rev. RNA* **2017**, *8*, 1413. [CrossRef] [PubMed]
88. Li, Y.; Zheng, Q.; Bao, C.; Li, S.; Guo, W.; Zhao, J.; Chen, D.; Gu, J.; He, X.; Huang, S. Circular RNA is enriched and stable in exosomes: A promising biomarker for cancer diagnosis. *Cell Res.* **2015**, *25*, 981–984. [CrossRef] [PubMed]
89. Xie, H.; Yao, J.; Wang, Y.; Ni, B. Exosome-transmitted circVMP1 facilitates the progression and cisplatin resistance of non-small cell lung cancer by targeting miR-524-5p-METTL3/SOX2 axis. *Drug Deliv.* **2022**, *29*, 1257–1271. [CrossRef]
90. Tan, Z.; Cao, F.; Jia, B.; Xia, L. Circ_0072088 promotes the development of non-small cell lung cancer via the miR-377-5p/NOVA2 axis. *Thorac. Cancer* **2020**, *11*, 2224–2236. [CrossRef]
91. Hu, S.; Zhang, Q.; Sun, J.; Xue, J.; Wang, C. Circular RNA circ_0000376 promotes paclitaxel resistance and tumorigenesis of non-small cell lung cancer via positively modulating KPNA4 by sponging miR-1298-5p. *Thorac. Cancer* **2023**, *14*, 2116–2126. [CrossRef] [PubMed]
92. Wang, L.; Zhao, L.; Wang, Y. Circular RNA circ_0020123 promotes non-small cell lung cancer progression by sponging miR-590-5p to regulate THBS2. *Cancer Cell Int.* **2020**, *20*, 387. [CrossRef] [PubMed]
93. Wei, D.; Zeng, J.; Rong, F.; Xu, Y.; Wei, R.; Zou, C. Circ_0020123 enhances the cisplatin resistance in non-small cell lung cancer cells partly by sponging miR-140-3p to regulate homeobox B5 (HOXB5). *Bioengineered* **2022**, *13*, 5126–5140. [CrossRef] [PubMed]
94. Wei, W.; Wang, C.; Wang, L.; Zhang, J. Circ_0020123 promotes cell proliferation and migration in lung adenocarcinoma via PDZD8. *Open Med.* **2022**, *17*, 536–549. [CrossRef] [PubMed]
95. Zhu, X.; Du, T.; Chen, X.; Hu, P. Circ-PDZD8 promotes cell growth and glutamine metabolism in non-small cell lung cancer by enriching LARP1 via sequestering miR-330-5p. *Thorac. Cancer* **2023**, *14*, 2187–2197. [CrossRef] [PubMed]
96. Zhang, H.; Huang, T.; Yuan, S.; Long, Y.; Tan, S.; Niu, G.; Zhang, P.; Yang, M. Circ_0020123 plays an oncogenic role in non-small cell lung cancer depending on the regulation of miR-512-3p/CORO1C. *Thorac. Cancer* **2022**, *13*, 1406–1418. [CrossRef] [PubMed]
97. Sun, F.; Yang, X.; Song, W.; Yu, N.; Lin, Q. Tanshinone IIA (TSIIA) represses the progression of non-small cell lung cancer by the circ_0020123/miR-1299/HMGB3 pathway. *Mol. Cell. Biochem.* **2023**, *478*, 1973–1986. [CrossRef] [PubMed]
98. De Fraipont, F.; Gazzeri, S.; Cho, W.C.; Eymin, B. Circular RNAs and RNA Splice Variants as Biomarkers for Prognosis and Therapeutic Response in the Liquid Biopsies of Lung Cancer Patients. *Front. Genet.* **2019**, *10*, 390. [CrossRef] [PubMed]
99. Dudekula, D.B.; Panda, A.C.; Grammatikakis, I.; De, S.; Abdelmohsen, K.; Gorospe, M. CircInteractome: A web tool for exploring circular RNAs and their interacting proteins and microRNAs. *RNA Biol.* **2016**, *13*, 34–42. [CrossRef] [PubMed]
100. Pedraz-Valdunciel, C.; Giannoukakos, S.; Gimenez-Capitan, A.; Fortunato, D.; Filipska, M.; Bertran-Alamillo, J.; Bracht, J.W.P.; Drozdowskyj, A.; Valarezo, J.; Zarovni, N.; et al. Multiplex Analysis of CircRNAs from Plasma Extracellular Vesicle-Enriched Samples for the Detection of Early-Stage Non-Small Cell Lung Cancer. *Pharmaceutics* **2022**, *14*, 2034. [CrossRef]
101. Pedraz-Valdunciel, C.; Giannoukakos, S.; Potie, N.; Gimenez-Capitan, A.; Huang, C.Y.; Hackenberg, M.; Fernandez-Hilario, A.; Bracht, J.; Filipska, M.; Aldeguer, E.; et al. Digital multiplexed analysis of circular RNAs in FFPE and fresh non-small cell lung cancer specimens. *Mol. Oncol.* **2022**, *16*, 2367–2383. [CrossRef] [PubMed]
102. Zhu, Y.; Shen, L.; Xia, Q.; Tao, H.; Liu, Z.; Wang, M.; Zhang, X.; Zhang, J.; Lv, J. Extracellular vesicle-derived circHIPK3: Novel diagnostic biomarker for lung cancer. *Adv. Med. Sci.* **2023**, *68*, 426–432. [CrossRef] [PubMed]
103. Zhang, F.; Jiang, J.; Qian, H.; Yan, Y.; Xu, W. Exosomal circRNA: Emerging insights into cancer progression and clinical application potential. *J. Hematol. Oncol.* **2023**, *16*, 67. [CrossRef] [PubMed]
104. Cammarata, G.; Barraco, N.; Giusti, I.; Gristina, V.; Dolo, V.; Taverna, S. Extracellular Vesicles-ceRNAs as Ovarian Cancer Biomarkers: Looking into circRNA-miRNA-mRNA Code. *Cancers* **2022**, *14*, 3404. [CrossRef] [PubMed]
105. Cui, J.; Wang, J.; Liu, L.; Zou, C.; Zhao, Y.; Xue, Z.; Sun, X.; Jiang, T.; Song, J. Presence and prospects of exosomal circRNAs in cancer (Review). *Int. J. Oncol.* **2023**, *62*, 5495. [CrossRef] [PubMed]

106. Wang, X.; Zhu, X.; Zhang, H.; Wei, S.; Chen, Y.; Chen, Y.; Wang, F.; Fan, X.; Han, S.; Wu, G. Increased circular RNA hsa_circ_0012673 acts as a sponge of miR-22 to promote lung adenocarcinoma proliferation. *Biochem. Biophys. Res. Commun.* **2018**, *496*, 1069–1075. [CrossRef] [PubMed]
107. Wang, J.; Li, H. CircRNA circ_0067934 silencing inhibits the proliferation, migration and invasion of NSCLC cells and correlates with unfavorable prognosis in NSCLC. *Eur. Rev. Med. Pharmacol. Sci.* **2018**, *22*, 3053–3060. [CrossRef]
108. Mo, W.L.; Deng, L.J.; Cheng, Y.; Yu, W.J.; Yang, Y.H.; Gu, W.D. Circular RNA hsa_circ_0072309 promotes tumorigenesis and invasion by regulating the miR-607/FTO axis in non-small cell lung carcinoma. *Aging* **2021**, *13*, 11629–11645. [CrossRef]
109. Wan, Z.; Jia, S.; Lu, J.; Ge, X.; Chen, Q. circ-ATAD1 as Competing Endogenous RNA for miR-191-5p Forces Non-small Cell Lung Cancer Progression. *Appl. Biochem. Biotechnol.* **2023**. [CrossRef]
110. Wang, L.; Zhang, Z.; Tian, H. Hsa_circ_0092887 targeting miR-490-5p/UBE2T promotes paclitaxel resistance in non-small cell lung cancer. *J. Clin. Lab. Anal.* **2023**, *37*, e24781. [CrossRef]
111. Jiang, M.M.; Mai, Z.T.; Wan, S.Z.; Chi, Y.M.; Zhang, X.; Sun, B.H.; Di, Q.G. Microarray profiles reveal that circular RNA hsa_circ_0007385 functions as an oncogene in non-small cell lung cancer tumorigenesis. *J. Cancer Res. Clin. Oncol.* **2018**, *144*, 667–674. [CrossRef] [PubMed]
112. Zhu, X.; Wang, X.; Wei, S.; Chen, Y.; Chen, Y.; Fan, X.; Han, S.; Wu, G. hsa_circ_0013958: A circular RNA and potential novel biomarker for lung adenocarcinoma. *FEBS J.* **2017**, *284*, 2170–2182. [CrossRef] [PubMed]
113. Wang, L.; Tong, X.; Zhou, Z.; Wang, S.; Lei, Z.; Zhang, T.; Liu, Z.; Zeng, Y.; Li, C.; Zhao, J.; et al. Circular RNA hsa_circ_0008305 (circPTK2) inhibits TGF-beta-induced epithelial-mesenchymal transition and metastasis by controlling TIF1gamma in non-small cell lung cancer. *Mol. Cancer* **2018**, *17*, 140. [CrossRef] [PubMed]
114. Wang, L.; Liang, Y.; Mao, Q.; Xia, W.; Chen, B.; Shen, H.; Xu, L.; Jiang, F.; Dong, G. Circular RNA circCRIM1 inhibits invasion and metastasis in lung adenocarcinoma through the microRNA (miR)-182/miR-93-leukemia inhibitory factor receptor pathway. *Cancer Sci.* **2019**, *110*, 2960–2972. [CrossRef] [PubMed]
115. Wang, L.; Liu, S.; Mao, Y.; Xu, J.; Yang, S.; Shen, H.; Xu, W.; Fan, W.; Wang, J. CircRNF13 regulates the invasion and metastasis in lung adenocarcinoma by targeting miR-93-5p. *Gene* **2018**, *671*, 170–177. [CrossRef] [PubMed]
116. Chao, F.; Zhang, Y.; Lv, L.; Wei, Y.; Dou, X.; Chang, N.; Yi, Q.; Li, M. Extracellular Vesicles Derived circSH3PXD2A Inhibits Chemoresistance of Small Cell Lung Cancer by miR-375-3p/YAP1. *Int. J. Nanomed.* **2023**, *18*, 2989–3006. [CrossRef] [PubMed]
117. Hoshino, A.; Kim, H.S.; Bojmar, L.; Gyan, K.E.; Cioffi, M.; Hernandez, J.; Zambirinis, C.P.; Rodrigues, G.; Molina, H.; Heissel, S.; et al. Extracellular Vesicle and Particle Biomarkers Define Multiple Human Cancers. *Cell* **2020**, *182*, 1044–1061.e1018. [CrossRef] [PubMed]
118. Jakobsen, K.R.; Paulsen, B.S.; Baek, R.; Varming, K.; Sorensen, B.S.; Jorgensen, M.M. Exosomal proteins as potential diagnostic markers in advanced non-small cell lung carcinoma. *J. Extracell. Vesicles* **2015**, *4*, 26659. [CrossRef] [PubMed]
119. Malla, R.R.; Pandrangi, S.; Kumari, S.; Gavara, M.M.; Badana, A.K. Exosomal tetraspanins as regulators of cancer progression and metastasis and novel diagnostic markers. *Asia-Pac. J. Clin. Oncol.* **2018**, *14*, 383–391. [CrossRef]
120. Taverna, S.; Pucci, M.; Giallombardo, M.; Di Bella, M.A.; Santarpia, M.; Reclusa, P.; Gil-Bazo, I.; Rolfo, C.; Alessandro, R. Amphiregulin contained in NSCLC-exosomes induces osteoclast differentiation through the activation of EGFR pathway. *Sci. Rep.* **2017**, *7*, 3170. [CrossRef]
121. Thuya, W.L.; Kong, L.R.; Syn, N.L.; Ding, L.W.; Cheow, E.S.H.; Wong, R.T.X.; Wang, T.; Goh, R.M.W.; Song, H.; Jayasinghe, M.K.; et al. FAM3C in circulating tumor-derived extracellular vesicles promotes non-small cell lung cancer growth in secondary sites. *Theranostics* **2023**, *13*, 621–638. [CrossRef]
122. Dou, X.; Hua, Y.; Chen, Z.; Chao, F.; Li, M. Extracellular vesicles containing PD-L1 contribute to CD8+ T-cell immune suppression and predict poor outcomes in small cell lung cancer. *Clin. Exp. Immunol.* **2022**, *207*, 307–317. [CrossRef]
123. Xu, J.; Wang, L.; Yin, N.; Chen, A.; Yi, J.; Tang, J.; Xiang, J. Proteomic profiling of extracellular vesicles and particles reveals the cellular response to cisplatin in NSCLC. *Thorac. Cancer* **2021**, *12*, 2601–2610. [CrossRef] [PubMed]
124. Kim, D.K.; Kang, B.; Kim, O.Y.; Choi, D.S.; Lee, J.; Kim, S.R.; Go, G.; Yoon, Y.J.; Kim, J.H.; Jang, S.C.; et al. EVpedia: An integrated database of high-throughput data for systemic analyses of extracellular vesicles. *J. Extracell. Vesicles* **2013**, *2*, 20384. [CrossRef] [PubMed]
125. Lai, H.; Li, Y.; Zhang, H.; Hu, J.; Liao, J.; Su, Y.; Li, Q.; Chen, B.; Li, C.; Wang, Z.; et al. exoRBase 2.0: An atlas of mRNA, lncRNA and circRNA in extracellular vesicles from human biofluids. *Nucleic Acids Res.* **2022**, *50*, D118–D128. [CrossRef]
126. Keerthikumar, S.; Chisanga, D.; Ariyaratne, D.; Al Saffar, H.; Anand, S.; Zhao, K.; Samuel, M.; Pathan, M.; Jois, M.; Chilamkurti, N.; et al. ExoCarta: A Web-Based Compendium of Exosomal Cargo. *J. Mol. Biol.* **2016**, *428*, 688–692. [CrossRef] [PubMed]
127. Rolfo, C.; Mack, P.C.; Scagliotti, G.V.; Baas, P.; Barlesi, F.; Bivona, T.G.; Herbst, R.S.; Mok, T.S.; Peled, N.; Pirker, R.; et al. Liquid Biopsy for Advanced Non-Small Cell Lung Cancer (NSCLC): A Statement Paper from the IASLC. *J. Thorac. Oncol. Off. Publ. Int. Assoc. Study Lung Cancer* **2018**, *13*, 1248–1268. [CrossRef]
128. Carvalho, A.S.; Moraes, M.C.S.; Hyun Na, C.; Fierro-Monti, I.; Henriques, A.; Zahedi, S.; Bodo, C.; Tranfield, E.M.; Sousa, A.L.; Farinho, A.; et al. Is the Proteome of Bronchoalveolar Lavage Extracellular Vesicles a Marker of Advanced Lung Cancer? *Cancers* **2020**, *12*, 3450. [CrossRef] [PubMed]
129. Lee, S.E.; Park, H.Y.; Hur, J.Y.; Kim, H.J.; Kim, I.A.; Kim, W.S.; Lee, K.Y. Genomic profiling of extracellular vesicle-derived DNA from bronchoalveolar lavage fluid of patients with lung adenocarcinoma. *Transl. Lung Cancer Res.* **2021**, *10*, 104–116. [CrossRef]

130. Hur, J.Y.; Kim, H.J.; Lee, J.S.; Choi, C.M.; Lee, J.C.; Jung, M.K.; Pack, C.G.; Lee, K.Y. Extracellular vesicle-derived DNA for performing EGFR genotyping of NSCLC patients. *Mol. Cancer* **2018**, *17*, 15. [CrossRef]
131. Park, J.; Lee, C.; Eom, J.S.; Kim, M.H.; Cho, Y.K. Detection of EGFR Mutations Using Bronchial Washing-Derived Extracellular Vesicles in Patients with Non-Small-Cell Lung Carcinoma. *Cancers* **2020**, *12*, 2822. [CrossRef] [PubMed]
132. Javadi, J.; Gorgens, A.; Vanky, H.; Gupta, D.; Hjerpe, A.; El-Andaloussi, S.; Hagey, D.; Dobra, K. Diagnostic and Prognostic Utility of the Extracellular Vesicles Subpopulations Present in Pleural Effusion. *Biomolecules* **2021**, *11*, 1606. [CrossRef] [PubMed]
133. Duma, N.; Santana-Davila, R.; Molina, J.R. Non-Small Cell Lung Cancer: Epidemiology, Screening, Diagnosis, and Treatment. *Mayo Clin. Proc.* **2019**, *94*, 1623–1640. [CrossRef] [PubMed]
134. Barta, J.A.; Powell, C.A.; Wisnivesky, J.P. Global Epidemiology of Lung Cancer. *Ann. Glob. Health* **2019**, *85*, 8. [CrossRef] [PubMed]
135. Planchard, D.; Popat, S.; Kerr, K.; Novello, S.; Smit, E.F.; Faivre-Finn, C.; Mok, T.S.; Reck, M.; Van Schil, P.E.; Hellmann, M.D.; et al. Metastatic non-small cell lung cancer: ESMO Clinical Practice Guidelines for diagnosis, treatment and follow-up. *Ann. Oncol. Off. J. Eur. Soc. Med. Oncol.* **2018**, *29*, iv192–iv237. [CrossRef] [PubMed]
136. Lee, C.K.; Wu, Y.L.; Ding, P.N.; Lord, S.J.; Inoue, A.; Zhou, C.; Mitsudomi, T.; Rosell, R.; Pavlakis, N.; Links, M.; et al. Impact of Specific Epidermal Growth Factor Receptor (EGFR) Mutations and Clinical Characteristics on Outcomes After Treatment with EGFR Tyrosine Kinase Inhibitors Versus Chemotherapy in EGFR-Mutant Lung Cancer: A Meta-Analysis. *J. Clin. Oncol. Off. J. Am. Soc. Clin. Oncol.* **2015**, *33*, 1958–1965. [CrossRef] [PubMed]
137. Ciardiello, F.; Hirsch, F.R.; Pirker, R.; Felip, E.; Valencia, C.; Smit, E.F. The role of anti-EGFR therapies in EGFR-TKI-resistant advanced non-small cell lung cancer. *Cancer Treat. Rev.* **2024**, *122*, 102664. [CrossRef]
138. Lei, Y.; Lei, Y.; Shi, X.; Wang, J. EML4-ALK fusion gene in non-small cell lung cancer. *Oncol. Lett.* **2022**, *24*, 277. [CrossRef]
139. Baglivo, S.; Ricciuti, B.; Ludovini, V.; Metro, G.; Siggillino, A.; De Giglio, A.; Chiari, R. Dramatic Response to Lorlatinib in a Heavily Pretreated Lung Adenocarcinoma Patient Harboring G1202R Mutation and a Synchronous Novel R1192P ALK Point Mutation. *J. Thorac. Oncol. Off. Publ. Int. Assoc. Study Lung Cancer* **2018**, *13*, e145–e147. [CrossRef]
140. Shaw, A.T.; Ou, S.H.; Bang, Y.J.; Camidge, D.R.; Solomon, B.J.; Salgia, R.; Riely, G.J.; Varella-Garcia, M.; Shapiro, G.I.; Costa, D.B.; et al. Crizotinib in ROS1-rearranged non-small-cell lung cancer. *N. Engl. J. Med.* **2014**, *371*, 1963–1971. [CrossRef]
141. Drilon, A.; Somwar, R.; Wagner, J.P.; Vellore, N.A.; Eide, C.A.; Zabriskie, M.S.; Arcila, M.E.; Hechtman, J.F.; Wang, L.; Smith, R.S.; et al. A Novel Crizotinib-Resistant Solvent-Front Mutation Responsive to Cabozantinib Therapy in a Patient with ROS1-Rearranged Lung Cancer. *Clin. Cancer Res. Off. J. Am. Assoc. Cancer Res.* **2016**, *22*, 2351–2358. [CrossRef] [PubMed]
142. Rudin, C.M.; Brambilla, E.; Faivre-Finn, C.; Sage, J. Small-cell lung cancer. *Nat. Rev. Dis. Primers* **2021**, *7*, 3. [CrossRef] [PubMed]
143. Wu, Z.; Su, J.; Li, F.L.; Chen, T.; Mayner, J.; Engler, A.; Ma, S.; Li, Q.; Guan, K.L. YAP silencing by RB1 mutation is essential for small-cell lung cancer metastasis. *Nat. Commun.* **2023**, *14*, 5916. [CrossRef] [PubMed]
144. Wildey, G.; Shay, A.M.; McColl, K.S.; Yoon, S.; Shatat, M.A.; Perwez, A.; Spainhower, K.B.; Kresak, A.M.; Lipka, M.; Yang, M.; et al. Retinoblastoma Expression and Targeting by CDK4/6 Inhibitors in Small Cell Lung Cancer. *Mol. Cancer Ther.* **2023**, *22*, 264–273. [CrossRef]
145. Paramananthan, A.; Asfiya, R.; Das, S.; McCully, G.; Srivastava, A. Extracellular Vesicle (EVs) Associated Non-Coding RNAs in Lung Cancer and Therapeutics. *Int. J. Mol. Sci.* **2022**, *23*, 13637. [CrossRef]
146. Beg, M.S.; Brenner, A.J.; Sachdev, J.; Borad, M.; Kang, Y.K.; Stoudemire, J.; Smith, S.; Bader, A.G.; Kim, S.; Hong, D.S. Phase I study of MRX34, a liposomal miR-34a mimic, administered twice weekly in patients with advanced solid tumors. *Investig. New Drugs* **2017**, *35*, 180–188. [CrossRef] [PubMed]
147. Hong, D.S.; Kang, Y.K.; Borad, M.; Sachdev, J.; Ejadi, S.; Lim, H.Y.; Brenner, A.J.; Park, K.; Lee, J.L.; Kim, T.Y.; et al. Phase 1 study of MRX34, a liposomal miR-34a mimic, in patients with advanced solid tumours. *Br. J. Cancer* **2020**, *122*, 1630–1637. [CrossRef] [PubMed]
148. Badami, E.; Carcione, C.; Chinnici, C.M.; Tinnirello, R.; Conaldi, P.G.; Iannolo, G. HCV Interplay with Mir34a: Implications in Hepatocellular Carcinoma. *Front. Oncol.* **2021**, *11*, 803278. [CrossRef]
149. Vakhshiteh, F.; Rahmani, S.; Ostad, S.N.; Madjd, Z.; Dinarvand, R.; Atyabi, F. Exosomes derived from miR-34a-overexpressing mesenchymal stem cells inhibit in vitro tumor growth: A new approach for drug delivery. *Life Sci.* **2021**, *266*, 118871. [CrossRef]
150. Shan, C.; Liang, Y.; Wang, K.; Li, P. Mesenchymal Stem Cell-Derived Extracellular Vesicles in Cancer Therapy Resistance: From Biology to Clinical Opportunity. *Int. J. Biol. Sci.* **2024**, *20*, 347–366. [CrossRef]
151. Sohrabi, B.; Dayeri, B.; Zahedi, E.; Khoshbakht, S.; Nezamabadi Pour, N.; Ranjbar, H.; Davari Nejad, A.; Noureddini, M.; Alani, B. Mesenchymal stem cell (MSC)-derived exosomes as novel vehicles for delivery of miRNAs in cancer therapy. *Cancer Gene Ther.* **2022**, *29*, 1105–1116. [CrossRef]
152. Wu, H.; Mu, X.; Liu, L.; Wu, H.; Hu, X.; Chen, L.; Liu, J.; Mu, Y.; Yuan, F.; Liu, W.; et al. Bone marrow mesenchymal stem cells-derived exosomal microRNA-193a reduces cisplatin resistance of non-small cell lung cancer cells via targeting LRRC1. *Cell Death Dis.* **2020**, *11*, 801. [CrossRef] [PubMed]
153. Chen, J.; Ding, C.; Yang, X.; Zhao, J. BMSCs-Derived Exosomal MiR-126-3p Inhibits the Viability of NSCLC Cells by Targeting PTPN9. *JBUON Off. J. Balk. Union Oncol.* **2021**, *26*, 1832–1841.
154. Li, X.; Wu, F. Mesenchymal stem cell-derived extracellular vesicles transfer miR-598 to inhibit the growth and metastasis of non-small-cell lung cancer by targeting THBS2. *Cell Death Discov.* **2023**, *9*, 3. [CrossRef] [PubMed]
155. Tian, W.; Yang, X.; Yang, H.; Lv, M.; Sun, X.; Zhou, B. Exosomal miR-338-3p suppresses non-small-cell lung cancer cells metastasis by inhibiting CHL1 through the MAPK signaling pathway. *Cell Death Dis.* **2021**, *12*, 1030. [CrossRef] [PubMed]

156. Zhou, W.; Xu, M.; Wang, Z.; Yang, M. Engineered exosomes loaded with miR-449a selectively inhibit the growth of homologous non-small cell lung cancer. *Cancer Cell Int.* **2021**, *21*, 485. [CrossRef] [PubMed]
157. Nie, H.; Xie, X.; Zhang, D.; Zhou, Y.; Li, B.; Li, F.; Li, F.; Cheng, Y.; Mei, H.; Meng, H.; et al. Use of lung-specific exosomes for miRNA-126 delivery in non-small cell lung cancer. *Nanoscale* **2020**, *12*, 877–887. [CrossRef] [PubMed]
158. Anthiya, S.; Ozturk, S.C.; Yanik, H.; Tavukcuoglu, E.; Sahin, A.; Datta, D.; Charisse, K.; Alvarez, D.M.; Loza, M.I.; Calvo, A.; et al. Targeted siRNA lipid nanoparticles for the treatment of KRAS-mutant tumors. *J. Control. Release Off. J. Control. Release Soc.* **2023**, *357*, 67–83. [CrossRef] [PubMed]
159. Huang, S.H.; Li, Y.; Zhang, J.; Rong, J.; Ye, S. Epidermal growth factor receptor-containing exosomes induce tumor-specific regulatory T cells. *Cancer Investig.* **2013**, *31*, 330–335. [CrossRef] [PubMed]
160. de Miguel-Perez, D.; Russo, A.; Arrieta, O.; Ak, M.; Barron, F.; Gunasekaran, M.; Mamindla, P.; Lara-Mejia, L.; Peterson, C.B.; Er, M.E.; et al. Extracellular vesicle PD-L1 dynamics predict durable response to immune-checkpoint inhibitors and survival in patients with non-small cell lung cancer. *J. Exp. Clin. Cancer Res. CR* **2022**, *41*, 186. [CrossRef] [PubMed]
161. Li, X.Q.; Liu, J.T.; Fan, L.L.; Liu, Y.; Cheng, L.; Wang, F.; Yu, H.Q.; Gao, J.; Wei, W.; Wang, H.; et al. Exosomes derived from gefitinib-treated EGFR-mutant lung cancer cells alter cisplatin sensitivity via up-regulating autophagy. *Oncotarget* **2016**, *7*, 24585–24595. [CrossRef]
162. Li, W.; Hu, Y.; Jiang, T.; Han, Y.; Han, G.; Chen, J.; Li, X. Rab27A regulates exosome secretion from lung adenocarcinoma cells A549: Involvement of EPI64. *APMIS Acta Pathol. Microbiol. Immunol. Scand.* **2014**, *122*, 1080–1087. [CrossRef] [PubMed]
163. Chen, T.; Guo, J.; Yang, M.; Zhu, X.; Cao, X. Chemokine-containing exosomes are released from heat-stressed tumor cells via lipid raft-dependent pathway and act as efficient tumor vaccine. *J. Immunol.* **2011**, *186*, 2219–2228. [CrossRef] [PubMed]
164. Hirschowitz, E.A.; Foody, T.; Kryscio, R.; Dickson, L.; Sturgill, J.; Yannelli, J. Autologous dendritic cell vaccines for non-small-cell lung cancer. *J. Clin. Oncol. Off. J. Am. Soc. Clin. Oncol.* **2004**, *22*, 2808–2815. [CrossRef] [PubMed]
165. Markov, O.; Oshchepkova, A.; Mironova, N. Immunotherapy Based on Dendritic Cell-Targeted/-Derived Extracellular Vesicles-A Novel Strategy for Enhancement of the Anti-tumor Immune Response. *Front. Pharmacol.* **2019**, *10*, 1152. [CrossRef] [PubMed]
166. Pitt, J.M.; Andre, F.; Amigorena, S.; Soria, J.C.; Eggermont, A.; Kroemer, G.; Zitvogel, L. Dendritic cell-derived exosomes for cancer therapy. *J. Clin. Investig.* **2016**, *126*, 1224–1232. [CrossRef] [PubMed]
167. Morse, M.A.; Garst, J.; Osada, T.; Khan, S.; Hobeika, A.; Clay, T.M.; Valente, N.; Shreeniwas, R.; Sutton, M.A.; Delcayre, A.; et al. A phase I study of dexosome immunotherapy in patients with advanced non-small cell lung cancer. *J. Transl. Med.* **2005**, *3*, 9. [CrossRef] [PubMed]
168. Andre, F.; Escudier, B.; Angevin, E.; Tursz, T.; Zitvogel, L. Exosomes for cancer immunotherapy. *Ann. Oncol. Off. J. Eur. Soc. Med. Oncol.* **2004**, *15* (Suppl. S4), iv141–iv144. [CrossRef]
169. Zitvogel, L.; Regnault, A.; Lozier, A.; Wolfers, J.; Flament, C.; Tenza, D.; Ricciardi-Castagnoli, P.; Raposo, G.; Amigorena, S. Eradication of established murine tumors using a novel cell-free vaccine: Dendritic cell-derived exosomes. *Nat. Med.* **1998**, *4*, 594–600. [CrossRef] [PubMed]
170. Kim, M.S.; Haney, M.J.; Zhao, Y.; Yuan, D.; Deygen, I.; Klyachko, N.L.; Kabanov, A.V.; Batrakova, E.V. Engineering macrophage-derived exosomes for targeted paclitaxel delivery to pulmonary metastases: In vitro and in vivo evaluations. *Nanomed. Nanotechnol. Biol. Med.* **2018**, *14*, 195–204. [CrossRef]
171. Kim, M.S.; Haney, M.J.; Zhao, Y.; Mahajan, V.; Deygen, I.; Klyachko, N.L.; Inskoe, E.; Piroyan, A.; Sokolsky, M.; Okolie, O.; et al. Development of exosome-encapsulated paclitaxel to overcome MDR in cancer cells. *Nanomed. Nanotechnol. Biol. Med.* **2016**, *12*, 655–664. [CrossRef] [PubMed]
172. Li, J.; Li, N.; Wang, J. M1 macrophage-derived exosome-encapsulated cisplatin can enhance its anti-lung cancer effect. *Minerva Medica* **2023**, *114*, 634–641. [CrossRef] [PubMed]
173. Srivastava, A.; Amreddy, N.; Babu, A.; Panneerselvam, J.; Mehta, M.; Muralidharan, R.; Chen, A.; Zhao, Y.D.; Razaq, M.; Riedinger, N.; et al. Nanosomes carrying doxorubicin exhibit potent anticancer activity against human lung cancer cells. *Sci. Rep.* **2016**, *6*, 38541. [CrossRef] [PubMed]
174. Lara, P.; Palma-Florez, S.; Salas-Huenuleo, E.; Polakovicova, I.; Guerrero, S.; Lobos-Gonzalez, L.; Campos, A.; Munoz, L.; Jorquera-Cordero, C.; Varas-Godoy, M.; et al. Gold nanoparticle based double-labeling of melanoma extracellular vesicles to determine the specificity of uptake by cells and preferential accumulation in small metastatic lung tumors. *J. Nanobiotechnol.* **2020**, *18*, 20. [CrossRef]
175. Aqil, F.; Kausar, H.; Agrawal, A.K.; Jeyabalan, J.; Kyakulaga, A.H.; Munagala, R.; Gupta, R. Exosomal formulation enhances therapeutic response of celastrol against lung cancer. *Exp. Mol. Pathol.* **2016**, *101*, 12–21. [CrossRef] [PubMed]
176. Munagala, R.; Aqil, F.; Jeyabalan, J.; Agrawal, A.K.; Mudd, A.M.; Kyakulaga, A.H.; Singh, I.P.; Vadhanam, M.V.; Gupta, R.C. Exosomal formulation of anthocyanidins against multiple cancer types. *Cancer Lett.* **2017**, *393*, 94–102. [CrossRef]
177. Agrawal, A.K.; Aqil, F.; Jeyabalan, J.; Spencer, W.A.; Beck, J.; Gachuki, B.W.; Alhakeem, S.S.; Oben, K.; Munagala, R.; Bondada, S.; et al. Milk-derived exosomes for oral delivery of paclitaxel. *Nanomed. Nanotechnol. Biol. Med.* **2017**, *13*, 1627–1636. [CrossRef] [PubMed]
178. Bari, E.; Ferrarotti, I.; Torre, M.L.; Corsico, A.G.; Perteghella, S. Mesenchymal stem/stromal cell secretome for lung regeneration: The long way through "pharmaceuticalization" for the best formulation. *J. Control. Release Off. J. Control. Release Soc.* **2019**, *309*, 11–24. [CrossRef] [PubMed]

179. Chinnici, C.M.; Russelli, G.; Bulati, M.; Miceli, V.; Gallo, A.; Busa, R.; Tinnirello, R.; Conaldi, P.G.; Iannolo, G. Mesenchymal stromal cell secretome in liver failure: Perspectives on COVID-19 infection treatment. *World J. Gastroenterol.* **2021**, *27*, 1905–1919. [CrossRef]
180. Yao, X.; Liao, B.; Chen, F.; Liu, L.; Wu, K.; Hao, Y.; Li, Y.; Wang, Y.; Fan, R.; Yin, J.; et al. Comparison of proteomic landscape of extracellular vesicles in pleural effusions isolated by three strategies. *Front. Bioeng. Biotechnol.* **2023**, *11*, 1108952. [CrossRef]
181. French, K.C.; Antonyak, M.A.; Cerione, R.A. Extracellular vesicle docking at the cellular port: Extracellular vesicle binding and uptake. *Semin. Cell Dev. Biol.* **2017**, *67*, 48–55. [CrossRef] [PubMed]
182. Mathieu, M.; Martin-Jaular, L.; Lavieu, G.; Thery, C. Specificities of secretion and uptake of exosomes and other extracellular vesicles for cell-to-cell communication. *Nat. Cell Biol.* **2019**, *21*, 9–17. [CrossRef] [PubMed]

Disclaimer/Publisher's Note: The statements, opinions and data contained in all publications are solely those of the individual author(s) and contributor(s) and not of MDPI and/or the editor(s). MDPI and/or the editor(s) disclaim responsibility for any injury to people or property resulting from any ideas, methods, instructions or products referred to in the content.

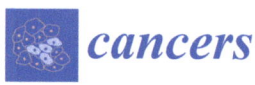 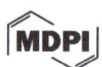

Review

Extracellular Vesicle-Related Non-Coding RNAs in Hepatocellular Carcinoma: An Overview

Giuseppa Augello [1,*], Alessandra Cusimano [1,2], Melchiorre Cervello [1] and Antonella Cusimano [1,*]

[1] Institute for Biomedical Research and Innovation, National Research Council (CNR), 90146 Palermo, Italy; alessandra.cusimano01@unipa.it (A.C.); melchiorre.cervello@irib.cnr.it (M.C.)
[2] Department of Biological, Chemical and Pharmaceutical Science and Technology (STEBICEF), University of Palermo, 90128 Palermo, Italy
* Correspondence: giuseppa.augello@irib.cnr.it (G.A.); antonella.cusimano@irib.cnr.it (A.C.)

Simple Summary: Hepatocellular carcinoma is a highly malignant tumor with increasing prevalence worldwide. Extracellular vesicles exert their biological functions via the delivery of different biomolecules, including non-coding RNAs. In this review, the diverse roles of the non-coding RNA cargo of hepatocellular carcinoma-derived extracellular vesicles will be discussed. Their function in tumor progression, immune escape, and drug resistance, as well as their potentialvalue as biomarkers of disease, will be summarized.

Abstract: Hepatocellular carcinoma (HCC) is the most common primary liver cancer. It is a major public health problem worldwide, and it is often diagnosed at advanced stages, when no effective treatment options are available. Extracellular vesicles (EVs) are nanosized double-layer lipid vesicles containing various biomolecule cargoes, such as lipids, proteins, and nucleic acids. EVs are released from nearly all types of cells and have been shown to play an important role in cell-to-cell communication. In recent years, many studies have investigated the role of EVs in cancer, including HCC. Emerging studies have shown that EVs play primary roles in the development and progression of cancer, modulating tumor growth and metastasis formation. Moreover, it has been observed that non-coding RNAs (ncRNAs) carried by tumor cell-derived EVs promote tumorigenesis, regulating the tumor microenvironment (TME) and playing critical roles in the progression, angiogenesis, metastasis, immune escape, and drug resistance of HCC. EV-related ncRNAs can provide information regarding disease status, thus encompassing a role as biomarkers. In this review, we discuss the main roles of ncRNAs present in HCC-derived EVs, including micro(mi) RNAs, long non-coding (lnc) RNAs, and circular (circ) RNAs, and their potential clinical value as biomarkers and therapeutic targets.

Keywords: hepatocellular carcinoma (HCC); non-coding RNAs; extracellular vesicles (EV); micro(mi) RNAs; long non-coding (lnc) RNAs; circular (circ) RNAs; tumor progression; immune escape; drug resistance; biomarkers

1. Introduction

Hepatocellular carcinoma (HCC) is a tumor with a typically poor prognosis [1]. Currently, it is the fourth main cause for cancer-associated death and has the sixth highest incidence of malignancy in the world, with 780,000 deaths and 1 million new cases per year, as of 2021 [1–3]. HCC is treated via hepatic resection only in its early stage, and patients with an early diagnosis often have a good prognosis, with a 5-year overall survival (OS) rate of 60–80% [4]. However, the intrahepatic and extrahepatic recurrence rate within 5 years of surgical resection remains high [4]. HCC usually lacks obvious symptoms, and 70% of patients are diagnosed at a late stage, when tumor resection is not possible [5]. HCC detection is based on abdominal ultrasonography (US) and elevated serum α-fetoprotein

(AFP) levels [6]. Although abdominal US is highly accurate, its ability to detect small nodules is limited, and measuring AFP levels is suboptimal for early detection due its sensitivity to early-stage tumors being very low [6]. Therefore, there is a need to discover novel markers for liver cancer diagnosis. In patients with advanced stage HCC, the Food and Drug Administration's (FDA) approved systemic treatment options are sorafenib, lenvatinib, cabozantinib, and immunotherapy (pembrolizumab and nivolumab); however, these treatments only partially improve the outcomes of these patients [7]. Indeed, long-term outcomes are still poor, and therefore new treatment strategies are urgently needed [7].

Extracellular vesicles (EVs) are a heterogeneous population of lipid bilayer-delimited particles naturally released from cells, and they are extensively distributed in various biological fluids [8,9]. Based mainly on their size, EVs can be grouped into exosomes (50–150 nm in diameter), ectosomes (100–1000 nm in diameter), apoptotic bodies (1–5 μm in diameter), and large oncosomes (1–10 μm in diameter) [10]. Exosome formation happens via the endocytosis of the cell membrane forming the early endosomes. Subsequently, early endosomes integrate active molecules and other substances forming multiple intraluminal vesicles (ILVs). Late endosomes mature into multivesicular bodies (MVBs), which can encapsulate cargoes derived from various organelles, including the trans-Golgi network (TGN) and endoplasmic reticulum (ER) compartments [11]. Subsequently, MVBs can fuse with lysosomes [12], and their content becomes degraded; some degradation products, such as amino acids, are made available for reuse by the cell. Furthermore, MVBs are translocated to the membrane and, upon fusion, release vesicles into the extracellular space [13]. In the extracellular space, small- (<200 nm) and medium-/large- (>200 nm) sized vesicles are released, collectively termed "extracellular vesicles". The EV membranes consist of a variable mixture of lipids and proteins. Besides membrane-inserted proteins, EVs can also contain biomolecules adsorbed onto their surface, also known as protein coronas [14].

Wolf et al. demonstrated that the protein corona on the surface of EVs can also promote normal angiogenesis in vivo [14]. Proteomic analysis highlighted an enrichment of proangiogenic factors in EVs, and the removal of the protein corona from EVs significantly reduced their angiogenic potential [15].

EVs are released by cells carrying a variety of biologically active molecules [16]. EVs can carry lipids, RNA molecules, DNA, soluble proteins (enzymes, cytokines, chemokines, growth factors), and other proteins, such as tumor suppressors, oncoproteins, and transcriptional and splicing regulators [16]. Furthermore, they are also used as "garbage bags" for discharging unwanted molecules [17].

EVs are natural transporters of various nutrients, as well as lipids and proteins, and other components, such as mineral compounds, which are necessary for tissue generation can be observed within them. In particular, osteoblasts shed EVs known as matrix vesicles [18] with enhanced ASMTL-AS1 expression, containing phosphatases, calcium, and inorganic phosphate, which are fundamental for hard tissue maturation [18]. These EVs play an important role in matrix mineralization; however, on the other hand, ectopic matrix vesicles pathologically promote undesirable calcification in vascular tissues [19].

EVs also carry a variety of regulatory proteins, such as proteins that remodel the extracellular matrix (ECM) [20], as well as mediate the intercellular signal transmission [21]. EVs play an important role in controlling the tumor microenvironment (TME), and they can control the development, immune escape, angiogenesis, invasion, and migration of certain cancers [22].

The isolation of EVs is a critical process, with the chosen method significantly impacting both the sample yield and purity [23,24]. The challenge in EV isolation stems not only from their nano-size, but also from potential contaminants, such as cellular debris, lipoproteins, protein complexes, albumin, argonaute protein complexes, vault viral particles, and aggregates carrying nucleic acids, which can be co-isolated with EVs [23–27].

Among the various protocols available, ultracentrifugation protocols, employing differential sequential cycles at 4 °C with forces up to 120,000 g, are widely used for EV isolation.

However, EVs isolated through ultracentrifugation may exhibit impaired functionality or form aggregates due to the forces exerted during high-speed centrifugation [28–30].

Another common method for EV isolation based on size is ultrafiltration, using membrane filters with specific size-exclusion limits [31–34]. However, preparations obtained via ultrafiltration often contain contaminants of similar diameters to EVs [31–34].

Size-exclusion chromatography is gaining popularity for EV isolation via fractionation, which yields high-purity preparations. This method filters samples through a porous stationary phase, based on hydrodynamic radii [29,35–38].

An alternative is precipitation methods, in which vesicle aggregates are formed by the addition of water-excluding polymers like polyethylene glycol (PEG) [39,40]. However, there is a risk of co-precipitating non-EV material. Commercial kits utilizing this method often include pre-isolation and post-isolation steps in order to minimize contamination [41–44].

Immunoaffinity techniques, exploiting surface proteins and receptors, have been developed to complement other isolation methods [45,46]. These techniques enhance efficiency, specificity, and integrity in recovering EVs from complex fluids, although challenges may arise from the antibody availability and marker presence across the entire EV population [47].

Recent advancements include isolation methods based on microfluidic technologies, which introduce innovative approaches to EV isolation [48,49].

After isolation, the second step in the study of EVs is their characterization in terms of physical and biochemical characteristics, as well as content [27]. The most common approach to defining the physicochemical and molecular characteristics of EVs is single-particle analysis [27,50]. The main single-particle analysis techniques used in the field of EVs are nanoparticle tracking analysis (NTA), electron microscopy, cryo-electron microscopy, atomic force microscopy, high-resolution microscopy, high-resolution flow cytometry, and Raman spectroscopy [50]. Such basic methods as protein quantification, Western Blot, qPCR, and omics analysis, including proteomics, lipidomic analysis, and RNA sequencing, are the main methodologies used to characterize EV cargoes [27].

EV secretion is an emerging mechanism by which tumor cells communicate with their surrounding environment [51]. Moreover, in cancer, EVs can transfer a variety of molecular factors to the target organ, inducing the inflammation necessary to create pre-metastatic niches [52]. In recent years, EVs have been increasingly recognized as important cancer biomarkers because of their high concentration in blood and other body fluids, and because of the bioinformation they carry from their cells of origin in the form of genes and proteins [53]. Compared to normal cells, cancer cells produce more EVs, and the number in the blood circulation of cancer patients is higher than the number in healthy people [53].

Non-coding RNA (ncRNA) is a nucleic acid that can be packaged within EVs and transferred among tumor cells [54]. The peculiar structure of EVs, with bilayer membranes, supports ncRNA transmission and protects them from degradation via circulatory nucleases. The most common types of ncRNAs are microRNA (miRNA), long non-coding RNA (lncRNA), and circular RNA (circRNA) [54]. In recent years, many reports have shown that EV-related ncRNAs play a pivotal role in many biological and pathological processes [55]. Studies regarding EV-related ncRNAs derived from HCC cells have been increasing, indicating that further knowledge of EV-related ncRNAs in liver cancer is significant for early diagnosis and treatment. In this review, the latest studies on various EV-related ncRNAs in HCC will be discussed, with a focus on their potential value as biomarkers of disease, as well as in tumor progression, drug resistance, and immune escape (Figure 1).

Figure 1 demonstrates some of the potential roles and applications that, to date, have been described in the literature following the analysis of the expression of different types of ncRNAs (miRNAs, lncRNAs, and circRNAs) in patients with HCC, or also in cell and animal models of this tumor.

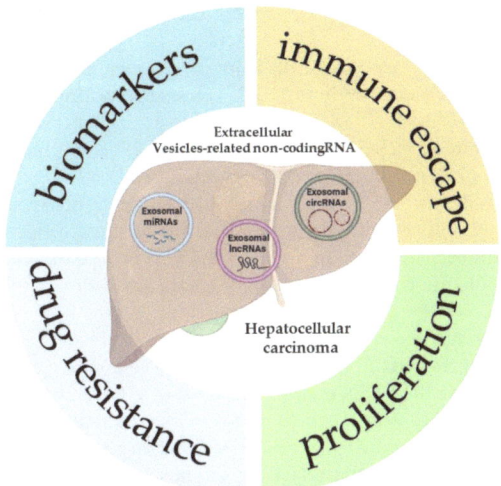

Figure 1. Extracellular vesicle-related non-coding RNAs in hepatocellular carcinoma. The illustration was created with BioRender.com, accessed on 9 January 2024.

2. miRNA-Extracellular Vesicles

miRNAs are small, non-coding, single-stranded RNA molecules, 19–25 nucleotides long, which have been implicated in the regulation of post-transcriptional gene expression via silencing messenger RNAs (mRNAs) [56]. miRNAs bind the 3′ untranslated region (3′ UTR) of the target mRNA, either blocking its translation or degrading it [56]. miRNAs play a crucial role in cell proliferation, differentiation, angiogenesis, metastasis, chemo-resistance to anticancer drugs, malignancy, and apoptosis; however, the information regarding these small non-coding RNAs in HCC-derived EVs is still limited [56,57] (Table 1).

Furthermore, miRNAs contained in HCC-derived EVs are found in biological fluids, meaning they can also be considered cancer biomarker candidates [58]. Different EV cargoes, including miRNAs, are associated with different tumor stages, allowing the early and late stages of the disease to be distinguished, highlighting their potentially important potential diagnostic and prognostic role [59].

2.1. miRNA-Extracellular Vesicles and Hepatocellular Carcinoma Progression

EVs are crucial mediators of both autocrine and paracrine cell communications among different types of liver cells (stellate cells, hepatocytes, and immune cells, including T and B cells, natural killer cells, and Kupffer cells), imperative for maintaining a physiological state. In a pathological state such as cancer, aberrantly expressed miRNAs contained in EVs may act as oncogenes in the absence of cell cycle control, similarly to in HCC, or they may act as tumor suppressors if miRNA blocks the expression of genes involved in cell proliferation [60–62].

Tang et al. found lower levels of exosomal miR-9-3p in the serum of HCC patients compared to control sera. Indeed, miR-9-3p binds and blocks HBGF-5 mRNA expression, which has been implicated in cell proliferation, as demonstrated by their subsequent studies in human HCC cell lines (SMMC-7721, HepG2, and QGY-7703). Furthermore, miR-9-3p decreases the expression of the ERK1/2 regulating cell cycle, cell proliferation, and cell development [62].

Conversely, as demonstrated by Cabiati et al. [57], EVs with high levels of miR-27a are more secreted by human HCC HepG2 cells than non-tumor hepatocytes. miR-27a promotes human HCC cell (HepG2, Bel-7402, and Bel-7404) proliferation through PPAR-γ suppression; in fact, miRNA overexpression is closely related to PPAR-γ downregulation.

PPAR-γ activation arrests the cell cycle via p21 and p53, as well as inducing apoptosis activating Fas [61].

High exosomal miR-429 expression in human HCC cells is involved in HCC progression, targeting Rb binding protein 4 (RBBP4) and activating E2F1, thus promoting POU class 5 homeobox 1 (POU5F1) expression [63,64].

SMMC-7721 cells secrete EVs containing miR-221, which targets the p27/Kip1 tumor suppressor gene, thus promoting tumor cell proliferation and migration [65].

The expression levels of exosomal miR-665 in the sera of 30 HCC patients were significantly increased when compared with a control group of healthy subjects. Indeed, Qu et al. demonstrated in vitro that miR-665 contained in human MHCC-97H- and MHCC-97L cell-derived EVs promotes cell proliferation and tumor growth via the activation of the MAPK/ERK pathway [66].

Zhou et al. indicated that HCC-derived exosomal miR-21 isolated from 97H and LM3 human liver cancer cell lines could convert normal HSCs (hepatic stellate cells) into CAFs (cancer-associated fibroblasts) by decreasing the PTEN expression, leading to the activation of the PDK1/AKT pathway. CAFs also promoted cancer progression, increasing the secretion of matrix metalloproteinase 2 (MMP2), MMP9, vascular endothelial growth factor (VEGF), tumor growth factor-β (TGF-β), and basic fibroblast growth factor (bFGF) [67].

miR-93 from human SKHEP1 and HuH7 cell-derived EVs promotes HCC proliferation and invasion via directly inhibiting TIMP2/TP53INP1/CDKN1A. Furthermore, the overexpression of miR-93 leads to poor prognosis in HCC patients [68].

Yang et al. demonstrated that human MHCC-97H cell-derived EVs with miR-3129 promoted HCC proliferation and epithelial-mesenchymal transition (EMT) in vitro, and they also promoted HCC growth and metastasis formation in vivo [69].

2.2. miRNA-Extracellular Vesicles and Immune Escape in Hepatocellular Carcinoma

In addition to tumor progression, HCC-derived EVs modulate many immune cells, thereby attenuating the anti-HCC immune response [60].

Macrophages play an important role in tumors because they participate in innate immunity. Tumor-associated macrophages (TAMs) consist of two subgroups, M1 and M2 [70]. M1 phenotype macrophages expressing pro-inflammatory cytokines inhibit cell proliferation, whereas the M2 phenotype produces anti-inflammatory cytokines, including TGF-β and IL-10, and demonstrates immunosuppressive and pro-tumoral effects [70,71].

In this context, Liu et al. found that human Hep3B and HepG2 cells transmit exosomal-miR-23a-3p to M2 macrophages, inhibiting PTEN expression and activating the PI3K/AKT signaling pathway; thus, PD-L1 expression increases, and T cell activities are inhibited. Therefore, miR-23a-3p performs a key role in tumor cell escapes from immune cytotoxicity [72].

miR-146a-5p, overexpressed in mouse Hepa1-6 cell-derived EVs, promotes the downregulation of TNF-α and the differentiation of CD206+ macrophages [73]. MiR-452-5p, secreted by human SNU-182 or Huh-7 cell-derived EVs, induces the polarization of M2 macrophages, accelerating HCC growth and metastasis by targeting the tumor suppressor TIMP3 [74]. Similarly, human HepG2 and HuH7 cell-derived exosomal miR-21-5p promotes M2 polarization, enhancing the production of pro-tumorous cytokines. Indeed, miR-21-5p is associated with poor prognosis in HCC [75].

Murine HCC H22 cells release EVs loaded with miRNA let-7b, which binds macrophages, blocking IL-6 production. Thus, this miRNA attenuates tumor inflammation [76].

miR-92b loaded in Hep3B cell-derived EVs downregulates CD69 expression in NK92 cells, influencing its activity against Hep3B cells [77].

2.3. miRNA-Extracellular Vesicles and Hepatocellular Carcinoma Drug Resistance

Drug resistance, occurring when cancer cells develop resistance to drugs, is the primary cause of chemotherapy failure [78,79]. The main mechanisms of resistance are the increased transport of efflux pumps, such as P-glycoprotein, the overexpression of multidrug resistance proteins, decreased drug uptake, increased resistance to apoptosis, and changes in drug target levels [78].

Sorafenib is an antineoplastic agent used to treat patients with advanced HCC [80]. It acts by inhibiting RAF kinases, the platelet-derived growth factor receptor (PDGFR-β), the vascular endothelial growth factor (VEGFR), and several other kinases [80]. Moreover, sorafenib may induce p53 expression, causing Forkhead box M1 (FOXM1) suppression. miR-25 in HepG2- and Huh7 cell-derived EVs blocks p53 expression in cancer cells, inducing the expression of FOXM1 and activating the HGF/Ras pathway. This results in the ineffective treatment of HCC with sorafenib [81].

Wang et al. [82] found that exosome-carried miR-744 l was decreased in both HepG2 cells when compared to LO2 cells, and in exosomes from the serum of HCC patients when compared with those derived from healthy individuals. These authors found that PAX2, highly expressed in HCC tissues compared to normal tissues, is a target of miR-744. When miR-744 is downregulated, the expression of PAX2 increases in HCC cells, promoting proliferation and sorafenib chemoresistance [82].

Human HCC cells (CSQT-2 and HCC-LM3) secrete exosomal miR-1247-3p, which decreases β-1,4-galactosyltransferase III (B4GALT3) expression, activating the β1-integrin/NF-κB pathway in fibroblasts that become CAFs [83]. CAFs activated by miR-1247-3p increase their secretion of IL-6 and IL-8, and other pro-inflammatory cytokines, thus leading to stemness, EMT, and chemoresistance to sorafenib [83,84].

2.4. miRNA-Extracellular Vesicles as Biomarkers in Hepatocellular Carcinoma

New non-invasive biomarkers, such as EV-loaded miRNAs, have been attracting the attention of the scientific community for HCC diagnosis, prognosis, and the prediction of therapy response [85,86].

There are several studies on EVs containing ncRNA as cancer biomarkers, but only recently has research on miRNAs as HCC biomarkers increased [86]. Many miRNAs are recognized for this role, such as miR-224, which is expressed at a significantly higher level in HepG2 and SKHEP1 cells than in healthy liver cells [87]. Similarly, serum exosomal miR-224 expression levels are higher in patients with HCC than in healthy controls. Furthermore, high exosomal expression of miR-224 in the serum of HCC patients is linked to large and advanced stage tumors [87].

miR-21-5p is upregulated more in plasma-derived exosomes from patients with HCC compared to patients with liver cirrhosis; instead, miR-92a3p is downregulated [88]. Moreover, Sorop et al. proposed a statistical model that integrates these two miRNAs with AFP as a novel screening tool to differentiate HCC from liver cirrhosis [88].

Cho et al. identified miR-4661-5p in HCC-derived EVs as a reliable biomarker of HCC at all stages [89]. The authors found that exosomal miR-4661-5p is a more effective and accurate serum biomarker for HCC diagnosis than serum AFP alone [89].

When analyzing the sera of 178 subjects, which included 28 healthy individuals, 27 patients with CHB (chronic hepatitis B), 33 patients with LC (liver cirrhosis), and 90 patients with HCC, exosomal miR-10b-5p was only present in high levels in HCC patients; therefore, it is considered a potential serum biomarker specifically in the early stages of HCC [90].

Exosomal miR-655, described above, may be considered a new biomarker for HCC diagnosis and prognosis [66].

EV-carried miR-3129 is more highly expressed in the plasma of HCC patients than in healthy subjects, and it is considered a potential new tool for HCC diagnosis [69].

Boonkawe et al. demonstrated that plasma-derived EV-miR-19-3p was significantly elevated in patients with HCC when compared to healthy individuals [91]. Therefore, this finding may allow exosomal miR-19-3p to be used as a valid biomarker for the early diagnosis of HCC [91].

High levels of miR-23a are associated with poor HCC prognosis. In fact, decreased levels of miR-23a block cell proliferation, as demonstrated by Bao et al. [92]. Cabiati et al.

also demonstrated that exosomal miR-23a, secreted by human HepG2 cells, is increased in HCC patients when compared to controls; therefore, it is used as a biomarker for the diagnosis of the early stages of HCC [57].

Finding HCC-derived EV-loaded miRNAs for use as new biomarkers will improve the performance of HCC surveillance systems and treatment in clinical practice. This is because several studies have demonstrated the great potential role of EV-miRNAs in cancer diagnosis, prognosis, tumor staging, and the prediction of therapy response [86].

Table 1. The biological functions and gene targets of exosomal miRNAs in HCC.

mRNA	Gene Target	Function	Type of Extraction	Reference
miR-9-3p	HBGF-5	cell proliferation	ultracentrifugation	[62]
miR-27°	PPAR-γ	cell proliferation	ultracentrifugation	[61]
miR-429	RBBP4	cell formation/progression	ultracentrifugation	[63]
miR-221	p27/Kip1	cell proliferation/development	ultracentrifugation	[65]
miR-665	MAPK/ERK	cell proliferation/biomarker	precipitation	[66]
miR-21	PTEN	cell proliferation/progression	ultracentrifugation	[67]
miR-93	TIMP2/TP53INP1/CDKN1A	cell proliferation/invasion	precipitation	[68]
miR-3129	TXNIP	cell proliferation/EMT/biomarker	ultracentrifugation	[69]
miR-23a-3p	PTEN	immune escape	-	[72]
miR-146a-5p	-	immune escape	ultracentrifugation	[73]
miR-452-5p	TIMP3	immune escape	gradient centrifugation	[74]
miR-21-5p	RhoB	immune escape/biomarker	ultrafiltration/ultracentrifugation/precipitation	[75,88]
miRNA let-7b	IL-6	immune escape	ultracentrifugation	[76]
miR-92b	CD69	immune escape/angiogenesis/metastasis	precipitation	[77]
miR-25	p53	drug resistance	ultracentrifugation	[81]
miR-744	PAX2	cell proliferation/drug resistance	ultracentrifugation	[82]
miR-1247-3p	B4GALT3	cell proliferation/EMT/drug resistance	ultracentrifugation	[83]
miR-224	GNMT	cell proliferation/biomarker	precipitation	[87]
miR-92°-3p	PTEN	cell proliferation/EMT/metastasis/biomarker	precipitation	[88]
miR-4661-5p	IL10	biomarker	precipitation	[89]
miR-10b-5p	-	biomarker	ultracentrifugation	[90]
miR-19-3-p	-	biomarker	precipitation	[91]
miR-23a	-	cell proliferation/biomarker	ultracentrifugation	[92]

3. lncRNA-Extracellular Vesicles

About 75% of the human genome is actively transcribed, but only 2% of this is represented by protein-encoding sequences [93]; the other sequences left are ncRNAs, which are RNAs that lack protein-coding capacity. Belonging to this latter group, lncRNAs are ncRNAs with a length of more than 200 nucleotides [94]. It has been demonstrated that lncRNAs play a pivotal role in various physiological and pathological processes like cancers, including HCC [95] (Table 2).

So far, more then 50,000 genes have been identified that transcribe lncRNAs [96]. The expression levels of lncRNAs vary depending on tissue type, and their expression is deregulated in pathological conditions [97]. lncRNAs are important intracellular regulators which can regulate gene expression via interacting with DNA binding promoters or distal regulatory elements and recruiting epigenetic modifiers [94].

lncRNAs can regulate mRNA stability by binding it. In addition, lncRNAs can also bind to miRNAs like molecular sponges, thus interfering with their activities.

lncRNAs have the ability to engage with proteins, contributing to the assembly of protein complexes, where they serve as a scaffold. Additionally, some lncRNAs have the capacity to encode small peptides, through which they exhibit their biological functions. lncRNAs can be packaged into exosomes to protect them from degradation [98].

3.1. lncRNA-Extracellular Vesicles and Hepatocellular Carcinoma Tumor Progression

The analysis of the autocrine effects of the EV contents released by tumor cells has highlighted the role of numerous EV-enriched lncRNAs.

lncRNA FAL1 improves liver cancer cell proliferation and migration by binding to miR-1236, which is a regulator of hypoxia-induced EMT and a cell metastasis biomarker [99].

lncRNA FAM138B (linc-FAM138B) is downregulated in HCC, and its low expression correlates with a poor prognosis [100]. linc-FAM138B can be packaged in exosomes (exo-FAM138B) and released by HCC cells. HCC cells treated with exo-FAM138B show reduced proliferation, migration, and invasion due to the inhibition of miR-765 levels [100]. In vivo data from a xenograft model confirmed that linc-Fam138B-EV suppresses tumor growth [100].

Plasma exosomal lncRNA RP11-85G21.1 (lnc85) stimulated HCC cellular proliferation and migration by targeting miR-324-5p [101].

Serum exosomal LINC00161 has been recognized as a potential biomarker for HCC [102]; however, in vitro exosomes derived from human HCC cells were able to stimulate the proliferation, migration, and angiogenesis of human umbilical vein endothelial (HUVEC) cells. In vivo experiments in mice showed that LINC00161 induces tumorigenesis and metastasis in HCC by targeting miR-590-3p and, consequently, activating its target, ROCK2 [102].

lncRNA ASMTL-AS1 is highly expressed in human HCC tissues and delivered by exosomes [103]. Enhanced ASMTL-AS1 expression induces cell proliferation and migration, along with promoting invasion and EMT in Huh7 cells via ASMTL-AS1/miR-342-3p/NLK/YAP axis [103].

Treatment with exosome-depleted lncH19 from human Huh7 cells inhibited proliferation, migration, and invasion, and induced apoptosis, in HCC cells, whereas exosomal lncH19 from untreated Huh7 cells promoted the proliferation and metastasis, and inhibited the apoptosis, of HCC cells [104]. Moreover, the authors found that the overexpression of miR-520a-3p reversed the effects of treatment with H19-Propofol-Huh7-exo [104]. These data, therefore, suggested that high levels of exosomal lncH19 enhanced tumor development in HCC sponging miR-520a-3p [104].

The lncRNA muskelin 1 antisense RNA (MKLN1-AS) has been demonstrated to play a growth-promoting role in HCC [105].

Special environmental conditions, such as hypoxia, can modulate the release of EVs and define specific cargos [106]. This is the case for linc-ROR, which is induced and enriched in exosomes produced by HCC cells under hypoxic stress [106]. Linc-ROR in recipient cells is able to induce the expression of hypoxia-inducible factor 1 α (HIF1a) and its downstream targets, such as pyruvate dehydrogenase kinase isozyme 1 (PDK1) [106].

lncRNA TUG1 presented in human CAF-secreted exosomes promoted migration, invasion, and glycolysis in human HepG2 cells [107].

In a model of DEN-induced HCC in rats, treatment with hepatic cancer stem cell (CSC)-derived exosomes upregulated the exosomal lncHEIH, lncHOTAIR, and lncTuc339 in rat liver cancer cells [108]. Conversely, the expression of these three lncRNAs was downregulated in livers treated with mesenchymal stem cell (MSC) exosomes derived from rat bone marrow [108]. Therefore, exosomes released from the two different stem cells have opposite effects on HCC: pro-tumoral for CSC-exosomes, and anti-tumoral for MSC-exosomes [108]. All three lncRNAs are involved in the regulation of cell proliferation and metastasis [109], and lncHOTAIR played a role in the transformation of normal liver stem cells into CSCs [110].

3.2. lncRNA-Extracellular Vesicles as Biomarkers in Hepatocellular Carcinoma

Numerous exosome-contained lncRNAs have been the subject of extensive research for their considerable diagnostic value as potential and promising liquid biopsy markers [98].

From the in silico analysis of human liver cancer tissue datasets, Su et al. identified a predictive signature based on five upregulated exosome-related lncRNAs (AC099850.3, LINC01138, MKLN1-AS, AL031985.3, and TMCC1-AS1) which have been associated with poor prognosis in liver cancer patients [111]. In the risk model created by the authors, the signature is correlated with the elevated expression of some crucial regulatory mechanisms of the immune system, and is related to the tumor immune microenvironment [111].

Kim et al. identified four serum EV-derived lncRNAs, SNHG1, MALAT1, HOTTIP, and DLEU2, which were significantly elevated in HCC patients when compared to non-HCC patients, and which significantly discriminated between the two groups [112].

Exosomal LINC00161 has been found to be upregulated in serum exosomes of HCC patients when compared to healthy subjects, and, as suggested by the authors, can be a valuable marker for the diagnosis of HCC [113].

The exosomal lncSENP3-EIF4A1 exhibits reduced expression in HCC patients compared to healthy controls [11]. Both in vitro and in vivo studies have demonstrated that the introduction of SENP3-EIF4A1 functions as a tumor suppressor, inhibiting the proliferation and migration of HCC cells and acting as a competitor of the miR-9-5p target [114].

Serum exosomal lncRNA CRNDE expression levels were shown to be higher in patients with HCC when compared to normal controls [115]. In addition, high levels of serum exosomal lncRNA CRNDE were reported to be correlated with poor prognosis in HCC patients [115]. In vitro, the inhibition of CRNDE expression in human HCC cells was associated with reduced cell proliferation, migration, and invasion [116].

Recently, Yao et al. demonstrated that plasmatic exosomal levels of PRKACA-202, H19-204, and THEMIS2-211 were upregulated in HCC patients when compared to normal controls [117]. In this study, the diagnostic value of the combination of exosomal levels of THEMIS2-211 and PRKACA-202 exceeded that of AFP for the diagnosis of early-stage HCC patients. Furthermore, at the molecular level, the authors demonstrated that THEMIS2-211, through its interaction with miR-940, has an oncogenic role in HCC and regulates proliferation, migration, invasion, and EMT via the modulation of the proteoglycan SPOK1 [117].

The exosome-derived lncRNAs CTD-2116N20.1 and RP11-136I14.5 have been recognized as potential biomarkers for predicting the survival rate of HCC patients [118]. Their presence is associated with an unfavorable prognosis in individuals with HCC. CTD-2116N20.1 is suggested to regulate proteins involved in cell proliferation and tumor metastasis [118].

The exosomal lncRNA RP11-583F2.2 was first identified via bioinformatic analysis and then validated in the serum of HCC patients [119]. Its expression is upregulated in HCC patients compared to viral hepatitis C patients and healthy people [119].

Similarly, exosomal lncRNA-HEIH expression levels allowed researchers to distinguish between chronic hepatitis C and hepatitis C virus (HCV)-associated HCC patients, as its expression only increased in exosomes from patients with HCV-related HCC [120].

Plasma exosomal lncRNA RP11-85G21.1 (lnc85) allowed AFP-negative HCC to be distinguished from liver cirrhosis patients and healthy controls [101].

The exosomal lncRNAs ENST00000440688.1, ENST00000457302.2, and ENSG00000248932.1 are differentially expressed in patients with metastatic HCC when compared to those with non-metastatic HCC [121]. LINC00635 and lncRNA ENSG00000258332.1 (LINC02394) were upregulated in HCC patients and, when combined with AFP, were able to distinguish HCC patients in an independent test of validation [122].

The expression of serum exosomal lncRNA-ATB, associated with exosomal miRNA-21, was inversely correlated with the overall survival and the progression-free survival rates of HCC patients [123].

The analysis of EVs derived from the serum of healthy individuals and individuals with hepatitis, cirrhosis, and HCC revealed the differential expressions of lncZEB2-19, lnc-GPR89B-15, lnc-EPC1-4, and lnc-FAM72D-3 among groups [124]. This functional study highlights that lnc-FAM72D-3 acts as an oncogene targeting hsa-miR-5787 expression, while lnc-EPC1-4 functions as a tumor suppressor gene targeting the influx transporters SLCO1B1v and miR-29b-1-5p [124].

3.3. lncRNA-Extracellular Vesicles and Immune Escape

Human PLC/PRF/5 and Hep3B HCC cell-derived exosomes were found to be enriched with lncTUC339, which is involved in modulating tumor cell growth and adhesion [109]. Exosome-derived TUC339 serves as a mechanism by which tumor cells influence and modify their surrounding environment; indeed, it can promote tumor growth [109] and modulate macrophage activation [125]. This study demonstrated that exosomes from HCC cells could be taken up by THP-1 cells, where TUC339 induced macrophage M1/M2 polarization, switching from a proinflammatory (M1) to an anti-inflammatory phenotype (M2). In addition, elevated levels of TUC339 were found in M(IL-4) macrophages [125].

The immunomodulatory capacity of HCC-released exosomal lncRNA has been demonstrated by other studies [126]. In HCC, the overexpression of PD ligands (PD-L1 and PD-L2) was linked to poor prognosis in HCC patients [127]. Fan et al. demonstrated that human HepG2 and Huh7 HCC cell lines released lncRNA PCED1B-AS1-containing exosomes, which enhanced PD-L expression in receipt HCC cells. PCED1B-AS1 induced PD-L expression via sponging hsa-mir-194-5p, which inhibited PD-L expression [126].

3.4. lncRNA-Extracellular Vesicles and Drug Resistance in Hepatocellular Carcinoma

lncRNA-ROR was found to be enriched in human HepG2 and PLC/PRF/5 HCC cell-derived exosomes, and seemed to be involved in the mechanisms of sorafenib resistance; indeed, lncRNA-ROR levels increased during sorafenib treatment, and inhibited sorafenib-induced cell death [128]. In the same way, lncRNA-VLDLR was involved in the resistance to drugs, such as camptothecin and doxorubicin, as well as sorafenib [129].

Table 2. The biological functions and gene targets of exosomal long non-coding (lnc) RNAs in HCC.

lncRNA	Gene Target	Function	Type of Extraction	Reference
lncRNA FAL1	miR-1236	cell proliferation/migration	precipitation	[99]
lncRNA FAM138B	miR-765	cell proliferation/migration/invasion	gradient centrifugation	[100]
lncRNA RP11-85G21.1 (lnc85)	miR-324-5p	cell proliferation/migration	precipitation	[101]
LINC00161	miR-590-3p	tumorigenesis/metastasis	precipitation	[102]
lncRNA ASMTL-AS1	miR-342-3p	cell proliferation/migration/invasion EMT	precipitation	[103]

Table 2. Cont.

lncRNA	Gene Target	Function	Type of Extraction	Reference
lncH19	miR-520a-3p	tumor development	precipitation	[104]
lncRNA MKLN1-AS	miR-22-3p	cell growth/angiogenesis/migration/	precipitation	[105,120]
Linc-ROR	HIF	regulate hypoxia condition/drug resistance	ultracentrifugation	[106]
lncRNA TUG1	PTEN	migration/invasion/glycolysis	ultracentrifugation	[107]
lnc HEIH		cell proliferation/metastasis/biomarker	ultracentrifugation and density gradient separation	[108,109,120]
lncTuc339		cell proliferation/metastasis Immune escape	ultracentrifugation and density gradient separation	[108,109]
Lnc HOTAIR		cell proliferation/metastasis	ultracentrifugation and density gradient separation	[108,110]
TMCC1-AS1, AL031985.3, LINC01138, AC099850.3		biomarkers	precipitation	[111]
DLEU2, HOTTIP, MALAT1, SNHG1		biomarkers	precipitation	[112]
lncSENP3-EIF4A1	miR-9-5p	immune escape	precipitation	[114]
lncRNA CRNDE		cell proliferation/migration/invasion biomarker	precipitation	[115]
THEMIS2-211	miR-940, modulation of proteoglycan SPOK1	proliferation/migration/invasion/EMT/biomarker	ultracentrifugation	[117]
PRKACA-202		biomarker	ultracentrifugation	[117]
CTD-2116N20.1		biomarker cell proliferation/tumor metastasis		[118]
RP11-136I14.5		biomarker		[118]
RP11-583F2.2	miR-1298	biomarker	precipitation	[119]
ENSG00000248932.1, ENST00000440688.1, ENST00000457302.2		biomarkers	precipitation	[121]
ENSG00000258332.1 (LINC02394), LINC00635		biomarkers	precipitation	[122]
lncRNA-ATB		biomarkers	precipitation	[123]
lnc-FAM72D-3, lnc-GPR89B-15, lncZEB2-19	Has-miR-5787	biomarkers/oncogene	ultracentrifugation	[124]
lnc-EPC1-4	SLCO1B1v and miR-29b-1-5p	biomarker/tumor suppressor	ultracentrifugation	[124]
lncRNA-VLDLR		drug resistance	ultracentrifugation	[129]

4. circRNA-Extracellular Vesicles

Circular RNAs (circRNAs) are endogenous non-coding products [130]. They were initially considered as a byproduct of splicing errors, but, thanks to a sequencing approach, it has been found that circRNAs are related to numerous diseases, including tumors [130,131]. circRNA has a closed circular structure, which is more stable and not easily degradable by exonuclease [132]. Moreover, being carried inside exosomes renders them difficult to be degraded by enzymes [133]. In the last few years, the role of circRNAs has been investigated; they play a vital role in biological functions, they are certainly known to function as competing endogenous RNA (ceRNA), and, together with miRNAs, they regulate the stability of target RNAs and gene expression [134,135]. Moreover, it was found that circRNAs, by interacting with proteins, can also function as protein decoys, scaffolds, and recruiters [136], with regulatory roles in different biological processes. Increasing evidence has confirmed the roles of circRNAs in early diagnosis, tumor progression and invasion, immune escape, and drug response in HCC (Table 3).

4.1. circRNA-Extracellular Vesicles and Hepatocellular Carcinoma Tumor Progression

Numerous studies have found that exosomal circRNAs may have a dual role, acting as promoter or suppressor of HCC progression, invasion, angiogenesis, metastasis, and EMT [137].

Dai et al. demonstrated that human normal hepatic epithelial (L02) cells exposed to arsenite release circRNA_100284 contained in exosomes [138]. CircRNA_00284 is able to activate the cell cycle and increase the proliferation of normal liver cells by interacting with miR-217 [138].

Exosomal circRNA Cdr1 was reported to be important for HCC cell proliferation and migration. Studies demonstrated that exosomes extracted from human HCC cells have elevated levels of Cdr1, and they can induce the proliferative and migratory capabilities of surrounding normal cells [139].

Yu et al. [140] found that Circ_0061395 induced HCC growth through the miR-877-5p/PIK3R3 pathway. They indicated that Circ_0061395 silencing inhibited HCC cell progression and induced cell cycle arrest and cell death in HCC cells.

Exosomal circTTLL5 was found to be more highly expressed in HCC tissues [141]. At the molecular level, the knockdown of circTTLL5 suppressed HCC cell proliferation in vitro, and, in vivo, inhibited tumor growth in mice [141]. Exosomal circRNAs also mediated the crosstalk between normal and cancer cells, thus regulating human HCC growth and metastasis [142].

EMT is a fundamental biological process for cancer cell invasion [143]. Exosome-circRNAs mediate the EMT of HCC cells. Zhang and colleagues showed that, in human cell lines and in mice xenograft models, circ_0003028, via an exosome pathway, controlled E-cadherin, N-cadherin, and vimentin, and induced the EMT transition [144]. Mechanically, circ_0003028 sponge miR-498, which controlled its downstream target ornithine decarboxylase 1 (ODC1) as well as the knockdown of circ_0003028, inhibited cell proliferation and metastasis, and also promoted apoptosis.

The exosome circWDR25 induced tumor progression and EMT through ALOX15 activation via the miR-4474-3p-sponge in SMMC-7721, Hep3B, and HCCLM3 human cell lines [145].

The overexpression of circ-0004277 enhanced the proliferation, migration, and EMT of HCC cells in nude mice and in human cell lines [146].

Higher levels of circ_002136 were shown to be contained in exosomes from HCC cell lines (HA22T and Huh7) rather than in a normal human liver-derived cell line (THLE-3) [147]. In vitro and nude mice experiments showed that silencing circ_002136 inhibited the growth of human HCC cells via the miR-19a-3p and RAB1A axis [147].

Lyu et al. found that circWHSC1, in addition to being associated with a worse overall survival rate in HCC patients, contributed to HCC growth via the elevation of homeobox A1 (HOXA1) expression through sponging miR-142-3p [148].

4.2. circRNA-Extracellular Vesicles and Immune Escape

Wang et al. have shown that circ_0074854 can be transferred from human HCC cells to human macrophages (THP-1 cells) through exosomes [149]. The downregulation of circ_0074854 in exosomes suppressed macrophage M2 polarization, then suppressing the invasion of HCC cells in in vitro and in vivo experiments [149].

Recently, Hu and colleagues reported that a conditioned medium from cultured HCC cells and plasma-exosomes from HCC patients showed high levels of circCCAR1 when compared to a normal human liver cell line and plasma-exosomes from healthy subjects [150]. The same authors have shown that exosomal circCCAR1 was adsorbed by CD8+ T cells, which induced their alteration by inhibiting proliferation, enhancing cell death, lowering cytokines secretion, and, in addition, stabilizing PD-1 protein expression on the cell surface. Thus, circCCAR1 would appear to promote resistance to anti-PD1 immunotherapy [150].

circUHRF1 was overexpressed in HCC cell-derived exosomes and induced NK cell exhaustion [151]. Exosomal circUHRF1 inhibited the secretion of IFN-γ and TNF-α via the induction of TIM-3 expression on NK cells [151]. Furthermore, HCC cell-derived exosomal circUHRF1 may promote the development of resistance to anti-PD1 therapy in a subgroup of HCC patients.

circASAP1, in addition to promoting proliferation and invasion in HCC cells, mediated macrophage infiltration via the miR-326 and miR-532-5p-CSF-1 axis [152].

A recent study found that human HCC cell-derived exosomal circGSE1 promoted the tumor immune escape process by expanding human T cells (Tregs) via the regulation of the miR-324-5p/TGFBR1/Smad3 axis [153]. As a result, the expansion of Tregs promoted the progression of HCC [153].

The ATP-adenosine metabolic pathway regulated by CD39/CD73 is an important immunosuppressive factor in HCC patients; in fact, it induces the culling of NK and T cells [154]. It was demonstrated in both in vitro and in vivo mice models that human macrophages absorb exosome circTMEM181, leading to the regulation of CD39 expression by sponging miR-488-3p [155]. CD39 expression, in synergy with CD73, activates the ATP–adenosine pathway and promotes HCC progression and resistance to anti-PD1 therapy [155]. In contrast, it has recently been shown that circTMEM181 is downregulated in HCC tissues, and decreased expression levels of circTMEM181 were associated with the shorter overall survival of HCC patients [156].

4.3. circRNA-Extracellular Vesicles and Drug Resistance in Hepatocellular Carcinoma

circRNAs play a crucial role in the development of drug resistance and radioresistance in different tumors, including HCC [157]. In human HCC, the cell-derived exosomal circRNA-SORE, also named circ_0087293 or circRNA_104797, controlled sorafenib resistance by stabilizing the oncoprotein YBX1 [158]. The research group's in vitro and in vivo results demonstrated that circRNA-SORE, by binding to YBX1, prevented proteasomal degradation via E3 ubiquitin ligase PRP19 [158].

Hao et al. demonstrated that circPAK1 was overexpressed in the Lenvatinib-resistant human cell lines, LM3 and Hep3B, and that exosomes from resistant cells can mediate the circPAK1 transfer to sensitive cells, thus inducing the lenvatinib resistance of receipt cells [159].

Other authors have demonstrated that circZFR was highly expressed in cisplatin-resistant human HCC cell lines (Huh7 and MHCC97L) and in CAFs [160]. Furthermore, human CAF-derived exosomes delivered circZFR to human HCC cells, inhibited the STAT3/NF-κB axis, and induced cisplatin resistance [160].

Finally, all circRNAs previously described as being involved in immune evasion have the potential to induce resistance to anti-PD1 therapy [156,160,161].

4.4. circRNA-Extracellular Vesicles as Biomarkers in Hepatocellular Carcinoma

In earlier works, Sun et al. found that three circRNAs, hsa_circ_0075792, hsa_circ_0004123, and hsa_circ_0004001, were upregulated in the blood samples of HCC patients, and that their expression was positively correlated with TNM stage and tumor size [161].

Other relevant evidence comes from the work of Lin et al., who found that circ_0072088 was highly expressed in human liver tumor tissues, as well as in exosomes isolated from serum of human patients with HCC [162]. Furthermore, its expression was correlated with unfavorable prognosis in HCC patients [162].

CircFBLIM1 has been shown to be upregulated in HCC serum exosomes [163]. CircFBLIM1 was shown to function as an miR-338 sponge [163]. In a mouse model of HCC tumorigenesis, its levels were correlated with HCC glycolysis and tumor progression induced by the circFBLIM1/miR-338/LRP6 axis [163].

Exosomal hsa_circ_0028861 and hsa_circ_0070396 were detected at higher levels in the serum of HCC patients when compared to sera from chronic HBV and cirrhosis individuals [164,165]. Of interest, the integration of hsa_circ_0028861 with AFP showed the best diagnostic capacity in HBV-derived HCC patients than each parameter alone.

In addition, Zhang et al. found that the levels of serum exosomal circTMEM45A were higher in HCC patients when compared to healthy controls, and its level was positively correlated with poor prognosis in patients [166]. In vitro and in vivo experiments demonstrated that circTMEM45A promoted cell mobility and tumorigenesis through the miR-665/IGF2 axis [166].

Recently, circANTXR1 was found at high levels in exosomes from the serum of HCC patients, and showed diagnostic value in distinguishing HCC patients from healthy controls [167]. Furthermore, circANTXR1, acting as an miR-532-5p sponge, promoted the progression of HCC through the upregulation of the DNA double-strand break repair gene XRCC5 [167]. Conversely, it was demonstrated that circ-0051443 contained in HCC tissues was significantly lower when compared to peritumoral tissue and normal tissues, suggesting that exosomal circ-0051443 is a potential biomarker and could be useful for distinguishing HCC tissue from adjacent normal tissues [168]. Furthermore, circ-0051443 was transferred from normal cells to HCC cells, and inhibited tumor progression by blocking the cell cycle and promoting the apoptosis of HCC cells [168].

Table 3. The biological functions, gene targets, and extraction types of exosomal circular RNAs in HCC.

circRNA	Gene Target	Function	Type of Extraction	Reference
circRNA_100284	miR-217	cell proliferation	precipitation	[138]
circRNA Cdr1	miR-1270	cell proliferation/invasion	precipitation	[139]
circ_0061395	miR-877	cell proliferation	precipitation	[140]
circTTLL5	miR-136-5p	cell proliferation	precipitation	[141]
circ_0003028	miR-498	cell proliferation/EMT	precipitation	[144]
circWDR25	miR-4474-3p	cell proliferation/EMT	ultracentrifugation	[145]
circ-0004277	ZO-1	cell proliferation/EMT	precipitation	[146]
circ_002136	miR-19a-3p	cell proliferation	precipitation	[147]
circWHSC1	miR-142-3p	cell proliferation	precipitation	[148]
circ_0074854	HuR	cell migration/immune escape	ultracentrifugation	[149]
circCCAR1	miR-127-5p	immune escape	precipitation	[150]
circUHRF1	miR-449c-5p	immune escape	precipitation	[151]
circASAP1	miR-326/ miR-532-5p	cell proliferation/ immune escape	precipitation	[152]
circGSE1	miR-324-5p	cell proliferation/immune scape	ultracentrifugation	[153]
circTMEM181	miR-488-3p	immune escape	ultracentrifugation	[155,156]
circRNA-SORE	miR-660-3p	drug resistance	-	[158]
circPAK1	14-3-3 ζ	cell proliferation/ drug resistance	ultracentrifugation	[159]
circ_0004001 circ_0004123 circ_0075792	-	biomarkers	-	[161]
circ_0072088	-	biomarkers	gradient centrifugation	[162]

5. Conclusions

Many studies have confirmed the significant role played by EVs in the pathophysiological processes of HCC. The cargo-based selection carried out in this review (Figure 2) also offers an analysis of the increasingly important role that ncRNAs play in the biology of HCC and the potential utility of these molecules in clinical applications.

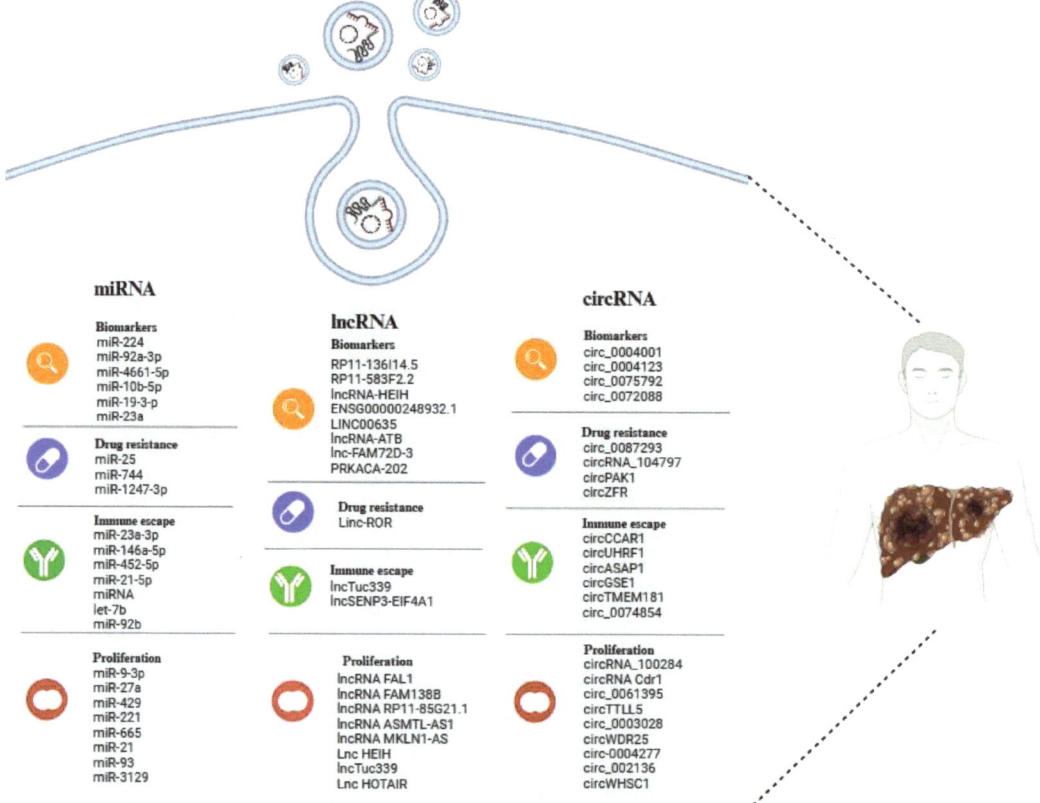

Figure 2. Overview of EV-related ncRNAs in HCC, displaying potential as biomarkers of disease, as well as indicators of tumor progression, drug resistance, and immune escape. The illustration was created with BioRender.com, accessed on 24 February 2024.

EVs and their ncRNA content perform an autocrine action, modulating the cell proliferation and tumorigenicity of the same cell that releases them; they have a paracrine action that conditions the entire tumor environment, modulating the behavior of other cell types, such as stem and immune cells. Finally, they seem to be related to drug resistance, although this aspect has not yet been extensively investigated.

The benefits of studying EVs come from the fact that exosomes originating from tumors contain diverse molecules, including proteins and ncRNA inherited from their parent cells. Consequently, they offer a precise representation of the characteristics exhibited by the tumor cells from which they originated [169]. This makes them crucial players in the fight against cancer, which we need to pay attention to as potential targets for future anti-tumor therapies.

In addition, their presence in biological fluids and the potential for the long-term storage of blood samples containing EVs in a biobank renders them good candidates as biomarkers and a precious tool for the diagnosis and prognosis of the disease. However, the primary obstacle in this context regards the technical challenges associated with the isolation of exosomes, which include a variety of different issues.

Furthermore, although technical challenges currently limit their clinical application, the data collected are promising, underscoring the need for further research in order to improve our understanding of exosomes and their potential significance as cancer biomarkers.

Author Contributions: G.A., A.C. (Alessandra Cusimano), M.C. and A.C. (Antonella Cusimano) participated in the conceptualization of the project, researched the various topic areas, and wrote multiple sections. All authors have read and agreed to the published version of the manuscript.

Funding: This research received no external funding.

Acknowledgments: We are grateful to Antonina Azzolina for support in preparing the figures and tables.

Conflicts of Interest: The authors declare no conflicts of interest.

References

1. Llovet, J.M.; Kelley, R.K.; Villanueva, A.; Singal, A.G.; Pikarsky, E.; Roayaie, S.; Lencioni, R.; Koike, K.; Zucman-Rossi, J.; Finn, R.S. Hepatocellular carcinoma. *Nat. Rev. Dis. Primers* **2021**, *7*, 6. [CrossRef]
2. Villanueva, A. Hepatocellular Carcinoma. *N. Engl. J. Med.* **2019**, *380*, 1450–1462. [CrossRef]
3. Llovet, J.M.; Pinyol, R.; Kelley, R.K.; El-Khoueiry, A.; Reeves, H.L.; Wang, X.W.; Gores, G.J.; Villanueva, A. Molecular pathogenesis and systemic therapies for hepatocellular carcinoma. *Nat. Cancer* **2022**, *3*, 386–401. [CrossRef]
4. Tampaki, M.; Papatheodoridis, G.V.; Cholongitas, E. Intrahepatic recurrence of hepatocellular carcinoma after resection: An update. *Clin. J. Gastroenterol.* **2021**, *14*, 699–713. [CrossRef]
5. Tsuchiya, N.; Sawada, Y.; Endo, I.; Saito, K.; Uemura, Y.; Nakatsura, T. Biomarkers for the Early Diagnosis of Hepatocellular Carcinoma. *World J. Gastroenterol.* **2015**, *21*, 10573–10583. [CrossRef]
6. Singal, A.G.; Lampertico, P.; Nahon, P. Epidemiology and Surveillance for Hepatocellular Carcinoma: New Trends. *J. Hepatol.* **2020**, *72*, 250–261. [CrossRef]
7. Cersosimo, R.J. Systemic targeted and immunotherapy for advanced hepatocellular carcinoma. *Am. J. Health Syst. Pharm.* **2021**, *78*, 187–202. [CrossRef]
8. Van de Wakker, S.I.; Meijers, F.M.; Sluijter, J.P.G.; Vader, P. Extracellular Vesicle Heterogeneity and Its Impact for Regenerative Medicine Applications. *Pharmacol. Rev.* **2023**, *75*, 1043–1061. [CrossRef]
9. Zhu, J.; Wang, S.; Yang, D.; Xu, W.; Qian, H. Extracellular vesicles: Emerging roles, biomarkers and therapeutic strategies in fibrotic diseases. *J. Nanobiotechnol.* **2023**, *21*, 164. [CrossRef]
10. Willms, E.; Cabañas, C.; Mäger, I.; Wood, M.J.A.; Vader, P. Extracellular Vesicle Heterogeneity: Subpopulations, Isolation Techniques, and Diverse Functions in Cancer Progression. *Front. Immunol.* **2018**, *9*, 738. [CrossRef]
11. Rezaee, M.; Mohammadi, F.; Keshavarzmotamed, A.; Yahyazadeh, S.; Vakili, O.; Milasi, Y.E.; Veisi, V.; Dehmordi, R.M.; Asadi, S.; Ghorbanhosseini, S.S.; et al. The landscape of exosomal non-coding RNAs in breast cancer drug resistance, focusing on underlying molecular mechanisms. *Front. Pharmacol.* **2023**, *14*, 1152672. [CrossRef] [PubMed]
12. Eitan, E.; Suire, C.; Zhang, S.; Mattson, M.P. Impact of lysosome status on extracellular vesicle content and release. *Ageing Res. Rev.* **2016**, *32*, 65–74. [CrossRef] [PubMed]
13. Xu, M.; Ji, J.; Jin, D.; Wu, Y.; Wu, T.; Lin, R.; Zhu, S.; Jiang, F.; Ji, Y.; Bao, B.; et al. The biogenesis and secretion of exosomes and multivesicular bodies (MVBs): Intercellular shuttles and implications in human diseases. *Genes Dis.* **2022**, *10*, 1894–1907. [CrossRef] [PubMed]
14. Wolf, M.; Poupardin, R.W.; Ebner-Peking, P.; Andrade, A.C.; Blöchl, C.; Obermayer, A.; Gomes, F.G.; Vari, B.; Maeding, N.; Eminger, E.; et al. A functional corona around extracellular vesicles enhances angiogenesis, skin regeneration and immunomodulation. *J. Extracell. Vesicles* **2022**, *11*, 12207. [CrossRef] [PubMed]
15. Sohal, I.S.; Kasinski, A.L. Emerging diversity in extracellular vesicles and their roles in cancer. *Front. Oncol.* **2023**, *13*, 1167717. [CrossRef] [PubMed]
16. Jin, Y.; Xing, J.; Xu, K.; Liu, D.; Zhuo, Y. Exosomes in the tumor microenvironment: Promoting cancer progression. *Front. Immunol.* **2022**, *13*, 1025218. [CrossRef] [PubMed]
17. Vidal, M. Exosomes: Revisiting their role as "garbage bags". *Traffic* **2019**, *20*, 815–828. [CrossRef] [PubMed]
18. Ansari, S.; de Wildt, B.W.M.; Vis, M.A.M.; de Korte, C.E.; Ito, K.; Hofmann, S.; Yuana, Y. Matrix Vesicles: Role in Bone Mineralization and Potential Use as Therapeutics. *Pharmaceuticals* **2021**, *14*, 289. [CrossRef]
19. Jing, L.; Li, L.; Sun, Z.; Bao, Z.; Shao, C.; Yan, J.; Pang, Q.; Geng, Y.; Zhang, L.; Wang, X.; et al. Role of Matrix Vesicles in Bone-Vascular Cross-Talk. *J. Cardiovasc. Pharmacol.* **2019**, *74*, 372–378. [CrossRef]
20. Rackov, G.; Garcia-Romero, N.; Esteban-Rubio, S.; Carrión-Navarro, J.; Belda-Iniesta, C.; Ayuso-Sacido, A. Vesicle-Mediated Control of Cell Function: The Role of Extracellular Matrix and Microenvironment. *Front. Physiol.* **2018**, *9*, 651. [CrossRef]

21. Berumen Sánchez, G.; Bunn, K.E.; Pua, H.H.; Rafat, M. Extracellular vesicles: Mediators of intercellular communication in tissue injury and disease. *Cell Commun. Signal.* **2021**, *19*, 104. [CrossRef] [PubMed]
22. Cavallari, C.; Camussi, G.; Brizzi, M.F. Extracellular Vesicles in the Tumour Microenvironment: Eclectic Supervisors. *Int. J. Mol. Sci.* **2020**, *21*, 6768. [CrossRef] [PubMed]
23. Ramirez, S.H.; Andrews, A.M.; Paul, D.; Pachter, J.S. Extracellular vesicles: Mediators and biomarkers of pathology along CNS barriers. *Fluids Barriers CNS* **2018**, *15*, 19. [CrossRef] [PubMed]
24. Ludwig, N.; Whiteside, T.L.; Reichert, T.E. Challenges in Exosome Isolation and Analysis in Health and Disease. *Int. J. Mol. Sci.* **2019**, *20*, 4684. [CrossRef] [PubMed]
25. Van Deun, J.; Mestdagh, P.; Sormunen, R.; Cocquyt, V.; Vermaelen, K.; Vandesompele, J.; Bracke, M.; De Wever, O.; Hendrix, A. The impact of disparate isolation methods for extracellular vesicles on downstream RNA profiling. *J. Extracell. Vesicles* **2014**, *3*, 24858. [CrossRef] [PubMed]
26. Lötvall, J.; Hill, A.F.; Hochberg, F.; Buzás, E.I.; Di Vizio, D.; Gardiner, C.; Gho, Y.S.; Kurochkin, I.V.; Mathivanan, S.; Quesenberry, P.; et al. Minimal experimental requirements for definition of extracellular vesicles and their functions: A position statement from the International Society for Extracellular Vesicles. *J. Extracell. Vesicles* **2014**, *3*, 26913. [CrossRef] [PubMed]
27. Théry, C.; Witwer, K.W.; Aikawa, E.; Alcaraz, M.J.; Anderson, J.D.; Andriantsitohaina, R.; Antoniou, A.; Arab, T.; Archer, F.; Atkin-Smith, G.K.; et al. Minimal information for studies of extracellular vesicles 2018 (MISEV2018): A position statement of the International Society for Extracellular Vesicles and update of the MISEV2014 guidelines. *J. Extracell. Vesicles* **2018**, *7*, 1535750. [CrossRef]
28. Zhang, X.; Borg EG, F.; Liaci, A.M.; Vos, H.R.; Stoorvogel, W. A novel three step protocol to isolate extracellular vesicles from plasma or cell culture medium with both high yield and purity. *J. Extracell. Vesicles* **2020**, *9*, 1791450. [CrossRef] [PubMed]
29. Mol, E.A.; Goumans, M.J.; Doevendans, P.A.; Sluijter, J.P.; Vader, P. Higher functionality of extracellular vesicles isolated using size-exclusion chromatography compared to ultracentrifugation. *Nanomedicine* **2017**, *13*, 2061–2065. [CrossRef]
30. Linares, R.; Tan, S.; Gounou, C.; Arraud, N.; Brisson, A.R. High-speed centrifugation induces aggregation of extracellular vesicles. *J. Extracell. Vesicles* **2015**, *4*, 29509. [CrossRef]
31. Grant, R.; Ansa-Addo, E.; Stratton, D.; Antwi-Baffour, S.; Jorfi, S.; Kholia, S.; Krige, L.; Lange, S.; Inal, J. A filtration-based protocol to isolate human plasma membrane-derived vesicles and exosomes from blood plasma. *J. Immunol. Methods* **2011**, *371*, 143–151. [CrossRef]
32. Lobb, R.J.; Becker, M.; Wen Wen, S.; Wong, C.S.; Wiegmans, A.P.; Leimgruber, A.; Möller, A. Optimized exosome isolation protocol for cell culture supernatant and human plasma. *J. Extracell. Vesicles* **2015**, *4*, 27031. [CrossRef] [PubMed]
33. Yu, L.L.; Zhu, J.; Liu, J.X.; Jiang, F.; Ni, W.K.; Qu, L.S.; Ni, R.Z.; Lu, C.H.; Xiao, M.B. A comparison of traditional and novel methods for the separation of exosomes from human samples. *BioMed Res. Int.* **2018**, *2018*, 3634563. [CrossRef] [PubMed]
34. Inal, J.M.; Kosgodage, U.; Azam, S.; Stratton, D.; Antwi-Baffour, S.; Lange, S. Blood/plasma secretome and microvesicles. *Biochim. Biophys. Acta* **2013**, *1834*, 2317–2325. [CrossRef]
35. Benedikter, B.J.; Bouwman, F.G.; Vajen, T.; Heinzmann, A.C.; Grauls, G.; Mariman, E.C.; Wouters EF, M.; Savelkoul, P.H.; Lopez-Iglesias, C.; Koenen, R.R.; et al. Ultrafiltration combined with size exclusion chromatography efficiently isolates extracellular vesicles from cell culture media for compositional and functional studies. *Sci. Rep.* **2017**, *7*, 15297. [CrossRef] [PubMed]
36. Foers, A.D.; Chatfield, S.; Dagley, L.F.; Scicluna, B.J.; Webb, A.I.; Cheng, L.; Hill, A.F.; Wicks, I.P.; Pang, K.C. Enrichment of extracellular vesicles from human synovial fluid using size exclusion chromatography. *J. Extrecell. Vesicles* **2018**, *7*, 1490145. [CrossRef]
37. Gamez-Valero, A.; Mongui_o-Tortajada, M.; Carreras-Planella, L.; Franquesa, M.; Beyer, K.; Borràs, F.E. Size-exclusion chromatography-based isolation minimally alters extracellular Vesicles' characteristics compared to precipitating agents. *Sci. Rep.* **2016**, *6*, 33641. [CrossRef]
38. Hirschberg, Y.; Schildermans, K.; van Dam, A.; Sterck, K.; Boonen, K.; Nelissen, I.; Vermeiren, Y.; Mertens, I. Characterizing extracellular vesicles from cerebrospinal fluid by a novel size exclusion chromatography method. *Alzheimer's Dement.* **2021**, *17*, e051264. [CrossRef]
39. García-Romero, N.; Madurga, R.; Rackov, G.; Palacín-Aliana, I.; Núñez-Torres, R.; Asensi-Puig, A.; Carri_on-Navarro, J.; Esteban-Rubio, S.; Peinado, H.; Gonz_alez-Neira, A.; et al. Polyethylene glycol improves current methods for circulating extracellular vesicle-derived DNA isolation. *J. Transl. Med.* **2019**, *17*, 75. [CrossRef]
40. Weng, Y.; Sui, Z.; Shan, Y.; Hu, Y.; Chen, Y.; Zhang, L.; Zhang, Y. Effective isolation of exosomes with polyethylene glycol from cell culture supernatant for in-depth proteome profiling. *Analyst* **2016**, *141*, 4640–4646. [CrossRef]
41. Ludwig, A.K.; de Miroschedji, K.; Doeppner, T.R.; Börger, V.; Ruesing, J.; Rebmann, V.; Durst, S.; Jansen, S.; Bremer, M.; Behrmann, E.; et al. Precipitation with polyethylene glycol followed by washing and pelleting by ultracentrifugation enriches extracellular vesicles from tissue culture supernatants in small and large scales. *J. Extracell. Vesicles* **2018**, *7*, 1528109. [CrossRef] [PubMed]
42. Baranyai, T.; Herczeg, K.; Onódi, Z.; Voszka, I.; Módos, K.; Marton, N.; Nagy, G.; Mäger, I.; Wood, M.J.; El Andaloussi, S.; et al. Isolation of exosomes from blood plasma: Qualitative and quantitative comparison of ultracentrifugation and size exclusion chromatography methods. *PLoS ONE* **2015**, *10*, e0145686. [CrossRef]
43. Brambilla, D.; Sola, L.; Ferretti, A.M.; Chiodi, E.; Zarovni, N.; Fortunato, D.; Criscuoli, M.; Dolo, V.; Giusti, I.; Murdica, V.; et al. EV separation: Release of intact extracellular vesicles immunocaptured on magnetic particles. *Anal. Chem.* **2021**, *93*, 5476–5483. [CrossRef]

44. Zarovni, N.; Corrado, A.; Guazzi, P.; Zocco, D.; Lari, E.; Radano, G.; Muhhina, J.; Fondelli, C.; Gavrilova, J.; Chiesi, A. Integrated isolation and quantitative analysis of exosome shuttled proteins and nucleic acids using immunocapture approaches. *Methods* 2015, *87*, 46–58. [CrossRef] [PubMed]
45. Gandham, S.; Su, X.; Wood, J.; Nocera, A.L.; Alli, S.C.; Milane, L.; Zimmerman, A.; Amiji, M.; Ivanov, A.R. Technologies and standardization in research on extracellular vesicles. *Trends Biotechnol.* 2020, *38*, 1066–1098. [CrossRef] [PubMed]
46. Paolini, L.; Zendrini, A.; Noto, G.D.; Busatto, S.; Lottini, E.; Radeghieri, A.; Dossi, A.; Caneschi, A.; Ricotta, D.; Bergese, P. Residual matrix from different separation techniques impacts exosome biological activity. *Sci. Rep.* 2016, *6*, 23550. [CrossRef]
47. Balaj, L.; Atai, N.A.; Chen, W.; Mu, D.; Tannous, B.A.; Breakefield, X.O.; Skog, J.; Maguire, C.A. Heparin affinity purification of extracellular vesicles. *Sci. Rep.* 2015, *5*, 10266. [CrossRef]
48. Chen, Z.; Yang, Y.; Yamaguchi, H.; Hung, M.C.; Kameoka, J. Isolation of cancer-derived extracellular vesicle subpopulations by a size-selective microfluidic platform. *Biomicrofluidics* 2020, *14*, 034113. [CrossRef] [PubMed]
49. Iliescu, F.S.; Vrtačnik, D.; Neuzil, P.; Iliescu, C. Microfluidic technology for clinical applications of exosomes. *Micromachines* 2019, *10*, 392. [CrossRef]
50. Chiang, C.Y.; Chen, C. Toward characterizing extracellular vesicles at a single-particle level. *J. Biomed. Sci.* 2019, *26*, 9. [CrossRef]
51. Bonner, S.E.; Willms, E. Intercellular communication through extracellular vesicles in cancer and evolutionary biology. *Prog. Biophys. Mol. Biol.* 2021, *165*, 80–87. [CrossRef] [PubMed]
52. Guo, Y.; Ji, X.; Liu, J.; Fan, D.; Zhou, Q.; Chen, C.; Wang, W.; Wang, G.; Wang, H.; Yuan, W.; et al. Effects of exosomes on pre-metastatic niche formation in tumors. *Mol. Cancer* 2019, *18*, 39. [CrossRef]
53. Bamankar, S.; Londhe, V.Y. The Rise of Extracellular Vesicles as New Age Biomarkers in Cancer Diagnosis: Promises and Pitfalls. *Technol. Cancer Res. Treat.* 2023, *22*, 15330338221149266. [CrossRef] [PubMed]
54. Xie, Y.; Dang, W.; Zhang, S.; Yue, W.; Yang, L.; Zhai, X.; Yan, Q.; Lu, J. The role of exosomal noncoding RNAs in cancer. *Mol. Cancer* 2019, *18*, 37. [CrossRef]
55. Wang, W.; Hao, L.P.; Song, H.; Chu, X.Y.; Wang, R. The Potential Roles of Exosomal Non-Coding RNAs in Hepatocellular Carcinoma. *Front. Oncol.* 2022, *12*, 790916. [CrossRef] [PubMed]
56. Wong, Q.W.; Lung, R.W.; Law, P.T.; Lai, P.B.; Chan, K.Y.; To, K.F.; Wong, N. MicroRNA-223 is commonly repressed in hepatocellular carcinoma and potentiates expression of Stathmin1. *Gastroenterology* 2008, *135*, 257–269. [CrossRef] [PubMed]
57. Cabiati, M.; Salvadori, C.; Basta, G.; Del Turco, S.; Aretini, P.; Cecchettini, A.; Del Ry, S. miRNA and long non-coding RNA transcriptional expression in hepatocellular carcinoma cell line-secreted extracellular vesicles. *Clin. Exp. Med.* 2022, *22*, 245–255. [CrossRef] [PubMed]
58. Kinoshita, T.; Yip, K.W.; Spence, T.; Liu, F.F. MicroRNAs in extracellular vesicles: Potential cancer biomarkers. *J. Hum. Genet.* 2017, *62*, 67–74. [CrossRef] [PubMed]
59. Lapitz, A.; Arbelaiz, A.; Olaizola, P.; Aranburu, A.; Bujanda, L.; Perugorria, M.J.; Banales, J.M. Extracellular Vesicles in Hepatobiliary Malignancies. *Front. Immunol.* 2018, *9*, 2270. [CrossRef]
60. Lee, Y.T.; Tran, B.V.; Wang, J.J.; Liang, I.Y.; You, S.; Zhu, Y.; Agopian, V.G.; Tseng, H.R.; Yang, J.D. The Role of Extracellular Vesicles in Disease Progression and Detection of Hepatocellular Carcinoma. *Cancers* 2021, *13*, 3076. [CrossRef]
61. Li, S.; Li, J.; Fei, B.Y.; Shao, D.; Pan, Y.; Mo, Z.H.; Sun, B.Z.; Zhang, D.; Zheng, X.; Zhang, M.; et al. MiR-27a promotes hepatocellular carcinoma cell proliferation through suppression of its target gene peroxisome proliferator-activated receptor γ. *Chin. Med. J.* 2015, *128*, 941–947. [CrossRef] [PubMed]
62. Tang, J.; Li, Y.; Liu, K.; Zhu, Q.; Yang, W.H.; Xiong, L.K.; Guo, D.L. Exosomal miR-9-3p suppresses HBGF-5 expression and is a functional biomarker in hepatocellular carcinoma. *Minerva Med.* 2018, *109*, 15–23. [CrossRef] [PubMed]
63. Yang, N.; Li, S.; Li, G.; Zhang, S.; Tang, X.; Ni, S.; Jian, X.; Xu, C.; Zhu, J.; Lu, M. The role of extracellular vesicles in mediating progression, metastasis and potential treatment of hepatocellular carcinoma. *Oncotarget* 2017, *8*, 3683–3695. [CrossRef] [PubMed]
64. Li, L.; Tang, J.; Zhang, B.; Yang, W.; Liu Gao, M.; Wang, R.; Tan, Y.; Fan, J.; Chang, Y.; Fu, J.; et al. Epigenetic modification of MiR-429 promotes liver tumour-initiating cell properties by targeting Rb binding protein 4. *Gut* 2015, *64*, 156–167. [CrossRef] [PubMed]
65. Xiong, W.; Sun, L.P.; Chen, X.M.; Li, H.Y.; Huang, S.A.; Jie, S.H. Comparison of microRNA expression profiles in HCC-derived microvesicles and the parental cells and evaluation of their roles in HCC. *J. Huazhong Univ. Sci. Technol. Med. Sci.* 2013, *33*, 346–352. [CrossRef] [PubMed]
66. Qu, Z.; Wu, J.; Wu, J.; Ji, A.; Qiang, G.; Jiang, Y.; Jiang, C.; Ding, Y. Exosomal miR-665 as a novel minimally invasive biomarker for hepatocellular carcinoma diagnosis and prognosis. *Oncotarget* 2017, *8*, 80666–80678. [CrossRef] [PubMed]
67. Zhou, Y.; Ren, H.; Dai, B.; Li, J.; Shang, L.; Huang, J.; Shi, X. Hepatocellular carcinoma-derived exosomal miRNA-21 contributes to tumor progression by converting hepatocyte stellate cells to cancer-associated fibroblasts. *J. Exp. Clin. Cancer Res.* 2018, *37*, 324. [CrossRef]
68. Xue, X.; Wang, X.; Zhao, Y.; Hu, R.; Qin, L. Exosomal miR-93 promotes proliferation and invasion in hepatocellular carcinoma by directly inhibiting TIMP2/TP53INP1/CDKN1A. *Biochem. Biophys. Res. Commun.* 2018, *502*, 515–521. [CrossRef]
69. Yang, Y.; Mao, F.; Guo, L.; Shi, J.; Wu, M.; Cheng, S.; Guo, W. Tumor cells derived-extracellular vesicles transfer miR-3129 to promote hepatocellular carcinoma metastasis by targeting TXNIP. *Dig. Liver Dis.* 2021, *53*, 474–485. [CrossRef]
70. Chen, S.; Saeed, A.F.U.H.; Liu, Q.; Jiang, Q.; Xu, H.; Xiao, G.G.; Rao, L.; Duo, Y. Macrophages in immunoregulation and therapeutics. *Signal Transduct. Target. Ther.* 2023, *8*, 207. [CrossRef]

71. Pan, Y.; Yu, Y.; Wang, X.; Zhang, T. Tumor-Associated Macrophages in Tumor Immunity. *Front. Immunol.* **2020**, *11*, 583084. [CrossRef]
72. Liu, J.; Fan, L.; Yu, H.; Zhang, J.; He, Y.; Feng, D.; Wang, F.; Li, X.; Liu, Q.; Li, Y.; et al. Endoplasmic Reticulum Stress Causes Liver Cancer Cells to Release Exosomal miR-23a-3p and Up-regulate Programmed Death Ligand 1 Expression in Macrophages. *Hepatology* **2019**, *70*, 241–258. [CrossRef]
73. Yin, C.; Han, Q.; Xu, D.; Zheng, B.; Zhao, X.; Zhang, J. SALL4-mediated upregulation of exosomal miR-146a-5p drives T-cell exhaustion by M2 tumor-associated macrophages in HCC. *Oncoimmunology* **2019**, *8*, 1601479. [CrossRef]
74. Zongqiang, H.; Jiapeng, C.; Yingpeng, Z.; Chuntao, Y.; Yiting, W.; Jiashun, Z.; Li, L. Exosomal miR-452-5p Induce M2 Macrophage Polarization to Accelerate Hepatocellular Carcinoma Progression by Targeting TIMP3. *J. Immunol. Res.* **2022**, *2022*, 1032106. [CrossRef]
75. Yu, H.; Pan, J.; Zheng, S.; Cai, D.; Luo, A.; Xia, Z.; Huang, J. Hepatocellular Carcinoma Cell-Derived Exosomal miR-21-5p Induces Macrophage M2 Polarization by Targeting RhoB. *Int. J. Mol. Sci.* **2023**, *24*, 4593. [CrossRef]
76. Li, D.; Jia, H.; Zhang, H.; Lv, M.; Liu, J.; Zhang, Y.; Huang, T.; Huang, B. TLR4 signaling induces the release of microparticles by tumor cells that regulate inflammatory cytokine IL-6 of macrophages via microRNA let-7b. *Oncoimmunology* **2012**, *1*, 687–693. [CrossRef]
77. Nakano, T.; Chen, I.H.; Wang, C.C.; Chen, P.J.; Tseng, H.P.; Huang, K.T.; Hu, T.H.; Li, L.C.; Goto, S.; Cheng, Y.F.; et al. Circulating exosomal miR-92b: Its role for cancer immunoediting and clinical value for prediction of posttransplant hepatocellular carcinoma recurrence. *Am. J. Transplant.* **2019**, *19*, 3250–3262. [CrossRef]
78. Maacha, S.; Bhat, A.A.; Jimenez, L.; Raza, A.; Haris, M.; Uddin, S.; Grivel, J.C. Extracellular vesicles-mediated intercellular communication: Roles in the tumor microenvironment and anti-cancer drug resistance. *Mol. Cancer* **2019**, *18*, 55. [CrossRef]
79. Davodabadi, F.; Sajjadi, S.F.; Sarhadi, M.; Mirghasemi, S.; Nadali Hezaveh, M.; Khosravi, S.; Kamali Andani, M.; Cordani, M.; Basiri, M.; Ghavami, S. Cancer chemotherapy resistance: Mechanisms and recent breakthrough in targeted drug delivery. *Eur. J. Pharmacol.* **2023**, *958*, 176013. [CrossRef] [PubMed]
80. Cabral, L.K.D.; Tiribelli, C.; Sukowati, C.H.C. Sorafenib Resistance in Hepatocellular Carcinoma: The Relevance of Genetic Heterogeneity. *Cancers* **2020**, *12*, 1576. [CrossRef]
81. Jaffar Ali, D.; He, C.; Xu, H.; Kumaravel, S.; Sun, B.; Zhou, Y.; Liu, R.; Xiao, Z. Microvesicles mediate sorafenib resistance in liver cancer cells through attenuating p53 and enhancing FOXM1 expression. *Life Sci.* **2021**, *271*, 119149. [CrossRef]
82. Wang, G.; Zhao, W.; Wang, H.; Qiu, G.; Jiang, Z.; Wei, G.; Li, X. Exosomal MiR-744 Inhibits Proliferation and Sorafenib Chemoresistance in Hepatocellular Carcinoma by Targeting PAX2. *Med. Sci. Monit.* **2019**, *25*, 7209–7217. [CrossRef]
83. Fang, T.; Lv, H.; Lv, G.; Li, T.; Wang, C.; Han, Q.; Yu, L.; Su, B.; Guo, L.; Huang, S.; et al. Tumor-derived exosomal miR-1247-3p induces cancer-associated fibroblast activation to foster lung metastasis of liver cancer. *Nat. Commun.* **2018**, *9*, 191. [CrossRef]
84. Kalluri, R.; Zeisberg, M. Fibroblasts in cancer. *Nat. Rev. Cancer* **2006**, *6*, 392–401. [CrossRef]
85. Sorop, A.; Constantinescu, D.; Cojocaru, F.; Dinischiotu, A.; Cucu, D.; Dima, S.O. Exosomal microRNAs as Biomarkers and Therapeutic Targets for Hepatocellular Carcinoma. *Int. J. Mol. Sci.* **2021**, *22*, 4997. [CrossRef]
86. Chen, Y.; Wu, T.; Zhu, Z.; Huang, H.; Zhang, L.; Goel, A.; Yang, M.; Wang, X. An integrated workflow for biomarker development using microRNAs in extracellular vesicles for cancer precision medicine. *Semin. Cancer Biol.* **2021**, *74*, 134–155. [CrossRef]
87. Cui, Y.; Xu, H.F.; Liu, M.Y.; Xu, Y.J.; He, J.C.; Zhou, Y.; Cang, S.D. Mechanism of exosomal microRNA-224 in development of hepatocellular carcinoma and its diagnostic and prognostic value. *World J. Gastroenterol.* **2019**, *25*, 1890–1898. [CrossRef]
88. Sorop, A.; Iacob, R.; Iacob, S.; Constantinescu, D.; Chitoiu, L.; Fertig, T.E.; Dinischiotu, A.; Chivu-Economescu, M.; Bacalbasa, N.; Savu, L.; et al. Plasma Small Extracellular Vesicles Derived miR-21-5p and miR-92a-3p as Potential Biomarkers for Hepatocellular Carcinoma Screening. *Front. Genet.* **2020**, *11*, 712. [CrossRef]
89. Cho, H.J.; Baek, G.O.; Seo, C.W.; Ahn, H.R.; Sung, S.; Son, J.A.; Kim, S.S.; Cho, S.W.; Jang, J.W.; Nam, S.W.; et al. Exosomal microRNA-4661-5p-based serum panel as a potential diagnostic biomarker for early-stage hepatocellular carcinoma. *Cancer Med.* **2020**, *9*, 5459–5472. [CrossRef]
90. Cho, H.J.; Eun, J.W.; Baek, G.O.; Seo, C.W.; Ahn, H.R.; Kim, S.S.; Cho, S.W.; Cheong, J.Y. Serum Exosomal MicroRNA, miR-10b-5p, as a Potential Diagnostic Biomarker for Early-Stage Hepatocellular Carcinoma. *J. Clin. Med.* **2020**, *9*, 281. [CrossRef]
91. Boonkaew, B.; Satthawiwat, N.; Pinjaroen, N.; Chuaypen, N.; Tangkijvanich, P. Circulating Extracellular Vesicle-Derived microRNAs as Novel Diagnostic and Prognostic Biomarkers for Non-Viral-Related Hepatocellular Carcinoma. *Int. J. Mol. Sci.* **2023**, *24*, 16043. [CrossRef]
92. Bao, L.; Zhao, J.; Dai, X.; Wang, Y.; Ma, R.; Su, Y.; Cui, H.; Niu, J.; Bai, S.; Xiao, Z.; et al. Correlation between miR-23a and onset of hepatocellular carcinoma. *Clin. Res. Hepatol. Gastroenterol.* **2014**, *38*, 318–330. [CrossRef]
93. ENCODE Project Consortium. An integrated encyclopedia of DNA elements in the human genome. *Nature* **2012**, *489*, 57–74. [CrossRef]
94. Geisler, S.; Coller, J. RNA in unexpected places: Long non-coding RNA functions in diverse cellular contexts. *Nat. Rev. Mol. Cell Biol.* **2013**, *14*, 699–712. [CrossRef]
95. Yang, Y.; Chen, L.; Gu, J.; Zhang, H.; Yuan, J.; Lian, Q.; Lv, G.; Wang, S.; Wu, Y.; Yang, Y.T.; et al. Recurrently deregulated lncRNAs in hepatocellular carcinoma. *Nat. Commun.* **2017**, *8*, 14421. [CrossRef]

96. Rosenbloom, K.R.; Dreszer, T.R.; Long, J.C.; Malladi, V.S.; Sloan, C.A.; Raney, B.J.; Cline, M.S.; Karolchik, D.; Barber, G.P.; Clawson, H.; et al. ENCODE whole-genome data in the UCSC Genome Browser: Update 2012. *Nucleic Acids Res.* **2012**, *40*, D912–D917. [CrossRef]
97. Tsagakis, I.; Douka, K.; Birds, I.; Aspden, J.L. Long non-coding RNAs in development and disease: Conservation to mechanisms. *J. Pathol.* **2020**, *250*, 480–495. [CrossRef]
98. Tellez-Gabriel, M.; Heymann, D. Exosomal lncRNAs: The newest promising liquid biopsy. *Cancer Drug Resist.* **2019**, *2*, 1002–1017. [CrossRef]
99. Li, B.; Mao, R.; Liu, C.; Zhang, W.; Tang, Y.; Guo, Z. LncRNA FAL1 promotes cell proliferation and migration by acting as a CeRNA of miR-1236 in hepatocellular carcinoma cells. *Life Sci.* **2018**, *197*, 122–129. [CrossRef]
100. Zhuo, C.; Yi, T.; Pu, J.; Cen, X.; Zhou, Y.; Feng, S.; Wei, C.; Chen, P.; Wang, W.; Bao, C.; et al. Exosomal linc-FAM138B from cancer cells alleviates hepatocellular carcinoma progression via regulating miR-765. *Aging* **2020**, *12*, 26236–26247. [CrossRef]
101. Huang, X.; Sun, L.; Wen, S.; Deng, D.; Wan, F.; He, X.; Tian, L.; Liang, L.; Wei, C.; Gao, K.; et al. RNA sequencing of plasma exosomes revealed novel functional long noncoding RNAs in hepatocellular carcinoma. *Cancer Sci.* **2020**, *111*, 3338–3349. [CrossRef]
102. You, L.N.; Tai, Q.W.; Xu, L.; Hao, Y.; Guo, W.J.; Zhang, Q.; Tong, Q.; Zhang, H.; Huang, W.K. Exosomal LINC00161 promotes angiogenesis and metastasis via regulating miR-590-3p/ROCK axis in hepatocellular carcinoma. *Cancer Gene Ther.* **2021**, *28*, 719–736. [CrossRef]
103. Ma, D.; Gao, X.; Liu, Z.; Lu, X.; Ju, H.; Zhang, N. Exosome-transferred long non-coding RNA ASMTL-AS1 contributes to malignant phenotypes in residual hepatocellular carcinoma after insufficient radiofrequency ablation. *Cell Prolif.* **2020**, *53*, e12795. [CrossRef]
104. Wang, D.; Xing, N.; Yang, T.; Liu, J.; Zhao, H.; He, J.; Ai, Y.; Yang, J. Exosomal lncRNA H19 promotes the progression of hepatocellular carcinoma treated with Propofol via miR-520a-3p/LIMK1 axis. *Cancer Med.* **2020**, *9*, 7218–7230. [CrossRef]
105. Pan, G.; Zhang, J.; You, F.; Cui, T.; Luo, P.; Wang, S.; Li, X.; Yuan, Q. ETS Proto-Oncogene 1-activated muskelin 1 antisense RNA drives the malignant progression of hepatocellular carcinoma by targeting miR-22-3p to upregulate ETS Proto-Oncogene 1. *Bioengineered* **2022**, *13*, 1346–1358. [CrossRef] [PubMed]
106. Takahashi, K.; Yan, I.K.; Haga, H.; Patel, T. Modulation of hypoxia-signaling pathways by extracellular linc-RoR. *J. Cell Sci.* **2014**, *127*, 1585–1594.
107. Lu, L.; Huang, J.; Mo, J.; Da, X.; Li, Q.; Fan, M.; Lu, H. Exosomal lncRNA TUG1 from cancer-associated fibroblasts promotes liver cancer cell migration, invasion, and glycolysis by regulating the miR-524-5p/SIX1 axis. *Cell Mol. Biol. Lett.* **2022**, *27*, 17. [CrossRef]
108. Alzahrani, F.A.; El-Magd, M.A.; Abdelfattah-Hassan, A.; Saleh, A.A.; Saadeldin, I.M.; El-Shetry, E.S.; Badawy, A.A.; Alkarim, S. Potential Effect of Exosomes Derived from Cancer Stem Cells and MSCs on Progression of DEN-Induced HCC in Rats. *Stem Cells Int.* **2018**, *2018*, 8058979. [CrossRef]
109. Kogure, T.; Yan, I.K.; Lin, W.-L.; Patel, T. Extracellular vesicle–mediated transfer of a novel long noncoding RNA TUC339: A mechanism of intercellular signaling in human hepatocellular cancer. *Genes Cancer* **2013**, *4*, 261–272. [CrossRef] [PubMed]
110. Ye, P.; Wang, T.; Liu, W.; Li, X.; Tang, L.; Tian, F. Enhancing HOTAIR/MiR-10b drives normal liver stem cells toward a tendency to malignant transformation through inducing epithelial-to-mesenchymal transition. *Rejuvenat. Res.* **2015**, *18*, 332–340. [CrossRef] [PubMed]
111. Su, D.; Zhang, Z.; Xu, Z.; Xia, F.; Yan, Y. A prognostic exosome-related LncRNA risk model correlates with the immune microenvironment in liver cancer. *Front. Genet.* **2022**, *13*, 965329. [CrossRef] [PubMed]
112. Kim, S.S.; Baek, G.O.; Son, J.A.; Ahn, H.R.; Yoon, M.K.; Cho, H.J.; Yoon, J.H.; Nam, S.W.; Cheong, J.Y.; Eun, J.W. Early detection of hepatocellular carcinoma via liquid biopsy: Panel of small extracellular vesicle-derived long noncoding RNAs identified as markers. *Mol. Oncol.* **2021**, *15*, 2715–2731. [CrossRef] [PubMed]
113. Sun, L.; Su, Y.; Liu, X.; Xu, M.; Chen, X.; Zhu, Y.; Guo, Z.; Bai, T.; Dong, L.; Wei, C.; et al. Serum and exosome long non coding RNAs as potential biomarkers for hepatocellular carcinoma. *J. Cancer* **2018**, *9*, 2631–2639. [CrossRef]
114. Wang, J.; Pu, J.; Zhang, Y.; Yao, T.; Luo, Z.; Li, W.; Xu, G.; Liu, J.; Wei, W.; Deng, Y. Exosome-transmitted long non-coding RNA SENP3-EIF4A1 suppresses the progression of hepatocellular carcinoma. *Aging* **2020**, *12*, 11550–11567. [CrossRef]
115. Wang, T.; Zhu, H.; Xiao, M.; Zhou, S. Serum exosomal long noncoding RNA CRNDE as a prognostic biomarker for hepatocellular carcinoma. *J. Clin. Lab. Anal.* **2021**, *35*, e23959. [CrossRef] [PubMed]
116. Lin, C.; Xiang, Y.; Sheng, J.; Liu, S.; Cui, M.; Zhang, X. Long non-coding RNA CRNDE promotes malignant progression of hepatocellular carcinoma through the miR-33a-5p/CDK6 axis. *J. Physiol. Biochem.* **2020**, *76*, 469–481. [CrossRef] [PubMed]
117. Yao, J.; Hua, X.; Shi, J.; Hu, X.; Lui, K.; He, K.; Mai, J.; Lan, T.; Lu, M. LncRNA THEMIS2-211, a tumor-originated circulating exosomal biomarker, promotes the growth and metastasis of hepatocellular carcinoma by functioning as a competing endogenous RNA. *FASEB J.* **2022**, *36*, e22238. [CrossRef]
118. Hou, Y.; Yu, Z.; Tam, N.L.; Huang, S.; Sun, C.; Wang, R.; Zhang, X.; Wang, Z.; Ma, Y.; He, X.; et al. Exosome-related lncRNAs as predictors of HCC patient survival: A prognostic model. *Am. J. Transl. Res.* **2018**, *10*, 1648–1662.
119. Matboli, M.; Labib, M.E.; Nasser, H.E.; El-Tawdi, A.H.F.; Habib, E.K.; Ali-Labib, R. Exosomal miR-1298 and lncRNA-RP11-583F2.2 Expression in Hepato-cellular Carcinoma. *Curr. Genom.* **2020**, *21*, 46–55. [CrossRef]

120. Zhang, C.; Yang, X.; Qi, Q.; Gao, Y.; Wei, Q.; Han, S. lncRNA-HEIH in serum and exosomes as a potential biomarker in the HCV-related hepatocellular carcinoma. *Cancer Biomark.* **2018**, *21*, 651–659. [CrossRef]
121. Lu, Y.; Duan, Y.; Xu, Q.; Zhang, L.; Chen, W.; Qu, Z.; Wu, B.; Liu, W.; Shi, L.; Wu, D.; et al. Circulating exosome-derived bona fide long non-coding RNAs predicting the occurrence and metastasis of hepatocellular carcinoma. *J. Cell Mol. Med.* **2020**, *24*, 1311–1318. [CrossRef]
122. Xu, H.; Chen, Y.; Dong, X.; Wang, X. Serum Exosomal Long Noncoding RNAs ENSG00000258332.1 and LINC00635 for the Diagnosis and Prognosis of Hepatocellular Carcinoma. *Cancer Epidemiol. Biomark. Prev.* **2018**, *27*, 710–716. [CrossRef]
123. Lee, Y.R.; Kim, G.; Tak, W.Y.; Jang, S.Y.; Kweon, Y.O.; Park, J.G.; Lee, H.W.; Han, Y.S.; Chun, J.M.; Park, S.Y.; et al. Circulating exosomal noncoding RNAs as prognostic biomarkers in human hepatocellular carcinoma. *Int. J. Cancer* **2019**, *144*, 1444–1452. [CrossRef] [PubMed]
124. Yao, Z.; Jia, C.; Tai, Y.; Liang, H.; Zhong, Z.; Xiong, Z.; Deng, M.; Zhang, Q. Serum exosomal long noncoding RNAs lnc-FAM72D-3 and lnc-EPC1-4 as diagnostic biomarkers for hepatocellular carcinoma. *Aging* **2020**, *12*, 11843–11863. [CrossRef] [PubMed]
125. Li, X.; Lei, Y.; Wu, M.; Li, N. Regulation of Macrophage Activation and Polarization by HCC-Derived Exosomal lncRNA TUC339. *Int. J. Mol. Sci.* **2018**, *10*, 2958. [CrossRef] [PubMed]
126. Fan, F.; Chen, K.; Lu, X.; Li, A.; Liu, C.; Wu, B. Dual targeting of PD-L1 and PD-L2 by PCED1B-AS1 via sponging hsa-miR-194-5p induces immunosuppression in hepatocellular carcinoma. *Hepatol. Int.* **2021**, *15*, 444–458. [CrossRef] [PubMed]
127. Jung, H.I.; Jeong, D.; Ji, S.; Ahn, T.S.; Bae, S.H.; Chin, S.; Chung, J.C.; Kim, H.C.; Lee, M.S.; Baek, M.J. Overexpression of PD-L1 and PD-L2 Is associated with poor prognosis in patients with hepatocellular carcinoma. *Cancer Res. Treat.* **2017**, *49*, 246–254. [CrossRef] [PubMed]
128. Takahashi, K.; Yan, I.K.; Kogure, T.; Haga, H.; Patel, T. Extracellular vesicle-mediated transfer of long non-coding RNA ROR modulates chemosensitivity in human hepatocellular cancer. *FEBS Open Bio* **2014**, *4*, 458–467. [CrossRef] [PubMed]
129. Takahashi, K.; Yan, I.K.; Wood, J.; Haga, H.; Patel, T. Involvement of Extracellular Vesicle long non-coding RNA (linc-VLDLR) in Tumor Cell Responses to Chemotherapy. *Mol. Cancer Res.* **2014**, *12*, 1377–1387. [CrossRef]
130. Vo, J.N.; Cieslik, M.; Zhang, Y.; Shukla, S.; Xiao, L.; Zhang, Y.; Wu, Y.M.; Dhanasekaran, S.M.; Engelke, C.G.; Cao, X.; et al. The landscape of circular RNA in cancer. *Cell* **2019**, *176*, 869–881. [CrossRef]
131. Fan, X.; Zhang, X.; Wu, X.; Guo, H.; Hu, Y.; Tang, F.; Huang, Y. Single-cell RNA-seq transcriptome analysis of linear and circular RNAs in mouse preimplantation embryos. *Genome Biol.* **2015**, *16*, 148. [CrossRef] [PubMed]
132. Wang, Y.; Li, Z.; Xu, S.; Guo, J. Novel potential tumor biomarkers: Circular RNAs and exosomal circular RNAs in gastrointestinal malignancies. *J. Clin. Lab. Anal.* **2020**, *34*, e23359. [CrossRef] [PubMed]
133. Hu, M.; Li, X.; Jiang, Z.; Xia, Q.; Hu, Y.; Guo, J.; Fu, L. Exosomes and circular RNAs: Promising partners in hepatocellular carcinoma from bench to bedside. *Discov. Oncol.* **2023**, *14*, 60. [CrossRef] [PubMed]
134. Memczak, S.; Jens, M.; Elefsinioti, A.; Torti, F.; Krueger, J.; Rybak, A.; Maier, L.; Mackowiak, S.D.; Gregersen, L.H.; Munschauer, M. Circular RNAs are a large class of animal RNAs with regulatory potency. *Nature* **2013**, *495*, 333–338. [CrossRef]
135. Hansen, T.B.; Jensen, T.I.; Clausen, B.H.; Bramsen, J.B.; Finsen, B.; Damgaard, C.K.; Kjems, J. Natural RNA circles function as efficient microRNA sponges. *Nature* **2013**, *495*, 384–388. [CrossRef] [PubMed]
136. Zhou, W.Y.; Cai, Z.R.; Liu, J.; Wang, D.S.; Ju, H.Q.; Xu, R.H. Circular RNA: Metabolism, functions and interactions with proteins. *Mol. Cancer* **2020**, *19*, 172. [CrossRef]
137. Zhao, Y.; Yao, J. The Biological Functions and Clinical Values of Exosomal Circular RNAs in Hepatocellular Carcinoma. *Front. Oncol.* **2022**, *12*, 885214. [CrossRef] [PubMed]
138. Dai, X.; Chen, C.; Yang, Q.; Xue, J.; Chen, X.; Sun, B.; Luo, F.; Liu, X.; Xiao, T.; Xu, H.; et al. Exosomal circRNA_100284 from arsenite-transformed cells, via microRNA-217 regulation of EZH2, is involved in the malignant transformation of human hepatic cells by accelerating the cell cycle and promoting cell proliferation. *Cell Death Dis.* **2018**, *9*, 454. [CrossRef]
139. Su, Y.; Lv, X.; Yin, W.; Zhou, L.; Hu, Y.; Zhou, A.; Qi, F. CircRNA Cdr1as functions as a competitive endogenous RNA to promote hepatocellular carcinoma progression. *Aging* **2019**, *11*, 8183–8203. [CrossRef]
140. Yu, Y.; Bian, L.; Liu, R.; Wang, Y.; Xiao, X. Circular RNA hsa_circ_0061395 accelerates hepatocellular carcinoma progression via regulation of the miR-877-5p/PIK3R3 axis. *Cancer Cell Int.* **2021**, *21*, 10. [CrossRef]
141. Liu, C.; Ren, C.; Guo, L.; Yang, C.; Yu, Q. Exosome-mediated circTTLL5 transfer promotes hepatocellular carcinoma malignant progression through miR-136-5p/KIAA1522 axis. *Pathol. Res. Pract.* **2023**, *241*, 154276. [CrossRef] [PubMed]
142. Liu, Y.; Wang, L.; Liu, W. Roles of circRNAs in the Tumorigenesis and Metastasis of HCC: A Mini Review. *Cancer Manag. Res.* **2022**, *14*, 1847–1856. [CrossRef]
143. Huang, Y.; Hong, W.; Wei, X. The molecular mechanisms and therapeutic strategies of EMT in tumor progression and metastasis. *J. Hematol. Oncol.* **2022**, *15*, 129. [CrossRef]
144. Zhang, T.; Sun, Q.; Shen, C.; Qian, Y. Circular RNA circ_0003028 regulates cell development through modulating miR-498/ornithine decarboxylase 1 axis in hepatocellular carcinoma. *Anticancer Drugs* **2023**, *34*, 507–518. [CrossRef]
145. Liu, L.; Liao, R.; Wu, Z.; Du, C.; You, Y.; Que, K.; Duan, Y.; Yin, K.; Ye, W. Hepatic stellate cell exosome-derived circWDR25 promotes the progression of hepatocellular carcinoma via the miRNA-4474-3P-ALOX-15 and EMT axes. *Biosci. Trends* **2022**, *16*, 267–281. [CrossRef] [PubMed]
146. Zhu, C.; Su, Y.; Liu, L.; Wang, S.; Liu, Y.; Wu, J. Circular RNA hsa_circ_0004277 Stimulates Malignant Phenotype of Hepatocellular Carcinoma and Epithelial-Mesenchymal Transition of Peripheral Cells. *Front. Cell Dev. Biol.* **2021**, *8*, 585565. [CrossRef] [PubMed]

147. Yuan, P.; Song, J.; Wang, F.; Chen, B. Exosome-transmitted circ_002136 promotes hepatocellular carcinoma progression by miR-19a-3p/RAB1A pathway. *BMC Cancer* **2022**, *22*, 1284. [CrossRef]
148. Lyu, P.; Zhai, Z.; Hao, Z.; Zhang, H.; He, J. CircWHSC1 serves as an oncogene to promote hepatocellular carcinoma progression. *Eur. J. Clin. Investig.* **2021**, *51*, e13487. [CrossRef]
149. Wang, Y.; Gao, R.; Li, J.; Tang, S.; Li, S.; Tong, Q.; Li, S. Downregulation of hsa_circ_0074854 Suppresses the Migration and Invasion in Hepatocellular Carcinoma via Interacting with HuR and via Suppressing Exosomes-Mediated Macrophage M2 Polarization. *Int. J. Nanomed.* **2021**, *16*, 2803–2818. [CrossRef]
150. Hu, Z.; Chen, G.; Zhao, Y.; Gao, H.; Li, L.; Yin, Y.; Jiang, J.; Wang, L.; Mang, Y.; Gao, Y.; et al. Exosome-derived circCCAR1 promotes CD8 + T-cell dysfunction and anti-PD1 resistance in hepatocellular carcinoma. *Mol. Cancer* **2023**, *22*, 55. [CrossRef]
151. Zhang, P.F.; Gao, C.; Huang, X.Y.; Lu, J.C.; Guo, X.J.; Shi, G.M.; Cai, J.B.; Ke, A.W. Cancer cell-derived exosomal circUHRF1 induces natural killer cell exhaustion and may cause resistance to anti-PD1 therapy in hepatocellular carcinoma. *Mol. Cancer* **2020**, *19*, 110. [CrossRef]
152. Hu, Z.Q.; Zhou, S.L.; Li, J.; Zhou, Z.J.; Wang, P.C.; Xin, H.Y.; Mao, L.; Luo, C.B.; Yu, S.Y.; Huang, X.W.; et al. Circular RNA Sequencing Identifies CircASAP1 as a Key Regulator in Hepatocellular Carcinoma Metastasis. *Hepatology* **2020**, *72*, 906–922. [CrossRef]
153. Huang, M.; Huang, X.; Huang, N. Exosomal circGSE1 promotes immune escape of hepatocellular carcinoma by inducing the expansion of regulatory T cells. *Cancer Sci.* **2022**, *113*, 1968–1983. [CrossRef] [PubMed]
154. Liu, T.; Tan, J.; Wu, M.; Fan, W.; Wei, J.; Zhu, B.; Guo, J.; Wang, S.; Zhou, P.; Zhang, H.; et al. High-affinity neoantigens correlate with better prognosis and trigger potent antihepatocellular carcinoma (HCC) activity by activating CD39$^+$CD8$^+$ T cells. *Gut* **2020**, *70*, 1965–1977. [CrossRef]
155. Lu, J.C.; Zhang, P.F.; Huang, X.Y.; Guo, X.J.; Gao, C.; Zeng, H.Y.; Zheng, Y.M.; Wang, S.W.; Cai, J.B.; Sun, Q.M.; et al. Amplification of spatially isolated adenosine pathway by tumor-macrophage interaction induces anti-PD1 resistance in hepatocellular carcinoma. *J. Hematol. Oncol.* **2021**, *14*, 200. [CrossRef]
156. Chen, B.; Li, Q.; Li, Y.; Li, Q.; Lai, H.; Huang, S.; Li, C.; Li, Y. circTMEM181 upregulates ARHGAP29 to inhibit hepatocellular carcinoma migration and invasion by sponging miR-519a-5p. *Hepatol. Res.* **2023**, *53*, 334–343. [CrossRef] [PubMed]
157. Ma, S.; Kong, S.; Wang, F.; Ju, S. CircRNAs: Biogenesis, functions, and role in drug-resistant Tumours. *Mol. Cancer* **2020**, *19*, 119. [CrossRef]
158. Xu, J.; Ji, L.; Liang, Y.; Wan, Z.; Zheng, W.; Song, X.; Gorshkov, K.; Sun, Q.; Lin, H.; Zheng, X.; et al. CircRNA-SORE mediates sorafenib resistance in hepatocellular carcinoma by stabilizing YBX1. *Signal Transduct. Target. Ther.* **2020**, *5*, 298. [CrossRef] [PubMed]
159. Hao, X.; Zhang, Y.; Shi, X.; Liu, H.; Zheng, Z.; Han, G.; Rong, D.; Zhang, C.; Tang, W.; Wang, X. CircPAK1 promotes the progression of hepatocellular carcinoma via modulation of YAP nucleus localization by interacting with 14-3-3ζ. *J. Exp. Clin. Cancer Res.* **2022**, *41*, 281. [CrossRef]
160. Zhou, Y.; Tang, W.; Zhuo, H.; Zhu, D.; Rong, D.; Sun, J.; Song, J. Cancer-associated fibroblast exosomes promote chemoresistance to cisplatin in hepatocellular carcinoma through circZFR targeting signal transducers and activators of transcription (STAT3)/nuclear factor-kappa B (NF-κB) pathway. *Bioengineered* **2022**, *13*, 4786–4797. [CrossRef]
161. Sun, X.H.; Wang, Y.T.; Li, G.F.; Zhang, N.; Fan, L. Serum-derived three-circRNA signature as a diagnostic biomarker for hepatocellular carcinoma. *Cancer Cell Int.* **2020**, *20*, 226. [CrossRef]
162. Lin, Y.; Zheng, Z.H.; Wang, J.X.; Zhao, Z.; Peng, T.Y. Tumor Cell-Derived Exosomal Circ-0072088 Suppresses Migration and Invasion of Hepatic Carcinoma Cells Through Regulating MMP-16. *Front. Cell Dev. Biol.* **2021**, *9*, 726323. [CrossRef]
163. Lai, Z.; Wei, T.; Li, Q.; Wang, X.; Zhang, Y.; Zhang, S. Exosomal circFBLIM1 Promotes Hepatocellular Carcinoma Progression and Glycolysis by Regulating the miR-338/LRP6 Axis. *Cancer Biother. Radiopharm.* **2020**, *38*, 674–683. [CrossRef] [PubMed]
164. Wang, Y.; Pei, L.; Yue, Z.; Jia, M.; Wang, H.; Cao, L.L. The Potential of Serum Exosomal has_circ_0028861 as the Novel Diagnostic Biomarker of HBV-Derived Hepatocellular Cancer. *Front. Genet.* **2021**, *12*, 703205. [CrossRef] [PubMed]
165. Lyu, L.; Yang, W.; Yao, J.; Wang, H.; Zhu, J.; Jin, A.; Liu, T.; Wang, B.; Zhou, J.; Fan, J.; et al. The diagnostic value of plasma exosomal hsa_circ_0070396 for hepatocellular carcinoma. *Biomark. Med.* **2021**, *15*, 359–371. [CrossRef] [PubMed]
166. Zhang, T.; Jing, B.; Bai, Y.; Zhang, Y.; Yu, H. Circular RNA circTMEM45A Acts as the Sponge of MicroRNA-665 to Promote Hepatocellular Carcinoma Progression. *Mol. Ther. Nucleic Acids* **2020**, *22*, 285–297. [CrossRef] [PubMed]
167. Huang, C.; Yu, W.; Wang, Q.; Huang, T.; Ding, Y. CircANTXR1 Contributes to the Malignant Progression of Hepatocellular Carcinoma by Promoting Proliferation and Metastasis. *J. Hepatocell. Carcinoma* **2021**, *8*, 1339–1353. [CrossRef] [PubMed]
168. Chen, W.; Quan, Y.; Fan, S.; Wang, H.; Liang, J.; Huang, L.; Chen, L.; Liu, Q.; He, P.; Ye, Y. Exosome-transmitted circular RNA hsa_circ_0051443 suppresses hepatocellular carcinoma progression. *Cancer Lett.* **2020**, *475*, 119–128. [CrossRef]
169. Czystowska-Kuzmicz, M.; Whiteside, T.L. The potential role of tumor-derived exosomes in diagnosis, prognosis, and response to therapy in cancer. *Expert. Opin. Biol. Ther.* **2021**, *21*, 241–258. [CrossRef]

Disclaimer/Publisher's Note: The statements, opinions and data contained in all publications are solely those of the individual author(s) and contributor(s) and not of MDPI and/or the editor(s). MDPI and/or the editor(s) disclaim responsibility for any injury to people or property resulting from any ideas, methods, instructions or products referred to in the content.

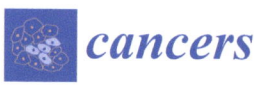 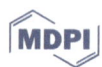

Review

Exploring the Potential of Non-Coding RNAs as Liquid Biopsy Biomarkers for Lung Cancer Screening: A Literature Review

Edoardo Garbo [1], Benedetta Del Rio [1], Giorgia Ferrari [1], Massimiliano Cani [1], Valerio Maria Napoli [1], Valentina Bertaglia [1], Enrica Capelletto [1], Christian Rolfo [2], Silvia Novello [1] and Francesco Passiglia [1,*]

[1] Department of Oncology, University of Turin, San Luigi Hospital, 10124 Orbassano, Italy; edoardo.garbo@unito.it (E.G.); benedetta.delrio@unito.it (B.D.R.); giorgia.ferrari@unito.it (G.F.); massimiliano.cani@unito.it (M.C.); valeriomaria.napoli@gmail.com (V.M.N.); valentina.bertaglia@gmail.com (V.B.); enrica.capelletto@gmail.com (E.C.); silvia.novello@unito.it (S.N.)

[2] Center for Thoracic Oncology, Tisch Cancer Institute, Mount Sinai Health System, Icahn School of Medicine at Mount Sinai, New York, NY 10029, USA; christian.rolfo@mssm.edu

* Correspondence: francesco.passiglia@unito.it

Simple Summary: Low-dose CT scan screening will be widely implemented on a large-scale base, aiming to reduce lung cancer related mortality in the high risk smoking population as already reported in multiple trials, in several countries. Recent evidence has suggested that the identification of liquid biopsy biomarkers may improve its accuracy in lung cancer early detection, reducing the false positive rate as well as overdiagnosis issues and potentially addressing one of the major obstacles in the implementation of Low-dose CT scan alone in this context. RNAs, particularly non-coding RNAs, are for sure the most studied and promising circulating biomarkers in this setting.

Abstract: Lung cancer represent the leading cause of cancer mortality, so several efforts have been focused on the development of a screening program. To address the issue of high overdiagnosis and false positive rates associated to LDCT-based screening, there is a need for new diagnostic biomarkers, with liquid biopsy ncRNAs detection emerging as a promising approach. In this scenario, this work provides an updated summary of the literature evidence about the role of non-coding RNAs in lung cancer screening. A literature search on PubMed was performed including studies which investigated liquid biopsy non-coding RNAs biomarker lung cancer patients and a control cohort. Micro RNAs were the most widely studied biomarkers in this setting but some preliminary evidence was found also for other non-coding RNAs, suggesting that a multi-biomarker based liquid biopsy approach could enhance their efficacy in the screening context. However, further studies are needed in order to optimize detection techniques as well as diagnostic accuracy before introducing novel biomarkers in the early diagnosis setting.

Keywords: lung cancer; screening; liquid biopsy; non-coding RNA

1. Introduction

Lung cancer remains nowadays the leading cause of cancer mortality accounting for 12% of overall cancer deaths worldwide. This is certainly linked to the peculiar biological behavior of this disease as well as to a significant diagnostic delay leading to advanced-stage diagnoses in about 50% of cases. For this reason, several efforts over the last years have been focused on the development of effective secondary prevention strategies, with different studies and metanalysis [1] showing that low-dose computed tomography (LDCT) is able to reduce lung cancer-related mortality in high-risk smoking subjects.

In detail, the National Lung Cancer Screening Trial (NLST) and The Dutch-Belgian Randomized Lung Cancer Screening Trial (NELSON) randomized studies demonstrated a significant reduction (around 20%) of lung cancer-related mortality in smoking populations undergoing LDCT as compared to either thorax RX or clinical observation [2,3], leading to the introduction of lung cancer screening in the United States since 2013. Among the different barriers limiting LDCT screening implementation in Europe, the high rate of overdiagnosis and false positive cases represent a relevant unmet need significantly impacting the subject management in real world scenarios. In addition to that, the potential exposure to the imaging radiation and the risk of overtreatment for indolent lung nodules further reduce subjects' compliance to the LDCT screening. In this context, the integration of tumor biomarkers through liquid biopsy could improve the diagnostic accuracy of LDCT screening in a non-invasive manner aiming to identify the high-risk population requiring further investigation, personalizing screening intervals and likely increasing subjects' compliance to the screening procedures. Furthermore, the possibility to perform a liquid biopsy in the peripheral hospitals near rural areas could allow to reach a larger smoking population who is usually recalcitrant to the LDCT, thus increasing the access rate to lung cancer screening in a different way and promoting personalized approaches.

A liquid biopsy is able to identify circulating tumor biomarkers that can be considered surrogates of the primary tumor as circulating tumor cells (CTCs), circulating tumor DNA (ctDNA), microRNA (miRNA), and exosomes. Liquid biopsies are already playing an important role in the clinical management of metastatic lung cancer patients through the evaluation of the tumor molecular profiling by ctDNA analysis, while also progressively extending to the early-stage disease in terms of minimal residual disease monitoring as well as cancer interception [4].

The role of CTCs in lung cancer screening has been investigated in several trials since cell dissemination is a relatively early event in tumor progression. These trials showed that CTCs detected in high-risk patients are able to anticipate the diagnosis of lung cancer, even years earlier than CT scans [5]. One of the main problems with using CTCs as a biomarker is represented by their rarity in peripheral blood.

Several studies have investigated the role of CtDNA and cell-free DNA (cfDNA) in screening encountering a fundamental issue: the concentration of cfDNA correlates with the disease burden of the tumor that is very low in early-stage disease, making it difficult to isolate. Despite this limitation, different studies have investigated the role of cfDNA in early diagnosis. To distinguish tumor from non-tumor cfDNA, they have looked at its concentration, genetic changes, or methylation as possible biomarkers [6]. In 2020 a study proposed the use of a cfDNA-based machine-learning method to improve the specificity of LDCT screening with interesting results [7].

Another interesting finding is the development of a blood-based multi-cancer early detection (MCED) test targeting a screening population. The test has been developed for the early detection of more than 50 types of cancer. The MCED test analyzed the methylation patterns of CtDNA and demonstrated high specificity (99.1%) and a positive predicted value of approximately 40% [8].

Only a small fraction (approximately 3%) of the genetic transcript is able to encode proteins, while the remaining part is defined as non-coding RNAs (ncRNAs). The definition of "coding" encompasses RNAs that encode proteins from DNA-derived information, such as mRNAs. Noncoding RNAs have a different role since they act as cellular regulators of gene expression at different transcriptional, post-transcriptional, and epigenetic levels. A few exceptions to this definition include some ncRNAs binding ribosomes encoding peptides exerting a modulator function on cellular activities [9]. It has become clear that ncRNAs also play an important role in the communication processes between cancer cells and tumor microenvironment and are crucial for regulating tumor growth [9]. In recent years the knowledge about ncRNAs roles in cancer process has exponentially grown [10], including diagnostic, prognostic, predictive, and therapeutical applications across different cancers and settings [11].

ncRNAs can be classified into two macro-categories: housekeeping ncRNAs and regulatory ncRNAs. Housekeeping ncRNAs regulate basic cellular functions and are ubiquitously expressed. Regulatory ncRNAs play a pivotal role in gene expression regulation and protein translation both at transcriptional and post-transcriptional levels. Increasing evidence points out their role in cancer development, regulation, and growth, making them a precious tool for cancer management at different stages [12,13].

Among the housekeeping ncRNAs, we encounter transfer RNA and ribosomal RNA. Regulatory ncRNAs, instead, can be divided into three major groups: circular RNAs (cricRNAs), long noncoding RNAs (>200 nt, lncRNAs), and small noncoding RNAs (<200 nt, sncRNAs) [13].

The ncRNAs can be found in different biofluids either as freely or encapsulated in extracellular vesicles [12,14], making them potentially stable biomarkers for clinical use, which have been explored also within LC screening clinical trials [13,15,16].

To date, among the different liquid biopsy biomarkers under clinical investigation in the lung cancer early detection setting, ncRNAs are for sure one of the most promising biomarkers to be implemented in the context of lung cancer screening. For this reason, this review will specifically focus on ncRNA role, describing biological function, available evidence, and clinical trials ongoing in this emerging setting.

2. Methods of Literature Search

An extensive literature search was performed on PubMed, using as cut-off date of 16 March 2023. Keywords included: noncoding RNA, lung cancer, screening. A total of 2538 articles were found and screened for eligibility, taking into account three major criteria of inclusion: (1) Single ncRNAs or ncRNA-based genomic signature; (2) biomarker analysis performed on blood or other biofluids; and (3) biomarker involvement in non-small cell lung cancer (NSCLC) screening or early diagnosis.

Both prospective and retrospective studies were considered. Only studies performed on humans were included, but they could include an in vitro/in vivo validation part. Only studies that involved a control group were considered. The control group could also have other pulmonary conditions or pulmonary nodules (PNs) that were retrospectively prospectively identified as benign lesions. Published abstracts without associated full articles were excluded from the analysis. Three independent reviewers collected data from the included articles, and another one subsequently reviewed all of the information.

To draw a clear overview of all clinical trials concerning LC screening that included a liquid biopsy part, we also performed research on clinicaltrials.gov using the following keywords: lung cancer and screening. A total of 601 trials were found and, among them, only those involving LDCT screening and encompassing biofluids collection for biomarkers research were included.

3. Results

3.1. Micro RNAs (miRNAs)

MiRNAs are fragments of single-stranded non-coding RNA with a length of approximately 20 ribonucleotides. Since they remain stable in biofluids, unlike other free RNA molecules, they can be detected in both serum and plasma. They regulate gene expression at the post-transcriptional level and are involved in the regulation of cell proliferation and apoptosis. In fact, their targets include oncogenes and tumor suppressor genes and their dysregulation can lead to malignant cell transformation across different tumor types [6,17].

miRNAs are one of the pivotal biomarkers explored in phase III trials of lung cancer screening, and our literature search identified studies that used both multi-miRNA signatures (>2 miRNA) and single miRNA approach for early NSCLC detection. In detail both the miR-test, a serum-based 13 miRNA signature, and the micro-RNA signature classifier (MSC), a plasma-based 24 miRNA risk score, showed very promising data for clinical use [18].

Overall, 32 studies evaluating the expression of multi-miRNA in early-stage NSCLC patients compared to healthy controls have been identified through our PubMed research. The identified signatures ranged from 2 to 24 miRNAs and were all validated on biological fluids that could be used for liquid biopsies purposes (Table 1). Almost all of the evaluated studies used plasma or serum for miRNA detection and the most used sequencing technique was quantitative real-time PCR (qRT-PCR). Among all of these studies matching our inclusion criteria, only six included a CT scan integrated to a specific miRNA signature for LC diagnosis.

Sozzi G. et al. [19] conducted a large retrospective analysis in this setting analyzing plasma samples from 939 participants to the Italian randomized MILD LC screening study (69 patients diagnosed with LC and 870 healthy individuals) using a 24-miRNA classifier. They identified a higher sensitivity (87%) and a similar specificity (81%) for LC detection, compared to LDCT alone (79% and 81%, respectively) with a false-positive rate of 3.7% vs. 19.4% with and without MSC integration.

In another prospective analysis conducted in the BIOMILD study, patients were [16] stratified into four different subgroups based on a miRNA signature classifier (MSC): 2 MSC+ with or without a positive CT scan and 2 MSC− with or without a positive CT scan. Individuals with a positive CT scan and an MSC− had a lower incidence of LC and individuals with both CT and MSC negative had a lower overall LC incidence at four years, interval cancer, stage I, and advanced stages diagnosis, as well as the lowest LC mortality rate at five years as compared to all other subgroups. So, the authors found out that the combined use of LDCT and MSC at baseline was able to predict individual LC incidence and mortality, with a major effect of MSC for LDCT-positive individuals.

Shun J et al. [20] applied a 3 miRNAs (miRs-21, 210, and 486-5p) plasma signature on healthy subjects, patients with benign pulmonary nodules (PNs), and malignant PNs. This approach achieved an area under the curve (AUC) of 0.855 for lung cancer detection in the testing cohort. The panel of the three mi RNA was then validated in an independent cohort of 156 patients who had solitary PNs, and this miRNAs signature produced a 76.32% sensitivity and 85% specificity in differentiating malignant from benign solitary PNs.

The same group [21] screened 10 miRNA differently expressed by LC and healthy smokers sputum and built a logistic regression model on a 2 miRNA combination (miR-31 and miR-210). This model generated an AUC of 0.83 in distinguishing LC patients from healthy smokers, moreover, the combination of CT scans and the 2 miRNA combination achieved an AUC of 0.95. In the validation cohort, the AUC dropped to 0.79, but the combination of miRNA and CT scans improved the specificity and sensitivity compared to CT scan alone.

Another plasma-based approach was conducted by Zheng D. et al. [22], who evaluated circulating small extracellular vesicle (EV) microRNAs in 208 patients with CT-detected PNs. Five miRNAs (let-7b-3p, miR-125b-5p, miR-150-5p, miR-101-3p, and miR-3168), included within the CirsEV-miR model were firstly tested in a small training cohort of 47 patients and then validated in a testing-cohort of 62 patients achieving an AUC for lung cancer detection of 0.920 and 0.760, respectively. This model was then validated in an external cohort of 92 patients (20 patients with benign PNs and 79 with malignant PNs), reaching an AUC of 0.781.

EVs and miRNAs were also tested in this setting by using NGS analysis [23]. They analyzed plasma from patients who had Lung-RADS4 PNs then confirmed as LC, versus over-diagnosed Lung-RADS4 PNs or high-risk Lung-RADS2 screening controls. They identified different expression levels of let-7b-5p, miR-184, and miR-22-3p as biomarkers for potentially discriminating cancer patients from high-risk controls. The multiple logistic regression analyses of the 3 EV miRNAs showed a combined ROC AUC value of 92.4%.

Other pulmonary pathological conditions, such as chronic obstructive pulmonary disease (COPD) and asthma, were included in some of the other studies and represent an interesting approach to eliminate some biases that could be created by smoking-related or pre-existing pulmonary conditions in the implementation of liquid biopsies within lung screening programs. Halvorsen A.R. et al. [24] used serum also from 16 COPD subjects to build their miRNA signature for their prediction model, showing a good performance in discriminating lung cancer from the control groups (AUC 0.89). Yang X et al. [25] used also serum of COPD, in their logistic regression model obtaining not only good performance in discriminating lung cancer patients from controls, but also a higher accuracy for adenocarcinoma (AC) patients rather than squamous cell carcinoma (SCC). Zaporozhchenko I.A. et al. [26] analyzed 179 miRNA in plasma samples obtained from patients with a non-cancerous lung disease (hyper- or metaplastic endobronchitis (EB)) and a cancer-free group of healthy volunteers. They found a 14 miRNA signature discriminating LC group and controls, but interestingly the performance of the model was largely unaffected by the presence of samples from patients with endobronchitis. A similar approach was led by Nadal E. et al. [27] analyzing also serum samples of patients with COPD and identifying a 4 miRNA signature for LC diagnosis, clustering also the discovery set into 2 different groups, characterized by different metastasis-free survival (MFS) and overall survival (OS). Fehlmann T. et al. [15], instead led a large multicenter retrospective cohort study, analyzing 3046 samples of LC patients (including NSCLC and small cell lung cancer, SCLC), and patients with other lung conditions (mostly COPD). A 14-miRNA signature derived from the training set was used to distinguish patients with lung cancer from patients with nontumor lung diseases both in the testing set (accuracy of 92.5%, sensitivity of 96.4%, and specificity of 88.6%) and in the validation set (accuracy of 95.9%, sensitivity of 76.3%, and specificity of 97.5%).

Some of the studies listed in Table 1, tested another interesting use of LB-based approach in the LC early-diagnosis setting which is LC histological subtype prediction. Lu S. et al. [28] conducted a miRNA analysis on plasma samples of a large cohort of patients (1132 samples, including healthy individuals and patients with NSCLC or SCLC) collected from five medical centers, developing a plasma miRNA panel capable to discriminate LC patients from healthy individuals, and SCLC from NSCLC (AUC 0.878 and 0.869 for training and validation cohort, respectively). Instead, a study by Powrózek T [29], et al., showed that miR-944 had a high diagnostic accuracy for operable squamous cell carcinoma detection (AUC 0.982), whereas miR-3662 for operable adenocarcinoma diagnosis (AUC 0.926). Jiang Y. et al. [30] used an NGS-based approach in analyzing plasma-derived EVs from healthy individuals, patients with early-stage SCLC, and patients with early-stage NSCLC, finding out that miRNA-483-3p derived from plasma EVs could be a potential biomarker for early-stage SCLC diagnosis, while both miRNA-152-3p and miRNA-1277-5p could be used for early-stage NSCLC diagnosis.

Other efforts of using miRNA-based liquid biopsy for lung cancer early detection were made by using single miRNAs as biomarkers such as miR-17-19 [31], miR-20 [32], miRNA-21 [33–42], miR-25 [43], miR-29 [44], miR-30 [45], miR-31 [46], miR-125, miR-126 [47–49], miR-135 [50], miR-143 [51], miR-145 [32], miR-148/152 family [52], miR-153, miR-155 [36,53,54], miR-182, miR-183 [47], miR-185 [55], miR-184 [56], miR-200 [57], miRNA-210 [47,58], miR-221 [32], miR-223 [32,59], miR-328 [60], miR-339 [61], miR-411 [62], miR-486 [63], miR-499 [64], miR-519 [65], miR-770 [66], mi-R762 [67], microRNA-2355 [68], hsa-miR2116, hsa-miR449c and hsa-miR2117 [69]. These single biomarker-based approaches led to similar results, but the heterogeneity of the study and the lack of a validation cohort make them likely less reliable for clinical implementation in the real-world setting.

Table 1. Multiparametric miRNAs studies.

Title	No. of Patients (LC vs. Others)	AUC	CT Combined	External Validation	Biofluid Used	miRNA
Circulating MicroRNAs as Non-Invasive Biomarkers for Early Detection of Non-Small-Cell Lung Cancer [70]	100 vs. 100	0.92 (95% CI: 0.87–0.95)	No	No	Plasma	24 miRNA signature
MicroRNA-based biomarkers for diagnosis of non-small cell lung cancer (NSCLC) [71]	76 vs. 72	0.91 (95% CI: 0.864–0.956)	No	Yes	Plasma and sputum	2 miRNAs (miRs-31-5p and 210-3p) in sputum + 3 miRNAs (miRs-21-5p, 210-3p, and 486-5p)
A unique set of 6 circulating microRNAs for early detection of non-small cell lung cancer [24]	38 vs. 32	0.89	No	Yes	Plasma	6 miRNA signature (miR-429, miR-205, miR-200b, miR-203, miR-125b and miR-34b)
Serum microRNA Signature Is Capable of Early Diagnosis for Non-Small Cell Lung Cancer [25]	63 vs. 15	0.93	No	No	Serum	5 miRNAs (miR-146b, miR-205, miR-29c, miR-30b, and miR-337)
Application of plasma circulating microRNA-448, 506, 4316, and 4478 analysis for non-invasive diagnosis of lung cancer [72]	90 vs. 85	0.896	No	No	Plasma	4 miRNAs (miRNA-448, 506, 4316, and 4478)
Increased micro-RNA 17, 21, and 192 gene expressions improve early diagnosis in non-small cell lung cancer [73]	60 vs. 30	Unk	No	No	Serum	2 miRNA + gene expression (micro-RNA 17, 21, and 192 gene expressions)
Baseline computed tomography screening and blood microRNA predict lung cancer risk and define adequate intervals in the BioMILD trial [16]	2664 vs. 1445	Unk	Yes	Prospective	Serum	13-miRNA serum signature (MSC)
Identifying circulating miRNA biomarkers for early diagnosis and monitoring of lung cancer [74]	48 vs. 984	0.9865	No	No	Serum	5 miRNA (miR-92, miR-140-5p, miR-331-3p, miR-223, miR-374a)
Profiling of 179 miRNA Expression in Blood Plasma of Lung Cancer Patients and Cancer-Free Individuals [26]	50 vs. 50	0.979	No	Yes	Serum and Plasma	14 miRNA
A novel circulating miRNA-based signature for the early diagnosis and prognosis prediction of non-small-cell lung cancer [75]	125 vs. 100	0.882	No	No	Serum	2 miRNA (miR-942 and serum miR-601)
Early Detection of Lung Cancer in Serum by a Panel of MicroRNA Biomarkers [76]	142 vs. 111	0.936	No	Yes	Serum	3 miRNAs (miR-125a-5p, miR-25, and miR-126)
Clinical Utility of a Plasma-Based miRNA Signature Classifier Within Computed Tomography Lung Cancer Screening: A Correlative MILD Trial Study [19]	86 vs. 870	Unk	Yes	Prospective	Serum	24 miRNA (MSC)
Identification of serum miRNAs by nano-quantum dots microarray as diagnostic biomarkers for early detection of non-small cell lung cancer [77]	164 vs. 112	0.93 (95% CI: 0.88, 0.96)	No	Yes	Serum	12 miRNA
External validation of a panel of plasma microRNA biomarkers for lung cancer [78]	471 vs. 489	0.963 (0.862–0.995)	No	Yes	Plasma	4 miRNA (miRs-126-3p, 145, 210-3p and 205-5p)
Two plasma microRNA panels for diagnosis and subtype discrimination of lung cancer [28]	539 vs. 456	0.873	No	Yes	Plasma	6 microRNAs (miR-17, miR-190b, miR-19a, miR-19b, miR-26b, and miR-375)
Circulating microRNA array (miR-182, 200b and 205) for the early diagnosis and poor prognosis predictor of non-small cell lung cancer [79]	50 vs. 30	0.883	No	No	Serum	3 miRNA (miR-182, miR-200b and miR-205)

Table 1. Cont.

Title	No. of Patients (LC vs. Others)	AUC	CT Combined	External Validation	Biofluid Used	miRNA
Potential circulating miRNA signature for early detection of NSCLC [80]	106 vs. 70	0.804	No	Yes	Serum	2 miRNA (miR-21, miR-141)
A Novel Serum 4-microRNA Signature for Lung Cancer Detection [27]	84 vs. 23	0.993	No	Yes	Serum	4 miRNA (miR-141, miR-200b, miR-193b and miR-301)
Sputum microRNA Biomarkers for Identifying Lung Cancer in Indeterminate Solitary Pulmonary Nodules [81]	203 vs. 210	0.92	No	Yes	Sputum	3 miRNA (miR-21, miR-31, miR-210)
Blood-borne miRNA profile-based diagnostic classifier for lung adenocarcinoma [82]	253 vs. 101	0.991	No	Yes	Serum	20 miRNA classifier
Plasma circulating microRNA-944 and microRNA-3662 as potential histologic type-specific early lung cancer biomarkers [29]	90 vs. 85	0.881	No	No	Plasma	2 miRNA (microRNA-944 and microRNA-3662)
Evaluation of circulating small extracellular vesicle-derived mRNAs as diagnostic biomarkers for differentiating between different pathological types of early lung cancer [30]	25 vs. 24	0.791	No	No	Plasma	2 miRNA (miR-152-3p and miR-1277-5p)
Plasma extracellular vesicle microRNA profiling and the identification of a diagnostic signature for stage I lung adenocarcinoma [83]	254 vs. 206	0.917	No	No	Plasma	4 miRNA (hsa-miR-106b-3p, hsa-miR-125a-5p, hsa-miR-3615, and hsa-miR-450b-5p
Evaluating the Use of Circulating MicroRNA Profiles for Lung Cancer Detection in Symptomatic Patients [15]	606 vs. 2440	0.944	No	No	Serum	14-miRNA
Analysis of MicroRNAs in Sputum to Improve Computed Tomography for Lung Cancer Diagnosis [21]	66 vs. 68	0.83	Yes	Yes	Sputum	2 miRNA (miR-31 and miR-210)
Identification and evaluation of circulating small extracellular vesicle microRNAs as diagnostic biomarkers for patients with indeterminate pulmonary nodules [22]	208 (nodules)	0.920	Yes	Yes	Plasma	CirsEV-miR model (let-7b-3p, miR-125b-5p, miR-150-5p, miR-101-3p, and miR-3168)
Diagnosis of lung cancer in individuals with solitary pulmonary nodules by plasma microRNA biomarkers [20]	108 vs. 142	0.855	Yes	Yes	Plasma	3 miRNAs (miRs-21, 210, and 486-5p)
Combining plasma extracellular vesicle Let-7b-5p, miR-184 and circulating miR-22-3p levels for NSCLC diagnosis and drug resistance prediction [23]	40 (nodules)	0.924	Yes	No	Plasma	3 miRNA (miR-184, and miR-22-3p) + EV (let-7b-5p)
Serum miR-1228-3p and miR-181a-5p as Noninvasive Biomarkers for Non-Small Cell Lung Cancer Diagnosis and Prognosis [84]	50 vs. 30	0.711	No	No	Serum	2 miRNA (miR-1228-3p, miR-181a-5p)
A six-microRNA panel in plasma was identified as a potential biomarker for lung adenocarcinoma diagnosis [85]	141 vs. 124	0.84	No	Yes	Serum	6 miRNA (miR-19b-3p, miR-21-5p, miR-221-3p, miR-409-3p, miR-425-5p and miR-584-5p)
Evaluation of Tumor-Derived Exosomal miRNA as Potential Diagnostic Biomarkers for Early-Stage Non-Small Cell Lung Cancer Using Next-Generation Sequencing [86]	46 vs. 42	0.899	No	No	Plasma	8 miRNA (miR-181-5p, miR-30a-3p, miR-30e-3p miR-361-5p, miR-10b-5p, miR-15b-5p, miR-320b)
Identification of a three-miRNA signature as a blood-borne diagnostic marker for early diagnosis of lung adenocarcinoma [87]	238 vs. 257	0.974	No	No	Plasma	3 miRNAs (miR-532, miR-628-3p and miR-425-3p)

3.2. Long Non Coding RNAs (lnc-RNAs)

LncRNAs look quite promising since they have been demonstrated to be stable in biofluids [88,89] and to be frequently dysregulated in NSCLC pathogenesis [90]. According to our literature search, a multi-lncRNA approach was conducted across 4 studies. Gupta C et al. [91], analyzed lncRNAs in the sputum of LC patients and cancer-free individuals demonstrating a good ability in discriminating the two groups through a panel containing SNHG1, H19, and HOTAIR (AUC 0.90). The second multi-lncRNA approach was conducted by Yuan S. et al. [92], who collected 528 plasma samples of patients with either LC, other lung conditions, or healthy volunteers. They identified a 4-lncRNA panel (RMRP, NEAT1, TUG1, and MALAT1) with a high diagnostic value for NSCLC (AUC 0.85 for AC and 0.93 for SCC in the expansion cohort). An alternative approach conducted by Li X et al. [93], aimed to search for lncRNAs in tumor-educated platelet (TEP), where a combined use of linc-GTF2H2-1, RP3-466P17.2, and lnc-ST8SIA4-12 achieved an AUC of 0.895. Ultimately in the analysis by Kamel L.M. et al [94], the combination of GAS5 and SOX2OT showed an AUC of 0.95 for distinguishing LC patients from healthy controls.

Single lncRNA-based studies were conducted for different lncRNAs obtaining lower performances similar to what has been observed with miRNAs until now [95–108], so limiting any clinical implementation in the real word setting.

3.3. Circular-RNAs (Circ-RNAs)

Circ-RNAs can be freely detected in biofluids (plasma and saliva) as well as in exosomes [109], and are aberrantly expressed in early-stage lung adenocarcinoma, making them a good biomarker for LC early detection [110]. Even though Yang X. et al. [111] meta-analysis, comparing circRNAs' expression in tissue and plasma/serum samples, showed that the diagnostic accuracy of tissue was higher (AUC 0.85 vs. 0.79), other evidence points out in the opposite direction. Falin C. et al. [112] validated a combination of circRNAs (hsa_circ_0001492, hsa_circ_0001346, hsa_circ_0000690, and hsa_circ_0001439) that were significantly upregulated in plasma exosomes of AC patients as compared to healthy controls. Hang D. et al. [113] adopted RNA sequencing (RNA-seq) and qRT-PCR approaches to explore cancer-related circRNAs expression, showing that circFARSA was increased in cancerous tissues, and was more abundant in the plasma of LC patients than controls. Other three circRNAs were tested as potential biomarkers for LC early detection with liquid biopsy showing a good diagnostic accuracy: hsa_circ_0023179 [114], hsa_circ_0006423 [115] and circFOXP1 [116].

3.4. Other Non-Coding RNAs and Combined Approaches

For what concerns small-nuclear RNAs we found three studies that tested the differences between LC patients and controls. Köhler J. et al. [117], determined RNU2-1f in the serum of patients with LC, chronic lung disease, and healthy controls, showing the ability to discriminate the LC group from others (AUC of 0.91). Moreover, the two isoforms of RNU2 (RNU2-1 and RNU2-2) were also tested in another study by Mazières J et al. [118], who demonstrated that miR-U2-1 was able to discriminate between patients with COPD and patients with COPD and lung cancer (AUC of 0.866). Dong et al. [119] used a tumor-platelet educated approach, finding out that TEP U1, U2, U5 were decreased in early-stage lung cancer patients compared with those in healthy subjects.

For what concerns piwiRNAs we found a study by Li J. et al. [120] demonstrating that piR-hsa-26925 and piR-hsa-5444 had a significantly higher level in serum exosome samples of AC patients than healthy controls.

No studies matching our inclusion criteria were found about ribosomal RNA (rRNA), transfer RNA (tRNA), and small nucleolar- RNAs (sno-RNAs) in the context of lung cancer screening.

Few studies were conducted using a combined ncRNAs approach, according to our inclusion criteria. In detail Peng H et al. [121] constructed a miRNA and MALAT1 non-coding RNA panel showing a good performance also in detecting stages I/II/III NSCLC.

A panel of seven small ncRNA pair ratios was tested by Dou Y. et al. [122] and could differentiate AC patients from other lung diseases of high-risk controls.

3.5. Ongoing Clinical Trials on Liquid Biopsy in Lung Cancer Screening

We also performed a study of ongoing clinical trials on clinicaltrials.gov using the keywords "lung cancer" and "screening". The data collection was completed on 16 March 2023 and identified a total of 601 ongoing trials related to lung cancer screening. Out of the 601 clinical trials identified, we selected 55 trials incorporating liquid biopsy and the analysis of biological samples for the detection of predictive biomarkers in the setting of LC screening (Table 2). The selected trials did not exclusively include healthy individuals at high risk of developing lung cancer, but also those with lung nodules, CT suspicion or pathologically confirmed lung cancer, as well as other benign lung diseases. Furthermore, a particularly noteworthy study included only never-smokers (defined as individuals with a lifetime exposure of less than 100 cigarettes) and Asian women (NCT05164757).

Among the 55 clinical trials shortlisted based on our inclusion criteria, 25 of them involved the use of chest CT or LDCT scans as a diagnostic tool for lung cancer screening. The HANSE trial (NCT04913155) also investigated other indicators such as coronary calcium score and emphysema score. One of the selected studies involved the use of chest MRI to assess the concordance of imaging features of nodules between LDCT and MRI in the study population (NCT05699213). Concluding, a small portion of these studies incorporates pulmonary function testing within their research protocols.

These selected trials also involved the collection and analysis of various biological samples to identify possible biomarkers for the early detection of lung cancer. Specifically, they included blood samples, different airways samples (bronchoalveolar lavage, BAL, bronchial biopsy and brushing samples, nasal swab, and brush samples), sputum samples, buccal swab samples, urine samples, and feces samples.

Among the 55 clinical trials that met our inclusion criteria, blood samples were collected in 52 trials, but only 33 of these explicitly state the specific biomarkers that were intended to be analyzed, including miRNA, epigenetic biomarkers, circulating free DNA (cfDNA), circulating tumor DNA (ctDNA), circulating tumor cells (CTC), Associated Macrophage-Like cells (CAMLs), exosome antigens, methylation changes in peripheral blood mononuclear cells (PBMC) and circulating tumor DNA, RNA integrity number (RIN), protein signatures, DNA methylation, whole-genome methylation, tumor antibodies, circulating nucleic acids, proteins, and genetic variation single nucleotide polymorphisms (SNPs), as well as DNA and RNA for germline analysis and whole-exome sequencing (WES). Specifically, only eight trials have a clear focus on the identification and analysis of miRNA. Moreover, 3 out of these 52 clinical trials involve the storage of blood samples in biobanks for potential future studies.

A small part of the clinical trials that met our inclusion criteria have already published results. We have already discussed the results of The Multicentric Italian Lung Detection (MILD) study, a prospective randomized controlled screening trial that compared the diagnostic performance of two different LDCT screening intervals in high-risk smoking populations. After a median active screening period of 6.2 years, the MILD trial concluded that biennial LDCT screening for lung cancer in individuals with a negative baseline LDCT can achieve a comparable clinical outcome to annual LDCT screening. The study, as already said, highlights the potential of circulating miRNAs as biomarkers for cancer detection and prognosis [19].

Table 2. Ongoing clinical trials investigating liquid biopsy non-coding RNA for lung cancer screening.

Trial (ClinicalTrials.gov Identifier/Name of Study)	Intervention	Description	Posted Results
NCT02247453 (BIOMILD)	Spirometry, blood samples for miRNA profiling	Plasma microRNA Profiling as First Line Screening Test for Lung Cancer Detection: a Prospective Study	Yes
NCT04913155 (HANSE)	Blood samples	HANSE-Holistic Implementation Study Assessing a Northern German Interdisciplinary Lung Cancer Screening Effort, Population-based Screening Study -Prospective, Randomized Comparator Controlled	No
NCT05452200 (ILYAD)	Spirometry, blood and breath samples	Pilot Study on Lung Cancer Screening Implementation Among Employees at Lyon Hospital	No
NCT02777996 (ITALUNG)	Blood and sputum samples	An Italian Randomized Trial for the Evaluation of the Efficacy of Lung Cancer Screening with Low Dose Computed Tomography	Yes
NCT05494021 (CLUS 3.0)	Blood samples	Lung Cancer Screening with Low-dose CT in China (CLUS Study) Version 3.0	No
NCT00103363	Sputum sample for cytology, spirometry, blood samples	Sputum Cytology in Screening Heavy Smokers for Lung Cancer	No
NCT03975504 (CLUS 2.0)	Blood samples	Community-based Lung Cancer Screening with Low-dose CT in China (CLUS Study) Version 2.0	No
NCT05384769	Liquid biopsy	Feasibility Study of Lung Cancer Screening Using Cell-Free DNA Liquid Biopsy at Home in High-Risk Current and Former Smokers	No
NCT00625690	Blood samples	Development of a Lung Cancer-Screening Program at the University of Nebraska Medical Center: A Feasibility Study	No
NCT04968548	Blood sample tested with Lung EpiCheck (Nucleix)	Determination and Validation of Lung EpiCheck®: A Multianalyte Assay for Lung Cancer Prediction. A Case-Control Study	No
NCT01687647 (AMORCE-CBP)	Blood and sputum samples	Interest of Morphometric Analysis of Sputum Cytology for Lung Cancer Screening in Workers Highly Exposed to Asbestos-Exploratory Analysis of Biomarkers Predictive for Lung Cancer	No
NCT03452514	Blood samples for miRNA profiling	Prospective Longitudinal Blinded Observational Diagnostic Study-Addition of microRNA Blood Test to Lung Cancer Screening Low Dose CT	No
NCT05174468	Breath samples	Analysis of Volatile Chemicals in Lung Cancer Screen-Eligible Subjects Using Infrared Spectroscopy	No
NCT00301119 (NYULCBC)	Blood and sputum samples, urine, BAL, lung tissue, buccal swab	Lung Cancer Biomarkers and Screening	No
NCT05306288 (DELFI-L201)	Blood samples for ctDNA detection using a DELFI-based test	Cancer Screening Assay Using DELFI; A Clinical Validation Study in Lung	No
NCT04204499 (ASCENT)	Blood samples for DNA/RNA germline analysis, tumor surplus collected for WES and RNA profiling	Analysis of Screen-detected Lung Cancers' Genomic Traits	No
NCT02500693 (AIR)	Blood samples for CTC analysis	Circulating Tumor Cells and Early Diagnosis of Lung Cancer in Patients with Chronic Obstructive Pulmonary Disease	No
NCT02611570	Blood samples, urine	Low Dose Computed Tomography Screening Study in Non-smokers with Risk Factors for Lung Cancer in Taiwan	No

Table 2. Cont.

Trial (ClinicalTrials.gov Identifier/ Name of Study)	Intervention	Description	Posted Results
NCT04315753	Blood samples for CTC analysis, exosome antigens and cfDNA mutational analysis	Circulating and Imaging Biomarkers to Improve Lung Cancer Management and Early Detection	No
NCT04409444 (qUEST)	Blood sample for analysis of CTC, circulating nucleic acid, proteins and genetic variations (SNPs); nasal swab and brush samples for the identification of inflammatory markers	An Observational Cohort Study Investigating the Impact of Community-based Lung Cancer Screening Across a Deprived Geographical Area and the Role of Biomarkers for the Early Detection of Lung Cancer	No
NCT05432128	Molecular typing early lung cancer, blood samples for peripheral blood ctDNA methylation testing	Molecular Typing System for Early Screening and Diagnosis of Lung Cancer Combined with Liquid Biopsy Technology	No
NCT00512746	Blood samples and sputtum samples for cytology and cytometry	A Randomised Controlled Trial of Surveillance for the Early Detection of Lung Cancer in an at Risk Group	No
NCT01475500	Blood and sputum samples, urine, nasal washings, buccal epithelium, endobronchial tissue, and BAL	Nashville Early Diagnosis Lung Cancer Project	No
NCT00420862 (DANTE Trial)	Blood and sputum samples	A Randomized Study on Lung Cancer Screening with Low-Dose Spiral Computed Tomography	Yes
NCT02504697 (DECAMP-2)	Blood, sputum and airway samples, urine	Detection of Early Lung Cancer Among Military Personnel Study 2 (DECAMP-2): Screening of Patients with Early Stage Lung Cancer or at High Risk for Developing Lung Cancer	No
NCT00899262 (MEDLUNG)	Sputum samples and endobronchial biopsy tissue specimens	Biomarkers for Early Detection of Lung Cancer in Patients with Lung Cancer, Participants at High-Risk for Developing Lung Cancer, or Healthy Volunteers	No
NCT05164757	Blood samples	New York Female Asian Nonsmoker Screening Study	No
NCT02837809 (MILD)	Blood samples for ctDNA detection and miRNA profiling	Early Lung Cancer Detection with Spiral Computed Tomography (CT), Positron Emission Tomography (PET) and Biomarkers: Randomized Trial in High Risk Individuals	Yes
NCT03628638	Blood samples for protein and nucleic acids analysis	Blood Sample Collection in Subjects Participating in a Lung Cancer Screening Program	No
NCT03934866 (SUMMIT)	Blood samples for cfNA analysis	The SUMMIT Study: Cancer Screening Study with or Without Low Dose Lung CT to Validate a Multi-cancer Early Detection Test	No
NCT03499678	Blood samples for the analysis of methylation changes in PBMC and ctDNA	Clinical Trials on Detection of Lung Cancer with Non-invasive Method Based on DNA Methylation of Circulated Tumor DNA, PBMC and T Cells	No
NCT01982149	Blood samples, urine, and airway epithelium	Incorporation of Genetic Expression of Airway Epithelium with CT Screening for Lung Cancer	No
NCT03181256	Blood samples, sputum, urine, nasal and buccal epithelium	Early Detection of Lung Cancer in the Medically Underserved Population	No
NCT04165564 (DECAMP 1 PLUS)	Blood and airway samples	DECAMP 1 PLUS: Prediction of Lung Cancer Using Noninvasive Biomarkers	No
NCT04957433	Blood and sputum samples	Lung Health Check Biomarker Study	No
NCT04558255	Blood samples	Plasma Biomarkers as a Non-invasive Approach for Early Diagnosis of Lung Cancer	No
NCT04323579 (CLEARLY)	Blood samples for the analysis of CTLs, miRNA signatures, exosome antigens and protein signatures	Validation of Multiparametric Models and Circulating and Imaging Biomarkers to Improve Lung Cancer EARLY Detection	No
NCT05462795	Blood samples for DNA methylation analysis	Liquid Biopsy to Distinguish Malignant from Benign Pulmonary Nodules and to Monitor Response to Therapy	No
NCT03791034	Blood samples for cfDNA analysis	Prospective Feasibility Study of Cell Free Circulating Tumor DNA for the Diagnosis and Treatment Monitoring in Early-stage Non-small Cell Lung Cancer	No
NCT04216511 (ECLC)	Blood samples for the detection of tumor autoantibody	Clinic Validation of Autoantibody Panel for Lung Cancer Diagnosis in Chinese Population	No

Table 2. *Cont.*

Trial (ClinicalTrials.gov Identifier/Name of Study)	Intervention	Description	Posted Results
NCT03633006	Blood samples	Blood Sample Collection in Subjects with Pulmonary Nodules or CT Suspicion of Lung Cancer or Pathologically Diagnosed Lung Cancer	No
NCT01925625 (ECLS)	Blood samples for autoantibodies detection using the EarlyCDT-Lung Test	Detection in Blood of Autoantibodies to Tumour Antigens as a Case-finding Method in Lung Cancer Using the EarlyCDT-Lung Test	No
NCT04825834 (DELFI-L101)	Blood samples for DNA based biomarkers analysis using the DELFI assay	DNA Evaluation of Fragments for Early Interception-Lung Cancer Training Study	No
NCT04156360	Blood samples for the detection of CTCs and CAMLs	Construction and Evaluation of the Liquid Biopsy-based Early Diagnostic Model for Lung Cancer	No
NCT04462185	Blood samples and nasal epithelium	A Prospective Cohort Study of Chinese Patients with Pulmonary Nodules: Prediction of Lung Cancer Using Noninvasive Biomarkers	No
NCT03293433	Blood samples for miRNA analysis	Quantification of microRNAs in Diagnosis of Pulmonary Nodules: Reproducibility Analysis of Intra- and Inter-observer and Inter-laboratory: Project miR-Nod	No
NCT03685669	Blood samples for ctDNA methylation analysis	Detection of Early-stage Lung Cancer by Using Methylation Signatures in Circulating Tumor DNA	No
NCT05227261 (K-DETEK)	Blood samples for ctDNA analysis	Assessment of a Novel Blood Test in Early Detection of the Five Common Cancers Based on the Investigation of the Circulating Tumour DNA	No
NCT03181490	Blood samples for ctDNA methylation profiles analysis	Multi-centers Validation of a Circulating Tumor DNA Assay to Differentiate Benign and Malignant Pulmonary Nodules Via Targeted High-throughput DNA Methylation Sequencing	No
NCT05415670	Blood sample for whole-genome methylation sequencing	Development a Pulmonary Nodules Diagnosis Classification Model for Benign/Malignant of Bronchoscopic Biopsy Specimens Based on High-throughput Whole-genome Methylation Sequencing (GM-seq)	No
NCT03989219	Blood samples for cfDNA methylation status analysis	Methylation of cfDNA in Diagnosing and Monitoring Benign and Malignant Pulmonary Nodule	No
NCT05724264 (SOLSTICE)	Blood samples for biomarker detection	SingapOre Lung Cancer Screening Through Integrating CT With Other biomarkErs	No
NCT05699213	Blood samples for biomarker detection	A Pilot Study Evaluating the Feasibility of Novel MRI Sequences and Blood-Based Biomarkers for Discriminating Nodules Found During Lung Cancer Screening	No
NCT05766046 (RISP)	Blood samples for miRNA analysis and biomarker detection	Early Diagnosis of Lung Cancer of the Italian Pulmonary Screening Network (RISP): Comparative Analysis for the Use of Low Dose Computed Tomography and Promotion of Primary Prevention Interventions in Subjects at High Risk for Lung Cancer	No
NCT05649046 (PREVALUNG ETOILE)	Blood samples and feces for microbiota analysis	Structuring of a Lung Cancer Screening Program Including Clinical, Radiological and Biological Phenotyping Useful for the Development of Individualized Risk Prediction Tools: PREVALUNG ETOILE	No

In this scenario, we previously illustrated also the results of the BioMILD trial [16] which is a large prospective study that aims to optimize the screening intensity for lung cancer through a combination of LDCT and a blood-based microRNA assay (MSC). The participants underwent baseline LDCT examination, spirometry, and miRNA profiling, and were followed for a median duration of 5.3 years. The study discovered that participants who were double-negative for LDCT and MSC had very low rates of lung cancer incidence and mortality. As a result, they were recommended to undergo LDCT screening once every three years. The results of the study confirmed that the combined use of LDCT and blood miRNAs at baseline can predict individual lung cancer incidence and mortality.

The New York University Lung Cancer Biomarker Center (NYULCBC) enrolled high-risk smokers and lung cancer patients into a screening cohort and a "rule-out lung cancer" cohort with the aim of identifying and validating biomarkers for the early detection of lung cancer. The participants completed a medical and respiratory symptom questionnaire, underwent pulmonary function testing, blood sampling, chest CT, and were followed up for nodule stability. Greenberg et al. [123] conducted a study to evaluate the levels of serum S-Adenosylmethionine (AdoMet) in participants enrolled in the NYULCBC trial from February to August 2004. The study found that patients with lung cancer had higher levels of serum AdoMet compared to healthy non-smokers and high-risk smokers with small noncalcified nodules. AdoMet level alone was able to differentiate patients with lung cancer from smokers with benign nodules with high sensitivity and specificity. When combined with nodule size, AdoMet level showed a sensitivity and specificity of 100% and 94%, respectively. The elevated AdoMet level in lung cancer patients may relate to the role of AdoMet in DNA methylation, as hypermethylation of the promoter regions of tumor suppressor genes in lung cancer and other malignancies has been reported. AdoMet could be a promising marker for early-stage lung cancer detection, but further studies are needed to confirm its efficacy in larger populations and its clinical utility for recurrence diagnosis.

Several clinical trials are investigating the effectiveness of incorporating new blood tests along with LDCT for lung cancer screening. The NCT01925625 trial tested whether using the EarlyCDT-Lung test and subsequent CT scanning to identify individuals at high risk of lung cancer could reduce the incidence of patients with advanced-stage lung cancer at diagnosis compared to standard clinical practice. The EarlyCDT-Lung test used an enzyme-linked immunosorbent assay (ELISA) to measure seven distinct autoantibodies, each having specificity for different tumor-associated antigens, including p53, NY-ESO-1, CAGE, GBU4-5, HuD, MAGE A4 and SOX2. At 2 years, the test showed high specificity (90.4%) and moderate sensitivity (32.1%) with a higher number of early-stage lung cancers detected in the intervention arm. However, no significant differences were observed in lung cancer and all-cause mortality between the intervention and control groups [124]. The study suggested that blood-based biomarkers followed by LDCT can detect early-stage lung cancer, but more research is required to determine the long-term impact and increase engagement.

Another test is Lung EpiCheck (Nucleix, Modi'in, Israel), which has been designed to detect hypermethylation status across six markers that are associated with lung cancer, by using cfDNA analysis. Recently, this test has been validated in European and Chinese patients samples and has demonstrated high accuracy rates, as well as an independent predictive capability for lung cancer detection, suggesting potential utility for improving screening access and compliance among high-risk populations [125]. In this scenario, the NCT04968548 trial is an observational study aimed at collecting blood samples and clinical data from individuals undergoing LDCT for lung cancer screening and those with confirmed lung cancer to determine and validate the Lung EpiCheck.

Furthermore, the NCT03452514 trial aims to validate the HMBDx microRNA Test by collecting blood samples from 400 individuals who are undergoing LDCT screening. The study plans to analyze microRNA signatures using a novel lung cancer test, compare the results with those obtained through CT scan findings and follow-up tests, and maintain a minimum follow-up period of 12 months post-enrollment.

Lastly, the primary objective of the NCT05306288 clinical trial is to validate the DELFI-based test for detecting lung cancer among individuals eligible for routine screening, using a genome-wide analysis technique called "DNA evaluation of fragments for early interception" (DELFI) to detect abnormalities in cfDNA [126]. Participants have blood collected and undergo medical record review at baseline and two additional time points. Presently, no conclusions are available as these last two clinical trials are still ongoing.

4. Discussion

Given the elevated incidence of overdiagnosis and false positive cases associated with LDCT screening, the identification of reliable biomarkers capable of improving the diagnostic accuracy, represents an unmet need. In this scenario, ncRNAs might be a potential reliable tool to stratify populations into precise categories of lung cancer risk. To date, microRNAs are those most investigated in large prospective trials for lung cancer screening purposes. As reported in the bioMILD trial, the implementation of miRNAs in NSCLC screening can reduce false positive rates and improve diagnostic accuracy of LDCT, thus opening the way for personalized screening approaches.

Furthermore, what emerged from our literature research is an extreme heterogeneity of the conducted studies using different methodologies of analyses and selecting various risk populations. This inevitably can be seen as a positive aspect, as in most of the studies presented, the results were consistent with the ability of ncRNAs to distinguish populations with lung cancer from those that were negative or might face overdiagnosis if subjected to LDCT. However, from a methodological point of view, it clearly constitutes a major issue to be addressed with further research in order to standardize a potential application of ncRNAs liquid biopsy in a real-world setting and safely implement them into our clinical practice.

Methodological limitations of analysis also emerged from this wide literature search, including the heterogeneity of ncRNA detection methods used across the different studies, mostly based on q-RT-PCR, but also on NGS limited panels, digital-droplet PCR, and RNA-seq, pointed out the issue of standardization methods to make ncRNAs part of clinical practice. In fact, from a practical point of view, detecting and sequencing this genetic material might be challenging for different reasons. Next-generation sequencing (NGS) is one of the high-throughput screening methods that can be implemented more efficiently into clinical research to validate panels of ncRNAs that can be used for LC screening research programs [127].

Some limits need also to be considered once we propose ncRNAs as a biofluid-based biomarker for LC screening but also in general for other purposes. First of all, the overall quantity of ncRNAs is generally lower in the intracellular, extracellular ambient, as well as in plasma or serum as compared to other genetic material, so it might be a challenge to detect them in patient-derived blood samples [128]. Another potential issue is related to the post-transcriptional modifications of ncRNA sequence making them similar to other ncRNAs of the same family (such as for micro RNAs, miRNAs), as well as to mRNAs sequence, making it difficult to distinguish each other. Another issue related to the use of ncRNAs liquid biopsy in LC screening context is the cost-effectiveness benefit that the real-world application of these techniques could imply. For now, large studies demonstrated a clear clinical benefit of LDCT-based screening programs [1], but it is not clear if the implementation of LB in this setting will be feasible from this point of view. In addition to that, further clinical trials testing the role of LB ncRNAs detection in non and light-smokers should be conducted.

Moreover, lung cancer heterogeneity is well-known and established across the board [129–131], limiting the use of single-biomarker based approaches. Conversely, the use of multiple biomarkers of the same class or multiple ncRNA class panels could improve diagnostic accuracy within screening programs, since the genetic variability among different tumors and individuals could be covered by different biomarkers working together at the same time.

5. Conclusions

In conclusion, the implementation of ncRNAs for LC screening purposes is one of the most promising biomarkers to integrate LB in the prevention setting. For this reason, standardization of protocols for LB ncRNAs detection and further prospective clinical trials with larger cohorts are needed to validate and introduce these novel biomarkers in the clinical arena. In addition, we believe that the use of ncRNAs belonging to multiple subcategories can further improve the ability to discriminate between negative and positive subjects, and therefore using expanded ncRNA panels for LC early detection should be one of the next implementations for LB studies in this research context. To date, clinicians should carefully interpret LB results coming from the early diagnosis studies and policymakers should push research to focus also on the implementation of liquid biopsy in the real-world setting.

Author Contributions: Conceptualization, F.P., E.G., G.F. and B.D.R.; methodology, F.P.; investigation, F.P., E.G., G.F. and B.D.R.; resources, F.P., E.G., G.F. and B.D.R.; data curation, F.P., E.G., G.F., B.D.R., M.C. and V.M.N.; writing—original draft preparation, F.P., E.G., G.F. and B.D.R.; writing—review and editing, F.P., M.C., V.M.N., E.G., G.F., V.B., C.R. and E.C.; visualization, E.G.; supervision, F.P. and S.N.; project administration, F.P. All authors have read and agreed to the published version of the manuscript.

Funding: This research received no external funding.

Conflicts of Interest: F.P. declared consultant/advisory fees from Astra Zeneca, Janssen, Sanofi, Amgen, Roche, Bristol Myer Squibb, Beigene, and Thermofisher Scientific. S.N. declared speaker bureau/advisor's fees from Boehringer Ingelheim, Roche, Merck Sharp, Dohme, Amgen, Thermo Fisher Scientific, Eli Lilly, GlaxoSmithKline, Merck, AstraZeneca, Janssen, Novartis, Takeda, Bayer, Pfizer. The other authors have no conflict of interest to declare.

References

1. Passiglia, F.; Cinquini, M.; Bertolaccini, L.; Del Facchinetti, R.M.F.; Ferrara, R.; Franchina, T.; Larici, A.; Malapelle, U.; Menis, J.; Passaro, A.; et al. Benefits and Harms of Lung Cancer Screening by Chest Computed Tomography: A Systematic Review and Meta-Analysis. *J. Clin. Oncol.* **2021**, *39*, 2575–2585. [CrossRef]
2. De Koning, H.J.; van der Aalst, C.M.; de Jong, P.A.; Scholten, E.T.; Nackaerts, K.; Heuvelmans, M.A.; Lammers, J.; Weenink, C.; Yousaf-Khan, U.; Horeweg, N.; et al. Reduced Lung-Cancer Mortality with Volume CT Screening in a Randomized Trial. *N. Engl. J. Med.* **2020**, *382*, 503–513. [CrossRef] [PubMed]
3. The National Lung Screening Trial Research Team. Reduced Lung-Cancer Mortality with Low-Dose Computed Tomographic Screening. *N. Engl. J. Med.* **2011**, *365*, 395–409. [CrossRef] [PubMed]
4. Serrano, M.J.; Garrido-Navas, M.C.; Diaz Mochon, J.J.; Cristofanilli, M.; Gil-Bazo, I.; Pauwels, P.; Malapelle, U.; Russo, A.; Lorente, J.; Ruiz-Rodriguez, A.; et al. Precision Prevention and Cancer Interception: The New Challenges of Liquid Biopsy. *Cancer Discov.* **2020**, *10*, 1635–1644. [CrossRef] [PubMed]
5. Ilie, M.; Hofman, V.; Long-Mira, E.; Selva, E.; Vignaud, J.M.; Padovani, B.; Mouroux, J.; Marquette, C.; Hofman, P. "Sentinel" Circulating Tumor Cells Allow Early Diagnosis of Lung Cancer in Patients with Chronic Obstructive Pulmonary Disease. *PLoS ONE* **2014**, *9*, e111597. [CrossRef] [PubMed]
6. Freitas, C.; Sousa, C.; Machado, F.; Serino, M.; Santos, V.; Cruz-Martins, N.; Teixeira, A.; Cunha, A.; Pereira, T.; Oliveira, H.; et al. The Role of Liquid Biopsy in Early Diagnosis of Lung Cancer. *Front. Oncol.* **2021**, *11*, 634316. [CrossRef] [PubMed]
7. Chabon, J.J.; Hamilton, E.G.; Kurtz, D.M.; Esfahani, M.S.; Moding, E.J.; Stehr, H.; Schroers-Martin, J.; Nabet, B.; Chen, B.; Chaudhuri, A.; et al. Integrating genomic features for non-invasive early lung cancer detection. *Nature* **2020**, *580*, 245–251. [CrossRef]
8. Nadauld, L.D.; McDonnell, C.H.; Beer, T.M.; Liu, M.C.; Klein, E.A.; Hudnut, A.; Whittington, R.; Taylor, B.; Oxnard, G.; Lipson, J.; et al. The PATHFINDER Study: Assessment of the Implementation of an Investigational Multi-Cancer Early Detection Test into Clinical Practice. *Cancers* **2021**, *13*, 3501. [CrossRef]
9. Liu, C.; Li, J. Coding or Noncoding, the Converging Concepts of RNAs. *Front. Genet.* **2019**, *10*, 496. [CrossRef]
10. Anastasiadou, E.; Jacob, L.S.; Slack, F.J. Non-coding RNA networks in cancer. *Nat. Rev. Cancer* **2017**, *18*, 5–18. [CrossRef]
11. Winkle, M.; El-daly, S.M.; Fabbri, M.; Calin, G.A. Noncoding RNA Therapeutics—Challenges and potential solutions. *Nat. Rev. Drug Discov.* **2021**, *20*, 629–645. [CrossRef]
12. Cammarata, G.; Miguel-perez DDe Russo, A.; Peleg, A.; Dolo, V.; Rolfo, C.; Taverna, S. Emerging noncoding RNAs contained in extracellular vesicles: Rising stars as biomarkers in lung cancer liquid biopsy. *Ther. Adv. Med. Oncol.* **2022**, *14*, 1–20. [CrossRef] [PubMed]

13. Slack, F.J.; Chinnaiyan, A.M. Review The Role of Non-coding RNAs in Oncology. *Cell* **2019**, *179*, 1033–1055. [CrossRef] [PubMed]
14. Szil, M.; Pös, O.; M, É.; Bugly, G. Circulating Cell-Free Nucleic Acids: Main Characteristics and Clinical Application. *Int. J. Mol. Sci.* **2020**, *21*, 6827.
15. Fehlmann, T.; Kahraman, M.; Ludwig, N.; Backes, C.; Galata, V.; Keller, V.; Geffers, L.; Mercaldo, N.; Hornung, D.; Weis, T.; et al. Evaluating the Use of Circulating MicroRNA Profiles for Lung Cancer Detection in Symptomatic Patients. *JAMA Oncol.* **2020**, *6*, 714–723. [CrossRef] [PubMed]
16. Pastorino, U.; Boeri, M.; Sestini, S.; Sabia, F.; Milanese, G.; Silva, M.; Suatoni, P.; Verri, C.; Cantarutti, A.; Sverzellati, N. Baseline computed tomography screening and blood microRNA predict lung cancer risk and define adequate intervals in the BioMILD trial. *Ann. Oncol.* **2022**, *33*, 395–405. [CrossRef] [PubMed]
17. Anfossi, S.; Babayan, A.; Pantel, K.; Calin, G.A. Clinical utility of circulating non-coding RNAs—An update. *Nat. Rev. Clin. Oncol.* **2018**, *15*, 541–563. [CrossRef]
18. Chu, G.C.W.; Lazare, K.; Sullivan, F. Serum and blood based biomarkers for lung cancer screening: A systematic review. *BMC Cancer* **2018**, *18*, 181. [CrossRef]
19. Sozzi, G.; Boeri, M.; Rossi, M.; Verri, C.; Suatoni, P.; Bravi, F.; Roz, L.; Conte, D.; Grassi, M.; Sverzellati, N.; et al. Clinical Utility of a Plasma-Based miRNA Signature Classifier Within Computed Tomography Lung Cancer Screening: A Correlative MILD Trial Study. *J. Clin. Oncol.* **2014**, *32*, 768–773. [CrossRef]
20. Shen, J.; Liu, Z.; Todd, N.W.; Zhang, H.; Liao, J.; Yu, L.; Guarnera, M.; Li, R.; Cai, L.; Zhan, M.; et al. Diagnosis of lung cancer in individuals with solitary pulmonary nodules by plasma microRNA biomarkers. *BMC Cancer* **2011**, *11*, 374. [CrossRef]
21. Shen, J.; Liao, J.; Guarnera, M.A.; Fang, H.; Cai, L.; Stass, S.A.; Jiang, F. Analysis of MicroRNAs in Sputum to Improve Computed Tomography for Lung Cancer Diagnosis. *J. Thorac. Oncol.* **2014**, *9*, 33–40. [CrossRef] [PubMed]
22. Zheng, D.; Zhu, Y.; Zhang, J.; Zhang, W.; Wang, H.; Chen, H.; Wu, C.; Ni, J.; Xu, X.; Nian, B.; et al. Identification and evaluation of circulating small extracellular vesicle microRNAs as diagnostic biomarkers for patients with indeterminate pulmonary nodules. *J. Nanobiotechnol.* **2022**, *20*, 172. [CrossRef] [PubMed]
23. Vadla, G.P.; Daghat, B.; Patterson, N.; Ahmad, V.; Perez, G.; Garcia, A.; Manjunath, Y.; Kaifi, J.; Li, G.; Chabu, C. Combining plasma extracellular vesicle Let-7b-5p, miR-184 and circulating miR-22-3p levels for NSCLC diagnosis and drug resistance prediction. *Sci. Rep.* **2022**, *12*, 6693. [CrossRef] [PubMed]
24. Halvorsen, A.R.; Bjaanæs, M.; LeBlanc, M.; Holm, A.M.; Bolstad, N.; Rubio, L.; Peñalver, J.; Cervera, J.; Mojarrieta, J.; López-Guerrero, J.; et al. A unique set of 6 circulating microRNAs for early detection of non-small cell lung cancer. *Oncotarget* **2016**, *7*, 37250. [CrossRef]
25. Yang, X.; Zhang, Q.; Zhang, M.; Su, W.; Wang, Z.; Li, Y.; Zhang, J.; Beer, D.; Yang, S.; Chen, G. Serum microRNA Signature Is Capable of Early Diagnosis for Non-Small Cell Lung Cancer. *Int. J. Biol. Sci.* **2019**, *15*, 1712–1722. [CrossRef]
26. Zaporozhchenko, I.A.; Morozkin, E.S.; Ponomaryova, A.A.; Rykova, E.Y.; Cherdyntseva, N.V.; Zheravin, A.A.; Pashkovskaya, O.; Pokushalov, E.; Vlassov, V.; Laktionov, P. Profiling of 179 miRNA Expression in Blood Plasma of Lung Cancer Patients and Cancer-Free Individuals. *Sci. Rep.* **2018**, *8*, 6348. [CrossRef]
27. Nadal, E.; Truini, A.; Nakata, A.; Lin, J.; Reddy, R.M.; Chang, A.C.; Ramnath, N.; Gotoh, N.; Beer, D.; Chen, G. A Novel Serum 4-microRNA Signature for Lung Cancer Detection. *Sci. Rep.* **2015**, *5*, 12464. [CrossRef]
28. Lu, S.; Kong, H.; Hou, Y.; Ge, D.; Huang, W.; Ou, J.; Yang, D.; Zhang, L.; Wu, G.; Song, Y.; et al. Two plasma microRNA panels for diagnosis and subtype discrimination of lung cancer. *Lung Cancer* **2018**, *123*, 44–51. [CrossRef]
29. Powrózek, T.; Krawczyk, P.; Kowalski, D.M.; Winiarczyk, K.; Olszyna-Serementa, M.; Milanowski, J. Plasma circulating microRNA-944 and microRNA-3662 as potential histologic type-specific early lung cancer biomarkers. *Transl. Res.* **2015**, *166*, 315–323. [CrossRef]
30. Jiang, Y.; Wei, S.; Geng, N.; Qin, W.; He, X.; Wang, X.; Qi, Y.; Song, S.; Wang, P. Evaluation of circulating small extracellular vesicle-derived miRNAs as diagnostic biomarkers for differentiating between different pathological types of early lung cancer. *Sci. Rep.* **2022**, *12*, 17201. [CrossRef]
31. Yang, C.; Jia, X.; Zhou, J.; Sun, Q.; Ma, Z. The MiR-17-92 Gene Cluster is a Blood-Based Marker for Cancer Detection in Non-Small-Cell Lung Cancer. *Am. J. Med. Sci.* **2020**, *360*, 248–260. [CrossRef]
32. Geng, Q.; Fan, T.; Zhang, B.; Wang, W.; Xu, Y.; Hu, H. Five microRNAs in plasma as novel biomarkers for screening of early-stage non-small cell lung cancer. *Respir. Res.* **2014**, *15*, 149. [CrossRef] [PubMed]
33. Abu-Duhier, F.M.; Javid, J.; Sughayer, M.A.; Mir, R.; Albalawi, T.; Alauddin, M.S. Clinical Significance of Circulatory miRNA-21 as an Efficient Non-Invasive Biomarker for the Screening of Lung Cancer Patients. *Asian Pac. J. Cancer Prev.* **2018**, *19*, 2607–2611. [PubMed]
34. Calvo-Lozano, O.; García-Aparicio, P.; Raduly, L.Z.; Estévez, M.C.; Berindan-Neagoe, I.; Ferracin, M.; Lechuga, L. One-Step and Real-Time Detection of microRNA-21 in Human Samples for Lung Cancer Biosensing Diagnosis. *Anal. Chem.* **2022**, *94*, 14659–14665. [CrossRef] [PubMed]
35. Sun, M.; Song, J.; Zhou, Z.; Zhu, R.; Jin, H.; Ji, Y.; Lu, Q.; Ju, H. Comparison of Serum MicroRNA21 and Tumor Markers in Diagnosis of Early Non-Small Cell Lung Cancer. *Dis. Markers* **2016**, *2016*, 3823121. [CrossRef]
36. Alexandre, D.; Teixeira, B.; Rico, A.; Valente, S.; Craveiro, A.; Baptista, P.V.; Cruz, C. Molecular Beacon for Detection miRNA-21 as a Biomarker of Lung Cancer. *Int. J. Mol. Sci.* **2022**, *23*, 3330. [CrossRef]

37. Wang, W.; Li, X.; Liu, C.; Zhang, X.; Wu, Y.; Diao, M.; Tan, S.; Huang, S.; Cheng, Y.; You, T. MicroRNA-21 as a diagnostic and prognostic biomarker of lung cancer: A systematic review and meta-analysis. *Biosci. Rep.* **2022**, *42*, BSR20211653. [CrossRef]
38. Qiu, F.; Gu, W.; Li, C.; Nie, S.; Yu, F. Analysis on expression level and diagnostic value of miR-19 and miR-21 in peripheral blood of patients with undifferentiated lung cancer. *Eur. Rev. Med. Pharmacol. Sci.* **2018**, *22*, 8367–8373.
39. Wang, H.; Xu, J.; Ding, L. MicroRNA-21 was a promising biomarker for lung carcinoma diagnosis: An update Meta-Analysis. *Thorac. Cancer* **2022**, *13*, 316–321. [CrossRef]
40. Yang, X.; Guo, Y.; Du, Y.; Yang, J.; Li, S.; Liu, S.; Li, K.; Zhang, D. Serum MicroRNA-21 as a Diagnostic Marker for Lung Carcinoma: A Systematic Review and Meta-Analysis. *PLoS ONE* **2014**, *9*, e97460. [CrossRef]
41. Chen, C.; Wang, J.; Lu, D.; You, R.; She, Q.; Chen, J.; Feng, S.; Lu, Y. Early detection of lung cancer via biointerference-free, target microRNA-triggered core–satellite nanocomposites. *Nanoscale* **2022**, *14*, 8103–8111. [CrossRef] [PubMed]
42. Qiao, F.; Luo, P.; Liu, C.; Fu, K.; Zhao, Y. Association between microRNA 21 expression in serum and lung cancer: A protocol of systematic review and meta-analysis. *Medicine* **2020**, *99*, e20314. [CrossRef] [PubMed]
43. Li, C.; Sun, L.; Zhou, H.; Yang, Y.; Wang, Y.; She, M.; Chen, J. Diagnostic value of microRNA-25 in patients with non-small cell lung cancer in Chinese population: A systematic review and meta-analysis. *Medicine* **2020**, *99*, e23425. [CrossRef]
44. Zhu, W.; He, J.; Chen, D.; Zhang, B.; Xu, L.; Ma, H.; Liu, H.; Zhang, Y. Expression of miR-29c, miR-93, and miR-429 as Potential Biomarkers for Detection of Early Stage Non-Small Lung Cancer. *PLoS ONE* **2014**, *9*, e87780. [CrossRef] [PubMed]
45. Liang, L.B.; Zhu, W.J.; Chen, X.M.; Luo, F.M. Plasma miR-30a-5p as an early novel noninvasive diagnostic and prognostic biomarker for lung cancer. *Future Oncol.* **2019**, *15*, 3711–3721. [CrossRef]
46. Ma, Y.; Chen, Y.; Lin, J.; Liu, Y.; Luo, K.; Cao, Y.; Wang, T.; Jin, H.; Su, Z.; Wu, H.; et al. Circulating miR-31 as an effective biomarker for detection and prognosis of human cancer: A meta-analysis. *Oncotarget* **2017**, *8*, 28660. [CrossRef] [PubMed]
47. Zhu, W.; Zhou, K.; Zha, Y.; Chen, D.; He, J.; Ma, H.; Liu, X.; Le, H.; Zhang, Y. Diagnostic Value of Serum miR-182, miR-183, miR-210, and miR-126 Levels in Patients with Early-Stage Non-Small Cell Lung Cancer. *PLoS ONE* **2016**, *11*, e0153046. [CrossRef]
48. Sun, L.; Zhou, H.; Yang, Y.; Chen, J.; Wang, Y.; She, M.; Li, C. Meta-analysis of diagnostic and prognostic value of miR-126 in non-small cell lung cancer. *Biosci. Rep.* **2020**, *40*, BSR20200349. [CrossRef]
49. Kim, J.E.; Eom, J.S.; Kim, W.; Jo, E.J.; Mok, J.; Lee, K.; Kim, K.; Park, H.; Lee, M.; Kim, M. Diagnostic value of microRNAs derived from exosomes in bronchoalveolar lavage fluid of early-stage lung adenocarcinoma: A pilot study. *Thorac. Cancer* **2018**, *9*, 911–915. [CrossRef]
50. Zou, Y.; Jing, C.; Liu, L.; Wang, T. Serum microRNA-135a as a diagnostic biomarker in non-small cell lung cancer. *Medicine* **2019**, *98*, e17814. [CrossRef]
51. Zengx, L.; Zhangs, Y.; Zhengj, F.; Wangy, Y. Altered miR-143 and miR-150 expressions in peripheral blood mononuclear cells for diagnosis of non-small cell lung cancer. *Chin. Med. J.* **2013**, *126*, 4510–4516.
52. Cheng, L.; Li, Q.; Tan, B.; Ma, D.; Du, G. Diagnostic value of microRNA-148/152 family in non-small-cell lung cancer (NSCLC): A systematic review and meta-analysis. *Medicine* **2021**, *100*, e28061. [CrossRef] [PubMed]
53. Shao, C.; Yang, F.; Qin, Z.; Jing, X.; Shu, Y.; Shen, H. The value of miR-155 as a biomarker for the diagnosis and prognosis of lung cancer: A systematic review with meta-analysis. *BMC Cancer* **2019**, *19*, 1103. [CrossRef] [PubMed]
54. Liu, X.; Tang, C.; Song, X.; Cheng, L.; Liu, Y.; Ding, F.; Xia, C.; Xue, L.; Xiao, J.; Huang, B. Clinical value of CTLA4-associated microRNAs combined with inflammatory factors in the diagnosis of non-small cell lung cancer. *Ann. Clin. Biochem.* **2020**, *57*, 151–161. [CrossRef]
55. Liu, J.; Han, Y.; Liu, X.; Wei, S. Serum miR-185 Is a Diagnostic and Prognostic Biomarker for Non-Small Cell Lung Cancer. *Technol. Cancer Res. Treat.* **2020**, *19*, 1533033820973276. [CrossRef]
56. Li, S.; Lin, Y.; Wu, Y.; Chen, H.; Huang, Z.; Lin, M.; Dong, J.; Wang, Y.; Yang, Z. The Value of Serum Exosomal miR-184 in the Diagnosis of NSCLC. *J. Health Eng.* **2022**, *2022*, 9713218. [CrossRef]
57. Wang, Y.; Lv, Y.; Li, G.; Zhang, D.; Gao, Z.; Gai, Q. Value of low-dose spiral CT combined with circulating miR-200b and miR-200c examinations for lung cancer screening in physical examination population. *Eur. Rev. Med. Pharmacol. Sci.* **2021**, *25*, 6123–6130.
58. Hu, X.; Peng, Q.; Zhu, J.; Shen, Y.; Lin, K.; Shen, Y.; Zhu, Y. Identification of miR-210 and combination biomarkers as useful agents in early screening non-small cell lung cancer. *Gene* **2020**, *729*, 144225. [CrossRef]
59. D'Antona, P.; Cattoni, M.; Dominioni, L.; Poli, A.; Moretti, F.; Cinquetti, R.; Gini, E.; Daffrè, E.; Noonan, D.; Imperatori, A.; et al. Serum miR-223: A Validated Biomarker for Detection of Early-Stage Non-Small Cell Lung Cancer. *Cancer Epidemiol. Biomark. Prev.* **2019**, *28*, 1926–1933. [CrossRef]
60. Ulivi, P.; Foschi, G.; Mengozzi, M.; Scarpi, E.; Silvestrini, R.; Amadori, D.; Zoli, W. Peripheral Blood miR-328 Expression as a Potential Biomarker for the Early Diagnosis of N.S.C.L.C. *Int. J. Mol. Sci.* **2013**, *14*, 10332–10342. [CrossRef]
61. Trakunram, K.; Chaniad, P.; Geater, S.L.; Keeratichananont, W.; Chittithavorn, V.; Uttayamakul, S.; Buya, S.; Raungrut, P.; Thongsuksai, P. Serum miR-339-3p as a potential diagnostic marker for non-small cell lung cancer. *Cancer Biol. Med.* **2020**, *17*, 652–663. [CrossRef]
62. Wang, S.; Li, Y.; Jiang, Y.; Li, R. Investigation of serum miR-411 as a diagnosis and prognosis biomarker for non-small cell lung cancer. *Eur. Rev. Med. Pharmacol. Sci.* **2017**, *21*, 4092–4097. [PubMed]
63. Li, W.; Wang, Y.; Zhang, Q.; Tang, L.; Liu, X.; Dai, Y.; Xiao, L.; Huang, S.; Chen, L.; Guo, Z.; et al. MicroRNA-486 as a Biomarker for Early Diagnosis and Recurrence of Non-Small Cell Lung Cancer. *PLoS ONE* **2015**, *10*, e0134220. [CrossRef]

64. Li, M.; Zhang, Q.; Wu, L.; Jia, C.; Shi, F.; Li, S.; Peng, A.; Zhang, G.; Song, X.; Wang, C. Serum miR-499 as a novel diagnostic and prognostic biomarker in non-small cell lung cancer. *Oncol. Rep.* **2014**, *31*, 1961–1967. [CrossRef] [PubMed]
65. Wang, A.; Zhang, H.; Wang, J.; Zhang, S.; Xu, Z. MiR-519d targets HER3 and can be used as a potential serum biomarker for non-small cell lung cancer. *Aging* **2020**, *12*, 4866–4878. [CrossRef]
66. Sun, B.; Liu, H.; Ding, Y.; Li, Z. Evaluating the diagnostic and prognostic value of serum miR-770 in non-small cell lung cancer. *Eur. Rev. Med. Pharmacol. Sci.* **2018**, *22*, 3061–3066.
67. Chen, L.; Li, Y.; Lu, J. Identification of Circulating miR-762 as a Novel Diagnostic and Prognostic Biomarker for Non-Small Cell Lung Cancer. *Technol. Cancer Res. Treat.* **2020**, *19*, 1533033820964222. [CrossRef] [PubMed]
68. Zhao, Y.; Zhang, W.; Yang, Y.; Dai, E.; Bai, Y. Diagnostic and prognostic value of microRNA-2355-3p and contribution to the progression in lung adenocarcinoma. *Bioengineered* **2021**, *12*, 4747–4756. [CrossRef]
69. Singh, A.; Kant, R.; Nandi, S.; Husain, N.; Naithani, M.; Mirza, A.A.; Saluja, T.; Srivastava, K.; Prakash, V.; Singh, S. Detection of differential expression of miRNAs in computerized tomography-guided lung biopsy. *J. Cancer Res. Ther.* **2022**, *18*, 231–239. [CrossRef]
70. Wozniak, M.B.; Scelo, G.; Muller, D.C.; Mukeria, A.; Zaridze, D.; Brennan, P. Circulating MicroRNAs as Non-Invasive Biomarkers for Early Detection of Non-Small-Cell Lung Cancer. *PLoS ONE* **2015**, *10*, e0125026. [CrossRef]
71. Liao, J.; Shen, J.; Leng, Q.; Qin, M.; Zhan, M.; Jiang, F. MicroRNA-based biomarkers for diagnosis of non-small cell lung cancer (NSCLC). *Thorac. Cancer* **2020**, *11*, 762–768. [CrossRef] [PubMed]
72. Powrózek, T.; Krawczyk, P.; Kowalski, D.M.; Kuźnar-Kamińska, B.; Winiarczyk, K.; Olszyna-Serementa, M.; Batura-Gabryel, H.; Milanowski, J. Application of plasma circulating microRNA-448, 506, 4316, and 4478 analysis for non-invasive diagnosis of lung cancer. *Tumor Biol.* **2016**, *37*, 2049–2055. [CrossRef] [PubMed]
73. Qi, Z.; Yang, D.Y.; Cao, J. Increased micro-RNA 17, 21, and 192 gene expressions improve early diagnosis in non-small cell lung cancer. *Med. Oncol.* **2014**, *31*, 195. [CrossRef] [PubMed]
74. Zhang, Y.H.; Jin, M.; Li, J.; Kong, X. Identifying circulating miRNA biomarkers for early diagnosis and monitoring of lung cancer. *Biochim. Biophys. Acta (BBA) Mol. Basis Dis.* **2020**, *1866*, 165847. [CrossRef]
75. Zhou, C.; Chen, Z.; Zhao, L.; Zhao, W.; Zhu, Y.; Liu, J.; Zhao, X. A novel circulating miRNA-based signature for the early diagnosis and prognosis prediction of non–small-cell lung cancer. *J. Clin. Lab. Anal.* **2020**, *34*, e23505. [CrossRef]
76. Wang, P.; Yang, D.; Zhang, H.; Wei, X.; Ma, T.; Cheng, Z.; Hong, Q.; Hu, J.; Zhuo, H.; Song, Y.; et al. Early Detection of Lung Cancer in Serum by a Panel of MicroRNA Biomarkers. *Clin. Lung Cancer* **2015**, *16*, 313–319.e1. [CrossRef]
77. Fan, L.; Qi, H.; Teng, J.; Su, B.; Chen, H.; Wang, C.; Xia, Q. Identification of serum miRNAs by nano-quantum dots microarray as diagnostic biomarkers for early detection of non-small cell lung cancer. *Tumor Biol.* **2016**, *37*, 7777–7784. [CrossRef]
78. Li, J.; Fang, H.; Jiang, F.; Ning, Y. External validation of a panel of plasma microRNA biomarkers for lung cancer. *Biomark. Med.* **2019**, *13*, 1557–1564. [CrossRef] [PubMed]
79. Zou, J.; Ma, L.; Li, X.; Xu, F.; Fei, X.; Liu, Q.; Bai, Q.; Dong, Y. Circulating microRNA array (miR-182, 200b and 205) for the early diagnosis and poor prognosis predictor of non-small cell lung cancer. *Eur. Rev. Med. Pharmacol. Sci.* **2019**, *23*, 1108–1115.
80. Arab, A.; Karimipoor, M.; Irani, S.; Kiani, A.; Zeinali, S.; Tafsiri, E.; Sheikhy, K. Potential circulating miRNA signature for early detection of N.S.C.L.C. *Cancer Genet.* **2017**, *216*, 150–158. [CrossRef]
81. Xing, L.; Su, J.; Guarnera, M.A.; Zhang, H.; Cai, L.; Zhou, R.; Stass, S.; Jiang, F. Sputum microRNA Biomarkers for Identifying Lung Cancer in Indeterminate Solitary Pulmonary Nodules. *Clin. Cancer Res.* **2015**, *21*, 484–489. [CrossRef]
82. Tai, M.C.; Yanagisawa, K.; Nakatochi, M.; Hotta, N.; Hosono, Y.; Kawaguchi, K.; Naito, M.; Taniguchi, H.; Wakai, K.; Yokoi, K.; et al. Blood-borne miRNA profile-based diagnostic classifier for lung adenocarcinoma. *Sci. Rep.* **2016**, *6*, 31389. [CrossRef]
83. Gao, S.; Guo, W.; Liu, T.; Liang, N.; Ma, Q.; Gao, Y.; Tan, F.; Xue, Q.; He, J. Plasma extracellular vesicle microRNA profiling and the identification of a diagnostic signature for stage I lung adenocarcinoma. *Cancer Sci.* **2022**, *113*, 648–659. [CrossRef] [PubMed]
84. Xue, W.; Zhang, M.; Li, R.; Liu, X.; Yin, Y.; Qu, Y. Serum miR-1228-3p and miR-181a-5p as Noninvasive Biomarkers for Non-Small Cell Lung Cancer Diagnosis and Prognosis. *Biomed. Res. Int.* **2020**, *2020*, 9601876. [CrossRef]
85. Zhou, X.; Wen, W.; Shan, X.; Zhu, W.; Xu, J.; Guo, R.; Cheng, W.; Wang, F.; Qi, L.; Chen, Y.; et al. A six-microRNA panel in plasma was identified as a potential biomarker for lung adenocarcinoma diagnosis. *Oncotarget* **2016**, *8*, 6513. [CrossRef]
86. Jin, X.; Chen, Y.; Chen, H.; Fei, S.; Chen, D.; Cai, X.; Liu, L.; Lin, B.; Su, H.; Zhao, L.; et al. Evaluation of Tumor-Derived Exosomal miRNA as Potential Diagnostic Biomarkers for Early-Stage Non–Small Cell Lung Cancer Using Next-Generation Sequencing. *Clin. Cancer Res.* **2017**, *23*, 5311–5319. [CrossRef] [PubMed]
87. Wang, Y.; Zhao, H.; Gao, X.; Wei, F.; Zhang, X.; Su, Y.; Wang, C.; Li, H.; Ren, X. Identification of a three-miRNA signature as a blood-borne diagnostic marker for early diagnosis of lung adenocarcinoma. *Oncotarget* **2016**, *7*, 26070. [CrossRef] [PubMed]
88. Arita, T.; Ichikawa, D.; Konishi, H.; Komatsu, S.; Shiozaki, A.; Shoda, K.; Kawaguchi, T.; Hirajima, S.; Nagata, H.; Kubota, T. Circulating Long Non-coding RNAs in Plasma of Patients with Gastric Cancer. *Anticancer Res.* **2013**, *33*, 3185–3193.
89. Chen, Y.; Zitello, E.; Chen, Y. The function of LncRNAs and their role in the prediction, diagnosis, and prognosis of lung cancer The function of LncRNAs and their role in the prediction, diagnosis, and prognosis of lung cancer. *Clin. Transl. Med.* **2021**, *11*, e367. [CrossRef]
90. Acha-Sagredo, A.; Uko, B.; Pantazi, P.; Bediaga, N.G.; Moschandrea, C.; Rainbow, L.; Marcus, M.; Davies, M.; Field, J.; Liloglou, T. Long non-coding RNA dysregulation is a frequent event in non-small cell lung carcinoma pathogenesis. *Br. J. Cancer* **2020**, *122*, 1050–1058. [CrossRef]

91. Gupta, C.; Su, J.; Zhan, M.; Stass, S.A.; Jiang, F. Sputum long non-coding RNA biomarkers for diagnosis of lung cancer. *Cancer Biomarkers* **2019**, *26*, 219–227. [CrossRef]
92. Yuan, S.; Xiang, Y.; Guo, X.; Zhang, Y.; Li, C.; Xie, W.; Wu, N.; Wu, L.; Cai, T.; Ma, X.; et al. Circulating Long Noncoding RNAs Act as Diagnostic Biomarkers in Non-Small Cell Lung Cancer. *Front. Oncol.* **2020**, *10*, 537120. [CrossRef] [PubMed]
93. Li, X.; Liu, L.; Song, X.; Wang, K.; Niu, L.; Xie, L.; Song, X. TEP linc-GTF2H2-1, RP3-466P17.2, and lnc-ST8SIA4-12 as novel biomarkers for lung cancer diagnosis and progression prediction. *J. Cancer Res. Clin. Oncol.* **2021**, *147*, 1609–1622. [CrossRef] [PubMed]
94. Kamel, L.M.; Atef, D.M.; Mackawy, A.M.H.; Shalaby, S.M.; Abdelraheim, N. Circulating long non-coding RNA GAS5 and SOX2OT as potential biomarkers for diagnosis and prognosis of non-small cell lung cancer. *Biotechnol. Appl. Biochem.* **2019**, *66*, 634–642. [CrossRef] [PubMed]
95. Li, Z.; Zhuo, Y.; Li, J.; Zhang, M.; Wang, R.; Lin, L. Long Non-Coding RNA SNHG4 Is a Potential Diagnostic and Prognostic Indicator in Non-Small Cell Lung Cancer. *Ann. Clin. Lab. Sci.* **2021**, *51*, 654–662.
96. Jiang, N.; Meng, X.; Mi, H.; Chi, Y.; Li, S.; Jin, Z.; Tian, H.; He, J.; Shen, W.; Tian, H.; et al. Circulating lncRNA XLOC_009167 serves as a diagnostic biomarker to predict lung cancer. *Clin. Chim. Acta* **2018**, *486*, 26–33. [CrossRef]
97. Li, W.; Li, N.; Kang, X.; Shi, K. Circulating long non-coding RNA AFAP1-AS1 is a potential diagnostic biomarker for non-small cell lung cancer. *Clin. Chim. Acta* **2017**, *475*, 152–156. [CrossRef]
98. Yang, Q.; Kong, S.; Zheng, M.; Hong, Y.; Sun, J.; Ming, X.; Gu, Y.; Shen, X.; Ju, S. Long intergenic noncoding RNA LINC00173 as a potential serum biomarker for diagnosis of non-small-cell lung cancer. *Cancer Biomark.* **2020**, *29*, 441–451. [CrossRef]
99. Tan, Q.; Zuo, J.; Qiu, S.; Yu, Y.; Zhou, H.; Li, N.; Wang, H.; Liang, C.; Yu, M.; Tu, J. Identification of circulating long non-coding RNA GAS5 as a potential biomarker for non-small cell lung cancer diagnosisnon-small cell lung cancer, long non-coding RNA, plasma, GAS5, biomarker. *Int. J. Oncol.* **2017**, *50*, 1729–1738. [CrossRef]
100. Pan, J.; Bian, Y.; Cao, Z.; Lei, L.; Pan, J.; Huang, J.; Cai, X.; Lan, X.; Zheng, H. Long noncoding RNA MALAT1 as a candidate serological biomarker for the diagnosis of non-small cell lung cancer: A meta-analysis. *Thorac. Cancer* **2020**, *11*, 329–335. [CrossRef]
101. Yao, X.; Wang, T.; Sun, M.Y.; Yuming, Y.; Guixin, D.; Liu, J. Diagnostic value of lncRNA HOTAIR as a biomarker for detecting and staging of non-small cell lung cancer. *Biomarkers* **2022**, *27*, 526–533. [CrossRef] [PubMed]
102. Li, N.; Wang, Y.; Liu, X.; Luo, P.; Jing, W.; Zhu, M.; Tu, J. Identification of Circulating Long Noncoding RNA HOTAIR as a Novel Biomarker for Diagnosis and Monitoring of Non–Small Cell Lung Cancer. *Technol. Cancer Res. Treat.* **2017**, *16*, 1060–1066. [CrossRef] [PubMed]
103. Min, L.; Zhu, T.; Lv, B.; An, T.; Zhang, Q.; Shang, Y.; Yu, Z.; Zheng, L.; Wang, Q. Exosomal LncRNA RP5-977B1 as a novel minimally invasive biomarker for diagnosis and prognosis in non-small cell lung cancer. *Int. J. Clin. Oncol.* **2022**, *27*, 1013–1024. [CrossRef] [PubMed]
104. Xian, J.; Zeng, Y.; Chen, S.; Lu, L.; Liu, L.; Chen, J.; Rao, B.; Zhao, Z.; Liu, J.; Xie, C.; et al. Discovery of a novel linc01125 isoform in serum exosomes as a promising biomarker for NSCLC diagnosis and survival assessment. *Carcinogenesis* **2021**, *42*, 831–841. [CrossRef] [PubMed]
105. Li, N.; Feng, X.B.; Tan, Q.; Luo, P.; Jing, W.; Zhu, M.; Liang, C.; Tu, J.; Ning, Y. Identification of Circulating Long Noncoding RNA Linc00152 as a Novel Biomarker for Diagnosis and Monitoring of Non-Small-Cell Lung Cancer. *Dis. Markers* **2017**, *2017*, 7439698. [CrossRef]
106. Cao, Y.; Zhang, H.; Tang, J.; Wang, R. Long non-coding RNA FAM230B is a novel prognostic and diagnostic biomarker for lung adenocarcinoma. *Bioengineered* **2022**, *13*, 7919–7925. [CrossRef]
107. Wang, H.; Lu, J.; Chen, W.; Gu, A. Upregulated lncRNA-UCA1 contributes to progression of lung cancer and is closely related to clinical diagnosis as a predictive biomarker in plasma. *Int. J. Clin. Exp. Med.* **2015**, *8*, 11824–11830.
108. He, C.; Huang, D.; Yang, F.; Huang, D.; Cao, Y.; Peng, J.; Luo, X. High Expression of lncRNA HEIH is Helpful in the Diagnosis of Non-Small Cell Lung Cancer and Predicts Poor Prognosis. *Cancer Manag. Res.* **2022**, *14*, 503–514. [CrossRef]
109. Li, C.; Zhang, L.; Meng, G.; Wang, Q.; Lv, X.; Zhang, J.; Li, J. Circular RNAs: Pivotal molecular regulators and novel diagnostic and prognostic biomarkers in non-small cell lung cancer. *J. Cancer Res. Clin. Oncol.* **2019**, *145*, 2875–2889. [CrossRef]
110. Zhao, J.; Li, L.; Wang, Q.; Han, H.; Zhan, Q.; Xu, M. CircRNA Expression Profile in Early-Stage Lung Adenocarcinoma Patients. *Cell. Physiol. Biochem.* **2017**, *44*, 2138–2146. [CrossRef]
111. Yang, X.; Tian, W.; Wang, S.; Ji, X.; Zhou, B. CircRNAs as promising biomarker in diagnostic and prognostic of lung cancer: An updated meta-analysis. *Genomics* **2021**, *113 Pt. 1*, 387–397. [CrossRef]
112. Chen, F.; Huang, C.; Wu, Q.; Jiang, L.; Chen, S.; Chen, L. Circular RNAs expression profiles in plasma exosomes from early - stage lung adenocarcinoma and the potential biomarkers. *J. Cell Biochem.* **2020**, *121*, 2525–2533. [CrossRef] [PubMed]
113. Hang, D.; Zhou, J.; Qin, N.; Zhou, W.; Ma, H.; Jin, G.; Hu, Z.; Dai, J.; Shen, H. A novel plasma circular RNA circFARSA is a potential biomarker for non-small cell lung cancer. *Cancer Med.* **2018**, *7*, 2783–2791. [CrossRef]
114. Zhang, Q.; Qin, S.; Peng, C.; Liu, Y.; Huang, Y.; Ju, S. Circulating circular RNA hsa_circ_0023179 acts as a diagnostic biomarker for non-small-cell lung cancer detection. *J. Cancer Res. Clin. Oncol.* **2022**, *149*, 3649–3660. [CrossRef]
115. Zhu, L.; Sun, L.; Xu, G.; Song, J.; Hu, B.; Fang, Z.; Dan, Y.; Li, N.; Shao, G. The diagnostic value of has_circ_0006423 in non-small cell lung cancer and its role as a tumor suppressor gene that sponges miR-492. *Sci. Rep.* **2022**, *12*, 13722. [CrossRef] [PubMed]
116. Luo, Y.; Zhang, Q.; Lv, B.; Shang, Y.; Li, J.; Yang, L.; Yu, Z.; Luo, K.; Deng, X.; Min, L.; et al. CircFOXP1: A novel serum diagnostic biomarker for non-small cell lung cancer. *Int. J. Biol. Markers* **2022**, *37*, 58–65. [CrossRef] [PubMed]

117. Köhler, J.; Schuler, M.; Gauler, T.C.; Nöpel-Dünnebacke, S.; Ahrens, M.; Hoffmann, A.C.; Kasper, S.; Nensa, F.; Gomez, B.; Hahnemann, M.; et al. Circulating U2 small nuclear RNA fragments as a diagnostic and prognostic biomarker in lung cancer patients. *J. Cancer Res. Clin. Oncol.* **2016**, *142*, 795–805. [CrossRef] [PubMed]
118. Mazières, J.; Catherinne, C.; Delfour, O.; Gouin, F.; Rouquette, I.; Delisle, M.B.; Delisle, M.; Prévot, G.; Escamilla, R.; Didier, A.; et al. Alternative Processing of the U2 Small Nuclear RNA Produces a 19–22nt Fragment with Relevance for the Detection of Non-Small Cell Lung Cancer in Human Serum. *PLoS ONE* **2013**, *8*, e60134. [CrossRef]
119. Dong, X.; Ding, S.; Yu, M.; Niu, L.; Xue, L.; Zhao, Y.; Xie, L.; Song, X.; Song, X. Small Nuclear RNAs (U1, U2, U5) in Tumor-Educated Platelets Are Downregulated and Act as Promising Biomarkers in Lung Cancer. *Front. Oncol.* **2020**, *10*, 1627. [CrossRef]
120. Li, J.; Wang, N.; Zhang, F.; Jin, S.; Dong, Y.; Dong, X.; Chen, Y.; Kong, X.; Tong, Y.; Mi, Q.; et al. PIWI-interacting RNAs are aberrantly expressed and may serve as novel biomarkers for diagnosis of lung adenocarcinoma. *Thorac. Cancer* **2021**, *12*, 2468–2477. [CrossRef]
121. Peng, H.; Wang, J.; Li, J.; Zhao, M.; Huang, S.; Gu, Y.; Li, Y.; Sun, X.; Yang, L.; Luo, Q.; et al. A circulating non-coding RNA panel as an early detection predictor of non-small cell lung cancer. *Life Sci.* **2016**, *151*, 235–242. [CrossRef] [PubMed]
122. Dou, Y.; Zhu, Y.; Ai, J.; Chen, H.; Liu, H.; Borgia, J.A.; Li, X.; Yang, F.; Jiang, B.; Wang, J.; et al. Plasma small ncRNA pair panels as novel biomarkers for early-stage lung adenocarcinoma screening. *BMC Genom.* **2018**, *19*, 545. [CrossRef] [PubMed]
123. Greenberg, A.K.; Rimal, B.; Felner, K.; Zafar, S.; Hung, J.; Eylers, E.; Phalan, B.; Zhang, M.; Goldberg, J.; Crawford, B.; et al. S-Adenosylmethionine as a Biomarker for the Early Detection of Lung Cancer. *Chest* **2007**, *132*, 1247–1252. [CrossRef]
124. Sullivan, F.M.; Mair, F.S.; Anderson, W.; Armory, P.; Briggs, A.; Chew, C.; Dorward, A.; Haughney, J.; Hogarth, F.; Kendrick, D.; et al. Earlier diagnosis of lung cancer in a randomised trial of an autoantibody blood test followed by imaging. *Eur. Respir. J.* **2021**, *57*, 2000670. [CrossRef] [PubMed]
125. Gaga, M.; Chorostowska-Wynimko, J.; Horváth, I.; Tammemagi, M.C.; Shitrit, D.; Eisenberg, V.H.; Liang, H.; Stav, D.; Faber, D.; Jansen, M.; et al. Validation of Lung EpiCheck, a novel methylation-based blood assay, for the detection of lung cancer in European and Chinese high-risk individuals. *Eur. Respir. J.* **2021**, *57*, 2002682. [CrossRef]
126. Cristiano, S.; Leal, A.; Phallen, J.; Fiksel, J.; Adleff, V.; Bruhm, D.C.; Jensen, S.; Medina, J.; Hruban, C.; White, J.; et al. Genome-wide cell-free DNA fragmentation in patients with cancer. *Nature* **2019**, *570*, 385–389. [CrossRef] [PubMed]
127. Grillone, K.; Riillo, C.; Scionti, F.; Rocca, R.; Tradigo, G.; Guzzi, P.H.; Alcaro, S.; Teresa, M.; Martino, D.; Tagliaferri, P.; et al. Non-coding RNAs in cancer: Platforms and strategies for investigating the genomic "dark matter". *J. Exp. Clin. Cancer Res.* **2020**, *39*, 117.
128. Pritchard, C.C.; Cheng, H.H.; Tewari, M. MicroRNA profiling: Approaches and considerations. *Nat. Publ. Group.* **2012**, *13*, 358–369. [CrossRef] [PubMed]
129. Jamal-Hanjani, M.; Wilson, G.A.; McGranahan, N.; Birkbak, N.J.; Watkins, T.B.K.; Veeriah, S.; Shafi, S.; Johnson, D.; Mitter, R.; Rosenthal, R.; et al. Tracking the Evolution of Non–Small-Cell Lung Cancer. *N. Engl. J. Med.* **2017**, *376*, 2109–2121. [CrossRef]
130. Karasaki, T.; Moore, D.A.; Veeriah, S.; Naceur-Lombardelli, C.; Toncheva, A.; Magno, N.; Ward, S.; Bakir, M.; Watkins, T.; Grigoriadis, K.; et al. Evolutionary characterization of lung adenocarcinoma morphology in TRACERx. *Nat. Med.* **2023**, *29*, 833–845. [CrossRef]
131. Frankell, A.M.; Dietzen, M.; Al Bakir, M.; Lim, E.L.; Karasaki, T.; Ward, S.; Veeriah, S.; Colliver, E.; Huebner, A.; Bunkum, A.; et al. The evolution of lung cancer and impact of subclonal selection in TRACERx. *Nature* **2023**, *616*, 525–533. [PubMed]

Disclaimer/Publisher's Note: The statements, opinions and data contained in all publications are solely those of the individual author(s) and contributor(s) and not of MDPI and/or the editor(s). MDPI and/or the editor(s) disclaim responsibility for any injury to people or property resulting from any ideas, methods, instructions or products referred to in the content.

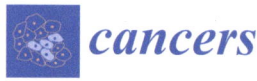 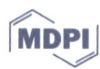

Review

Cystic Fibrosis and Cancer: Unraveling the Complex Role of CFTR Gene in Cancer Susceptibility

Giuseppe Fabio Parisi [1,*], Maria Papale [1], Giulia Pecora [1], Novella Rotolo [1], Sara Manti [2], Giovanna Russo [3] and Salvatore Leonardi [1]

[1] Pediatric Respiratory Unit, Department of Clinical and Experimental Medicine, San Marco Hospital, University of Catania, Viale Carlo Azeglio Ciampi sn, 95121 Catania, Italy; mariellapap@yahoo.it (M.P.); giupec87@hotmail.it (G.P.); rotolo@policlinico.unict.it (N.R.); leonardi@unict.it (S.L.)
[2] Pediatric Unit, Department of Human and Pediatric Pathology "Gaetano Barresi", AOUP G. Martino, University of Messina, Via Consolare Valeria, 1, 98124 Messina, Italy; sara.manti@unime.it
[3] Pediatric Hematology and Oncology Unit, Department of Clinical and Experimental Medicine, University of Catania, 95123 Catania, Italy; diberuss@unict.it
* Correspondence: gf.parisi@policlinico.unict.it; Tel.: +39-0954794181

Simple Summary: Cystic fibrosis (CF) is a genetic condition that affects the lungs, digestion, and other body systems. People with CF have a higher chance of developing certain types of cancer. The reason for this is related to a gene called CFTR, which is altered in CF patients. This gene normally helps regulate the movement of substances in and out of cells. When it does not work properly, it can lead to changes in cells that make them more likely to become cancerous. The cancers most commonly associated with CF are colorectal, pancreatic, and respiratory cancers. By understanding how CFTR and cancer are connected, doctors can develop better ways to screen for and treat these cancers in people with CF. More research is needed to fully understand this link and improve care for CF patients.

Abstract: Cystic fibrosis (CF) is a genetic disorder affecting multiple organs, primarily the lungs and digestive system. Over the years, advancements in medical care and treatments have significantly increased the life expectancy of individuals with CF. However, with this improved longevity, concerns about the potential risk of developing certain types of cancers have arisen. This narrative review aims to explore the relationship between CF, increased life expectancy, and the associated risk for cancers. We discuss the potential mechanisms underlying this risk, including chronic inflammation, immune system dysregulation, and genetic factors. Additionally, we review studies that have examined the incidence and types of cancers seen in CF patients, with a focus on gastrointestinal, breast, and respiratory malignancies. We also explore the impact of CFTR modulator therapies on cancer risk. In the gastrointestinal tract, CF patients have an elevated risk of developing colorectal cancer, pancreatic cancer, and possibly esophageal cancer. The underlying mechanisms contributing to these increased risks are not fully understood, but chronic inflammation, altered gut microbiota, and genetic factors are believed to play a role. Regular surveillance and colonoscopies are recommended for early detection and management of colorectal cancer in CF patients. Understanding the factors contributing to cancer development in CF patients is crucial for implementing appropriate surveillance strategies and improving long-term outcomes. Further research is needed to elucidate the molecular mechanisms involved and develop targeted interventions to mitigate cancer risk in individuals with CF.

Keywords: cystic fibrosis; CFTR gene; cancer risk; life expectancy; genetic factors; colorectal cancer; pancreatic cancer; breast cancer; respiratory cancers; CFTR modulator therapies

1. Introduction

Cystic fibrosis (CF) is a complex genetic disorder that primarily affects the respiratory and digestive systems. It is caused by mutations in the cystic fibrosis transmembrane conductance regulator (CFTR) gene, resulting in dysfunctional CFTR protein [1,2]. CF's hallmark is its impact on the production of thick, sticky mucus, which obstructs airways, leading to recurrent respiratory infections and impaired lung function. Additionally, the digestive tract's secretions are affected, causing challenges in nutrient absorption and digestive processes [3].

While CF is well-known for its impact on lung function and digestive processes, the increase in life expectancy with the introduction of new highly effective CFTR modulator (HEMT) therapy and recent evidence suggests a potential association between CF and an increased risk of developing certain types of cancers [4–9]. In recent years, research efforts have focused on elucidating the underlying mechanisms and understanding the implications of this relationship.

The genetic basis of CF lies in the CFTR gene, which regulates the flow of chloride ions across cell membranes. Mutations in the CFTR gene lead to impaired ion transport, resulting in the characteristic symptoms of CF. However, these mutations have also been implicated in various cellular processes that influence cancer development and progression [10,11]. Recent studies have focused on the potential impact of CFTR dysfunction on key pathways involved in carcinogenesis, such as cell proliferation, apoptosis, and DNA repair mechanisms [7–9]. Understanding these molecular mechanisms is crucial for unraveling the link between CF and cancer risk [12].

In addition to the genetic and molecular aspects, CF is characterized by chronic inflammation and dysregulated immune responses. The chronic inflammatory state in CF is primarily driven by the dysfunctional CFTR protein and is evident in both the respiratory and digestive systems [13]. This chronic inflammation can create a pro-tumorigenic microenvironment that promotes the initiation and progression of cancers [14]. Recent research has shed light on the role of inflammatory mediators, immune cells, and altered immune responses in the context of CF-related cancers [15,16]. Exploring the immunological aspects of CF and their influence on cancer development is essential for a comprehensive understanding of the disease.

Several specific types of cancer have been associated with CF, including colorectal, pancreatic, breast, and respiratory malignancies [7–9]. Epidemiological studies have consistently shown an increased incidence of some of these cancers in individuals with CF compared to the general population [17]. The specific mechanisms underlying the increased risk remain the subject of ongoing research. Factors such as chronic inflammation, altered immune response, gut microbiota dysbiosis, and CFTR dysfunction likely contribute to the development of these cancers in individuals with CF [18].

The implications of these findings extend beyond understanding the association between CF and cancer risk. They have significant clinical implications for the management of individuals with CF, including screening, surveillance, and treatment strategies. Tailored screening protocols are necessary to facilitate early detection, while surveillance for specific cancers should be incorporated into routine CF care. Furthermore, collaborations between CF care teams and oncology specialists are vital for providing comprehensive care to individuals with CF-related cancers [19].

This comprehensive review aims to accomplish the following objectives:

- Synthesize Current Knowledge: Summarize and consolidate the existing literature on the relationship between CF, the CFTR gene, and cancer susceptibility.
- Examine Specific Cancer Associations: Investigate the associations between CFTR gene mutations and the risk of specific cancer types, including pancreatic, respiratory, colorectal, breast, liver, esophageal, and gastric cancers.
- Explore Underlying Mechanisms: Explore the molecular and cellular mechanisms by which CFTR gene mutations may influence cancer susceptibility, encompassing factors such as chronic inflammation, impaired DNA repair, hormonal imbalances, and other cellular processes.

- Highlight Emerging Research: Highlight recent advancements and emerging research that shed light on the complex interplay between CF, CFTR gene mutations, and cancer development.
- Identify Knowledge Gaps: Identify gaps in the current understanding of the CFTR–cancer relationship, pinpointing areas that require further research and investigation.
- Clinical Implications: Discuss the potential clinical implications of the CFTR–cancer connection, including its impact on cancer surveillance, early detection, and potential therapeutic interventions.
- Inform Future Research Directions: Propose future research directions and methodologies that could elucidate the intricate mechanisms underlying the association between CFTR gene mutations and cancer susceptibility.

2. Methods

This comprehensive review of the association between CF and cancers was conducted using a narrative approach to gather and analyze relevant literature over the past decade. A comprehensive search of electronic databases, including PubMed, Scopus, and Web of Science, was conducted to identify relevant articles published in English. The search strategy incorporated keywords related to cystic fibrosis, cancer, malignancy, CFTR, and associated terms. The search was limited to articles published from 1990.

The initial search yielded a large number of articles (>500). Duplicate articles were removed, and titles and abstracts were screened for relevance. Full-text articles of potentially relevant studies were retrieved and assessed for eligibility. The inclusion criteria encompassed studies that investigated the association between CF and cancers. Review articles, original research papers, and case reports were considered.

Data from selected articles were extracted systematically. The following information was collected: author(s), publication year, study design, study population, cancer type, sample size, methods used for data collection, and key findings related to the association between CF and cancers. Additionally, data on the genetic, molecular, and immunological aspects of CF that contribute to cancer risk were extracted.

The extracted data were synthesized to provide a comprehensive overview of recent findings. The information was organized thematically, focusing on the genetic, molecular, and immunological aspects of CF, as well as specific types of cancer associated with CF, such as colorectal, pancreatic, breast, and respiratory malignancies. Key findings were summarized, and relevant concepts were discussed in detail.

The included studies were critically evaluated for their methodological quality and potential biases. Any limitations or gaps in the current literature were identified and discussed. The strengths and weaknesses of the studies were taken into account during the interpretation of the results.

The information gathered from the data synthesis and critical analysis was used to develop the manuscript. The review was structured to provide a comprehensive overview of recent findings regarding the association between CF and cancers. The introduction, methods, results, and discussion sections were written, highlighting the key aspects and implications of the findings.

3. Role of CFTR in Cancers

The role of CFTR in cancer is an intriguing area of investigation that has gained substantial interest in recent years. Initially recognized for its involvement in CF, CFTR has emerged as a potential player in cancer development and progression [20].

One of the key aspects of CFTR's role in cancer is its influence on ion transport and cellular homeostasis. CFTR acts as a chloride channel, regulating the movement of chloride ions and water across cell membranes. Dysregulation of CFTR can disrupt ion transport, leading to altered cellular homeostasis. This disruption has been associated with changes in cellular pH regulation and metabolism, both of which have significant implications for cancer cell growth and survival [21]. For example, CFTR dysfunction may disturb the balance of intracellular chloride and bicarbonate ions, affecting pH levels and influencing critical metabolic processes in cancer cells [22]. Furthermore, CFTR has been implicated in the regulation of epithelial–mesenchymal transition (EMT), a fundamental process involved in cancer metastasis. EMT is characterized by the loss of epithelial cell characteristics and the acquisition of a more mesenchymal-like phenotype, enabling cells to invade surrounding tissues and metastasize to distant sites. CFTR has been shown to modulate EMT through various mechanisms. CFTR dysfunction can lead to alterations in ion transport, calcium signaling, and the activity of signaling pathways such as transforming growth factor-beta (TGF-β) and Wnt/β-catenin, all of which play crucial roles in EMT regulation [23]. These changes in EMT-related pathways can contribute to increased invasiveness and metastatic potential of cancer cells.

Inflammation is a well-established driver of cancer development, and CFTR dysfunction has been associated with elevated levels of inflammation in various tissues. CFTR mutations can result in increased production of pro-inflammatory cytokines and chemokines, creating a pro-tumorigenic microenvironment [24]. Moreover, CFTR dysfunction may impact immune responses, influencing the infiltration and activation of immune cells within the tumor microenvironment. The dysregulated immune response in the presence of CFTR dysfunction may further contribute to cancer progression [25].

CFTR also appears to be involved in cellular proliferation and survival pathways. CFTR dysfunction can modulate the activity of signaling pathways such as phosphoinositide 3-kinase (PI3K)/Akt and mitogen-activated protein kinase (MAPK), which are crucial for cell growth and survival [23,26]. Additionally, CFTR may interact with other proteins involved in cell cycle regulation and apoptosis, influencing the behavior and survival of cancer cells [27]. These molecular interactions and alterations in signaling pathways can contribute to uncontrolled cellular proliferation and resistance to cell death mechanisms.

Furthermore, CFTR has been implicated in drug resistance in certain cancers [28]. The activity of CFTR can affect the response of cancer cells to chemotherapeutic agents by influencing drug uptake, efflux, and intracellular concentration. CFTR-mediated drug resistance can impact the effectiveness of cancer treatment and pose challenges in achieving successful outcomes.

In summary, CFTR plays a multifaceted role in cancer, influencing various aspects of tumor biology, including ion transport, EMT, inflammation, cellular proliferation, and drug response (Figure 1). Dysregulation of CFTR can have profound effects on cancer development and progression, further elucidating the molecular mechanisms underlying CF.

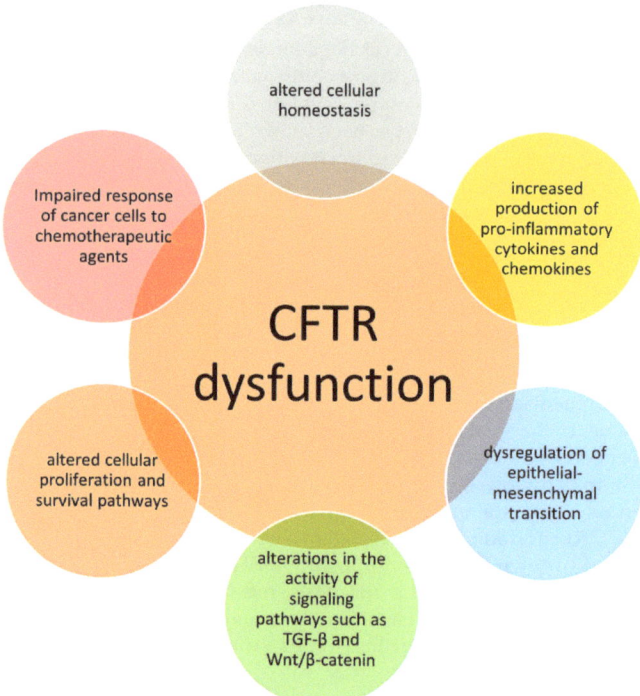

Figure 1. CFTR dysfunction and mechanisms related to predisposition to cancers. CFTR dysfunction in CF triggers chronic inflammation, impaired DNA repair, and hormonal imbalances. These mechanisms collectively predispose individuals to various cancers, highlighting the intricate interplay between CF and cancer susceptibility.

4. CF and Gastrointestinal Cancers

Gastrointestinal cancers encompass a range of malignancies affecting the digestive tract, including the esophagus, stomach, small intestine, colon, rectum, pancreas, and liver. Understanding the link between CF and gastrointestinal cancers is important for improving patient care, implementing appropriate surveillance and screening measures, and identifying potential therapeutic interventions.

4.1. Esophageal Cancer

Esophageal cancer is a relatively rare but aggressive malignancy that poses significant challenges to patients and healthcare providers. While the exact molecular mechanisms linking CF and esophageal cancers are not yet fully understood, several factors have been proposed to contribute to this association [7].

One potential mechanism is chronic inflammation resulting from CFTR dysfunction. The thickened mucus and impaired clearance in the respiratory and digestive systems of CF patients create an environment conducive to chronic inflammation. Chronic inflammation is known to play a key role in carcinogenesis, and it has been suggested that long-term inflammation in the esophagus may increase the risk of developing esophageal cancer in individuals with CF [29].

Additionally, CFTR mutations may impact the composition of the esophageal microbiota. Dysbiosis, an imbalance of bacterial species in the esophagus, has been associated with an increased risk of esophageal diseases, including esophageal cancer. CF patients may have altered esophageal microbiota due to the effects of CFTR dysfunction, and this dysbiosis could potentially contribute to the development of esophageal malignancies [30].

Moreover, CF patients often face nutritional challenges due to malabsorption and malnutrition. These nutritional issues may lead to deficiencies in key vitamins and minerals, which are essential for maintaining cellular health and DNA repair mechanisms. Such deficiencies could increase the susceptibility to cellular damage and the risk of developing esophageal cancers [31].

Furthermore, recent studies have implicated specific molecular pathways in the association between CFTR dysfunction and esophageal cancer development. For example, it has been suggested that CFTR mutations may lead to alterations in calcium signaling pathways, which play a critical role in cell proliferation, differentiation, and apoptosis. Dysregulation of calcium signaling can contribute to uncontrolled cell growth and the development of cancer [32].

Another potential molecular mechanism involves the disruption of epithelial cell homeostasis in the esophagus. CFTR dysfunction may impair the transport of bicarbonate ions, which are important for maintaining the proper pH balance in the esophageal epithelium. This disruption can lead to cellular stress, DNA damage, and increased susceptibility to carcinogenesis [33,34].

Finally, adults with CF have a higher risk of developing Barret's esophagus, which is a precursor for esophageal cancer [35].

Despite these potential associations and molecular mechanisms, the exact link between CF and esophageal cancers remains an active area of research. The relative risk of esophageal cancer in patients with CF is not well-established due to limited available data. As of now, there is a lack of consensus on the specific relative risk values for esophageal cancer in CF patients. The rarity of esophageal cancer in CF patients and the complexity of its underlying mechanisms make it challenging to draw definitive conclusions. Further studies are needed to elucidate the precise molecular pathways connecting CFTR dysfunction and the development of esophageal malignancies.

4.2. Gastric Cancer

Gastric cancer, also known as stomach cancer, is a malignant tumor that develops in the stomach lining. CFTR dysfunction in the stomach can lead to the accumulation of thick mucus, impairing mucociliary clearance. The retained mucus creates a favorable environment for bacterial colonization, resulting in chronic gastritis and inflammation. Chronic inflammation, characterized by the release of pro-inflammatory cytokines, chemokines, and growth factors, can promote genetic mutations, stimulate cellular proliferation, and enhance angiogenesis, ultimately contributing to the development and progression of gastric cancer [36,37].

CFTR plays a role in regulating chloride and bicarbonate ion transport, which impacts gastric acid secretion. CFTR dysfunction can lead to altered gastric acid production and pH levels. Reduced gastric acid secretion may increase the risk of gastric cancer by impairing microbial defense mechanisms and promoting the growth of Helicobacter pylori, a bacterium implicated in gastric cancer development. Moreover, altered gastric pH can affect the digestion and absorption of dietary factors that may modulate gastric carcinogenesis [38,39].

In addition to CFTR mutations, CF-related genetic variations may contribute to the increased risk of gastric cancer. Genome-wide association studies have identified certain genetic variants associated with both CF and gastric cancer susceptibility. These genetic variations may affect immune response, DNA repair mechanisms, or other processes involved in gastric carcinogenesis, highlighting potential shared genetic pathways between CF and gastric cancer [40,41].

Various other molecular pathways have been implicated in the association between CFTR dysfunction and gastric cancer development. For instance, CFTR dysfunction may lead to altered calcium signaling, affecting cell proliferation, differentiation, and apoptosis, which are critical processes in gastric carcinogenesis. Disruption of epithelial cell homeostasis, impaired bicarbonate ion transport, and subsequent cellular stress and DNA damage may also contribute to the development of gastric cancer in CF [42,43].

Therefore, the association between CF, CFTR, and gastric cancer involves complex molecular mechanisms. Chronic inflammation, altered gastric acid secretion, CF-related malnutrition, genetic variations, and disrupted cellular pathways collectively contribute to the increased risk of gastric cancer in individuals with CF.

Similar to esophageal cancer, the relative risk of gastric cancer in patients with CF is not well-defined. The available data on the association between CF and gastric cancer are limited, making it challenging to estimate precise relative risk values for this specific cancer type.

Further research is needed to fully elucidate these mechanisms and their interplay in the development and progression of gastric cancer in CF patients.

4.3. Pancreatic Cancer

Pancreatic cancer is a devastating disease characterized by its aggressiveness and poor prognosis. CF patients have an increased relative risk of developing pancreatic cancer. Studies have reported relative risk values ranging from 5 to 10 times higher in CF patients compared to the general population [17,19,44,45]. CFTR dysfunction caused by mutations in the CFTR gene leads to abnormal ion transport across epithelial cells, including those lining the pancreatic ducts. The resulting impaired CFTR function leads to altered fluid secretion and increased viscosity of pancreatic secretions, ultimately leading to ductal obstruction. The accumulation of thickened secretions creates a microenvironment conducive to inflammation, fibrosis, and cellular damage, potentially predisposing individuals with CF to pancreatic cancer [44,45].

CFTR dysfunction and pancreatic duct obstruction trigger chronic inflammation in the pancreas. Inflammatory processes involve the release of pro-inflammatory cytokines, chemokines, and reactive oxygen species, leading to cellular damage and genetic mutations. Prolonged inflammation can induce DNA damage, dysregulate cellular signaling pathways, and disturb cell growth and survival mechanisms, all of which are implicated in pancreatic cancer development [46].

CF-related pancreatic insufficiency often coexists with bile duct abnormalities and impaired bile flow. These conditions can result in increased exposure of pancreatic tissue to bile acids, digestive enzymes, and duodenal reflux. The duodenal refluxate, consisting of bile acids and other duodenal contents, can cause cellular injury, inflammation, and oxidative stress in the pancreas. Sustained exposure to these damaging factors may contribute to the initiation and progression of pancreatic cancer [47,48].

In addition to CFTR mutations, CF-related genetic factors have been implicated in pancreatic cancer development. Genome-wide association studies have identified specific genetic variants associated with both CF and pancreatic cancer susceptibility. These variants may affect immune response, cellular metabolism, or other pathways involved in pancreatic carcinogenesis. Investigating these shared genetic factors can provide valuable insights into the molecular mechanisms connecting CF and pancreatic cancer [49,50].

Growing evidence suggests that alterations in the gut microbiota, known as dysbiosis, may play a role in pancreatic cancer development. CF-related pancreatic insufficiency, altered bile flow, and impaired digestive processes can disrupt the gut microbial ecosystem. Dysbiosis in CF patients may result in the production of harmful metabolites, chronic inflammation, and perturbation of the host–microbiota interaction, which may contribute to pancreatic carcinogenesis [51,52].

In conclusion, the association between CF, CFTR, and pancreatic cancer involves intricate molecular mechanisms. CFTR dysfunction, pancreatic duct obstruction, chronic inflammation, altered bile flow, CFTR-related genetic factors, impaired nutrient absorption, and microbiota dysbiosis collectively contribute to the increased risk of pancreatic cancer in individuals with CF. Further research is necessary to fully elucidate these molecular mechanisms and their interplay in the development and progression of pancreatic cancer in CF patients.

4.4. Liver Cancer

CFTR dysfunction resulting from CF-associated mutations disrupts chloride and bicarbonate transport, leading to impaired bile secretion and altered bile composition. This disturbance in bile flow can cause cholestasis and subsequent hepatic fibrosis [53]. Prolonged fibrotic changes in the liver microenvironment create a pro-inflammatory milieu and promote cellular proliferation, thereby increasing the risk of hepatocellular carcinoma (HCC). Studies have shown that CF patients with liver cirrhosis have an increased risk of developing HCC [54,55].

CFTR dysfunction contributes to chronic inflammation and oxidative stress in the liver. Impaired CFTR function leads to the accumulation of bile acids, which can induce oxidative damage and activate inflammatory pathways. Chronic inflammation and oxidative stress create a favorable environment for the development of hepatic cancer by promoting DNA damage, genomic instability, and cellular proliferation. Studies have demonstrated increased levels of pro-inflammatory markers and oxidative stress in CF-related liver disease [56,57].

CFTR has been shown to play a role in liver regeneration. During liver injury, CFTR expression is upregulated, suggesting its involvement in the regenerative process. CFTR-deficient mice exhibit impaired liver regeneration, suggesting that altered CFTR expression and function may disrupt the regenerative capacity of liver cells. Impaired liver regeneration can contribute to the development of hepatic cancer [58,59].

In addition to CFTR mutations, other CF-related genetic factors have been associated with an increased risk of hepatic cancer. Genetic variations in CFTR modifier genes, such as the Solute Carrier Organic Anion Transporter (SLCO) family, have been implicated in hepatocarcinogenesis. These variations may affect drug metabolism, transport, and cellular pathways involved in liver cancer development. Studies have identified associations between CFTR-related genetic variations and increased susceptibility to liver cancer in CF patients [60,61].

CF patients may have a slightly elevated risk of developing liver cancer, although the relative risk values vary across studies. Relative risk values around 1.5 to 2.0 have been suggested [17,19].

In summary, there has been growing evidence supporting a link between CF, CFTR dysfunction, and the development of hepatic cancer. The molecular mechanisms underlying this association involve CFTR dysfunction-related hepatic fibrosis, chronic inflammation, oxidative stress, impaired liver regeneration, CFTR-related genetic factors, and nutritional deficiencies.

4.5. Intestinal Cancers

4.5.1. Colorectal Cancer

Colorectal cancer (CRC) is a malignant neoplasm that arises from the epithelial cells lining the colon or rectum. Patients with CF are at a 6-fold higher risk for CRC [19,37,62]. The mechanisms underlying this association are not yet fully understood, but several factors have been implicated.

CFTR dysfunction in the intestinal epithelium leads to persistent inflammation and oxidative stress. The impaired CFTR function affects ion transport, mucus clearance, and the integrity of the intestinal barrier [63,64]. These disruptions create an environment conducive to chronic inflammation and oxidative stress, which can promote the development of CRC. Inflammation and oxidative stress induce DNA damage, genomic instability, and cellular proliferation, key factors in carcinogenesis.

Recent studies have highlighted the role of pro-inflammatory cytokines, such as interleukin-6 (IL-6) and tumor necrosis factor-alpha (TNF-α), in CRC development. Increased expression of these cytokines has been observed in CF patients, indicating a potential link between CF-associated inflammation and CRC [65,66]. Additionally, oxidative stress resulting from impaired CFTR function can lead to the accumulation of reactive oxygen species (ROS), causing DNA damage and favoring the initiation and progression of CRC [67,68].

CF patients often exhibit dysbiosis, an imbalance in the composition and function of the gut microbiota. Dysbiosis in CF is characterized by a reduction in beneficial bacteria, such as Bifidobacterium and Lactobacillus species, and an increase in potentially harmful bacteria, including Enterobacteriaceae and Pseudomonas aeruginosa. Dysbiosis can contribute to inflammation, impaired intestinal barrier function, and increased susceptibility to CRC. The specific dysbiosis patterns associated with CRC in CF patients warrant further investigation [69,70].

Recent studies have highlighted the potential role of specific bacterial species in CRC development. For example, Fusobacterium nucleatum, a common member of the gut microbiota, has been associated with CRC progression by promoting inflammation and impairing immune surveillance [71,72]. In CF patients, dysbiosis and altered microbial composition may create a microenvironment conducive to the growth of pathogenic bacteria, further contributing to the development of CRC.

In addition to CFTR mutations, CF-related genetic factors may influence the risk of CRC development in CF patients. Modifier genes that interact with CFTR, such as those involved in inflammation, immune response, and cellular proliferation, may play a role in CRC susceptibility. Variations in these genes can modify the disease phenotype and influence the development of CRC in CF patients [73,74].

Recent studies have identified genetic polymorphisms associated with both CF and CRC, suggesting a potential genetic link between the two conditions. For example, the TNF-α gene polymorphism has been implicated in both CF and CRC susceptibility [75]. These genetic factors may modulate the inflammatory response, alter immune cell function, and contribute to the development of CRC in CF patients.

Current guidelines recommend CRC surveillance for CF patients starting at the age of 40 or 10 years before the youngest affected relative's diagnosis (whichever comes first). The surveillance typically involves periodic colonoscopies with the aim of detecting precancerous polyps or early-stage CRC. Additionally, individuals with CF who present with concerning symptoms such as unexplained gastrointestinal bleeding or persistent change in bowel habits should undergo timely evaluation [76,77].

4.5.2. Small Bowel Adenocarcinoma

Small bowel adenocarcinoma (SBA) is a rare but aggressive form of intestinal cancer that can occur in CF patients. The underlying mechanisms linking CF and SBA are not yet fully elucidated, but several factors may contribute to its development.

Several tumor suppressor genes have been implicated in SBA development, including TP53, APC, and SMAD4. TP53, commonly known as the "guardian of the genome", plays a crucial role in DNA repair and cell cycle regulation. CFTR dysfunction could potentially affect TP53 function, compromising its ability to suppress tumor formation and progression in the small intestine [78,79]. Further studies are needed to elucidate the specific molecular interactions between CFTR and tumor suppressor genes in the context of SBA development.

5. Breast Cancer

The prevalence of breast cancer in CF patients is generally not higher than that in the general population. However, with advancements in CF treatments, individuals with CF are living longer, and there is a growing population of women with CF reaching the age at which breast cancer becomes more common [9].

Estrogens play a significant role in both the pathophysiology of CF and breast cancer. However, their effects on these two conditions are distinct and require separate considerations. In the context of CF, estrogen has been shown to exert beneficial effects on lung function and disease progression. CF is characterized by abnormal ion transport due to mutations in the cystic fibrosis transmembrane conductance regulator (CFTR) gene. Estrogen has been found to enhance CFTR function and increase chloride secretion in the airways, leading to improved mucus clearance and lung function [80,81]. Estrogen's protective effects on lung function may be attributed to its ability to stimulate CFTR expression and activity through various signaling pathways, including cyclic adenosine monophosphate (cAMP)-dependent mechanisms [82].

In contrast, estrogen plays a complex role in the pathophysiology of breast cancer. Estrogen receptor (ER) signaling is known to promote the growth and proliferation of breast cancer cells. In hormone receptor-positive breast cancers, estrogen binds to ERs, leading to the activation of downstream signaling pathways that drive tumor cell growth and survival. Estrogen also promotes angiogenesis, the formation of new blood vessels, which is crucial for tumor growth and metastasis [83–85].

It is worth noting that the use of hormone replacement therapy (HRT) in CF patients needs careful consideration. While HRT may have potential benefits for improving lung function and bone health in postmenopausal CF women, it also carries potential risks, including the promotion of hormone-sensitive cancers such as breast cancer [86]. The decision to use HRT should be made on an individual basis, taking into account the patient's overall health status and the potential benefits and risks.

While there is limited data on breast cancer risk specifically in CF, it is important to consider appropriate screening strategies for CF patients. Following general breast cancer screening guidelines is recommended, including regular clinical breast exams, mammography, and breast self-examinations (American Cancer Society). Screening mammograms typically begin at age 40 and continue annually for women at average risk of breast cancer [87].

CF-related factors may present challenges in breast cancer screening and management. CF-related lung disease can make it difficult for patients to undergo mammography due to positioning and breathing difficulties. In such cases, alternative imaging modalities such as breast ultrasound or magnetic resonance imaging (MRI) may be considered [88]. Collaborating with healthcare providers experienced in managing breast cancer screening in individuals with CF can help develop appropriate and effective screening strategies.

Breast cancer screening and management should be integrated into the comprehensive care of CF patients. A multidisciplinary approach involving CF specialists, oncologists, genetic counselors, and other healthcare providers is crucial to address the unique needs and challenges of CF patients regarding breast cancer. Close coordination and communication among the different healthcare professionals involved are important to ensure comprehensive and coordinated care.

Psychosocial support should also be provided throughout the breast cancer screening and management process. CF patients may already face significant physical and emotional burdens related to their condition, and breast cancer screening and potential diagnosis can add additional emotional challenges. Counseling services, support groups, and resources can help CF patients navigate the emotional aspects of breast cancer screening and potential diagnosis.

6. Lung Cancers

Lung cancer is one of the most common malignancies worldwide, and individuals with CF have an increased, although still not quantifiable, risk of developing certain types of lung cancers. The role of the CFTR in CF and its relationship to lung cancer have been the focus of scientific investigation. Epidemiologic data reveal that individuals with CF have an increased risk of developing certain types of lung cancers compared to the general population [89,90]. One notable subtype of lung cancer that is more prevalent in CF patients is bronchial gland carcinoma, which arises from the mucous glands in the airways. While bronchial gland carcinomas are relatively rare in the general population, they occur more frequently in CF patients [91,92]. The specific mechanisms underlying this increased susceptibility to bronchial gland carcinomas in CF are still being investigated.

In addition to bronchial gland carcinomas, CF patients also have a heightened risk of other lung malignancies, such as squamous cell carcinoma and adenocarcinoma [17,93]. These types of lung cancers are commonly associated with smoking, and CF patients who smoke face an even higher risk of developing lung cancer compared to non-smoking CF patients. Therefore, smoking cessation is strongly encouraged in CF patients to reduce the risk of lung cancer and other smoking-related health complications [94,95].

Several factors contribute to the increased risk of lung cancer in CF patients. Chronic inflammation and tissue damage in the lungs, often caused by chronic bacterial infections like Pseudomonas aeruginosa, play a crucial role. These infections lead to persistent inflammation and oxidative stress, creating an environment that promotes tumor development. Moreover, the genetic mutations in the CFTR gene, resulting in CFTR dysfunction, may also contribute to an altered cellular environment that favors the development of lung cancer [90,93].

It is important to note that despite the increased risk, the overall incidence of lung cancer in CF patients remains relatively low compared to the general population. The improved survival and enhanced quality of life in CF patients due to advancements in CF treatments and therapies may contribute to the increased likelihood of reaching an age where lung cancer becomes more common. Regular monitoring and screening for lung cancer are crucial in CF patients, particularly those with additional risk factors like smoking, as early detection can lead to improved outcomes.

7. Other Emerging Cancers

Although rare, cases of thyroid tumors, melanomas, ovarian cancers, and brain tumors have been reported [17,62,90,96].

Other emerging cancers in CF, including bone cancer, soft tissue sarcoma, bladder cancer, prostate cancer, and uterine cancer, have limited data available [91]. The potential impact of CFTR dysfunction on these cancers requires more comprehensive studies to establish a clearer association.

It is important to note that the epidemiologic data for emerging cancers in CF are limited, and further research is necessary to better understand the prevalence and molecular mechanisms involved. Advancements in research will contribute to improved screening, prevention, and management strategies for cancer in patients with CF.

8. Highly Effective CFTR Modulator Therapy (HEMT) and Cancers

CFTR modulator therapy has revolutionized the treatment landscape for CF by targeting the underlying defect in the CFTR gene [97,98]. However, little is known about the possible long-term effects and their potential impact on cancer risk. At present, the available data on the long-term effects of modulator therapies on cancer risk in CF patients are limited due to the relatively recent introduction of these drugs and the need for long-term follow-up studies. However, based on the current knowledge and studies conducted thus far, there is no conclusive evidence to suggest that modulator therapy increases the overall risk of cancer in CF patients [99–104].

9. Conclusions

The role of the CFTR gene in the development and progression of cancers in patients with CF is an emerging area of research (Table 1). Although CF primarily affects the respiratory and gastrointestinal systems, evidence suggests that CFTR gene mutations may also increase the risk of specific cancers in CF patients.

Table 1. Main cancers associated with cystic fibrosis.

Cancer Type	Molecular Mechanisms	Relative Risk
Esophageal cancer	<ul><li>Chronic inflammation</li><li>Altered composition of esophageal microbiota</li><li>Alterations in calcium signaling pathways</li><li>Disruption of epithelial cell homeostasis</li><li>Higher risk of developing Barret's esophagus</li></ul>	not well-established
Gastric cancer	<ul><li>Chronic inflammation</li><li>Altered gastric acid production and pH levels</li><li>Alterations in calcium signaling pathways</li><li>Disruption of epithelial cell homeostasis</li></ul>	not well-established
Pancreatic cancer	<ul><li>Chronic inflammation</li><li>Altered bile flow</li><li>Oxidative stress</li></ul>	5–10
Liver cancer	<ul><li>Chronic inflammation</li><li>Altered bile flow</li><li>Impaired liver regeneration</li><li>Genetic variations in modifier genes, such as the Solute Carrier Organic Anion Transporter (SLCO) family</li></ul>	1.5–2
Intestinal cancers	<ul><li>Chronic inflammation</li><li>Oxidative stress</li><li>Altered composition of intestinal microbiota</li><li>Genetic polymorphisms</li><li>Implications of tumor suppressor genes</li></ul>	6
Breast cancer	<ul><li>Hormonal imbalances, such as increased estrogen levels</li></ul>	not well-established
Lung cancer	<ul><li>Chronic inflammation</li><li>Altered mucociliary clearance</li></ul>	not well-established

In the gastrointestinal tract, CF patients have an elevated risk of developing colorectal cancer, pancreatic cancer, and possibly esophageal cancer. The underlying mechanisms contributing to these increased risks are not fully understood, but chronic inflammation, altered gut microbiota, and genetic factors are believed to play a role. Regular surveillance and colonoscopies are recommended for early detection and management of colorectal cancer in CF patients.

The advent of CFTR modulator therapies has significantly improved the clinical outcomes of CF patients by correcting CFTR dysfunction. However, concerns have been raised about the potential long-term effects of CFTR modulator therapy on cancer risk. Further research is needed to clarify the relationship between CFTR modulator therapy and cancer development in CF patients.

In conclusion, the CFTR gene, responsible for the pathogenesis of CF, may also play a role in the development and progression of certain cancers in CF patients. Understanding the molecular mechanisms underlying these associations and identifying effective surveillance and management strategies are crucial for optimizing the care of CF patients and mitigating cancer risks. Continued research in this field will contribute to the development of personalized approaches to cancer prevention, screening, and treatment in individuals with CF. The possible clinical implications of these observations are profound, as they pave the way for enhanced cancer surveillance, tailored early detection strategies, and potential targeted therapies, ensuring comprehensive care for individuals with both CF and cancer predisposition.

Author Contributions: Conceptualization G.F.P., M.P., and G.P.; methodology S.M. and M.P.; validation, G.F.P. and S.L.; formal analysis, G.F.P., S.M., and G.R.; investigation, N.R. and M.P.; resources, G.F.P.; data curation, G.F.P., G.P., S.M., and G.R.; writing—original draft preparation, G.F.P., M.P., and G.P.; writing—review and editing, S.M., N.R., G.R., and S.L.; visualization, S.L.; supervision, G.R. and S.L. All authors have read and agreed to the published version of the manuscript.

Funding: This research received no external funding.

Conflicts of Interest: The authors declare no conflict of interest.

References

1. Elborn, J.S. Cystic fibrosis. *Lancet* **2016**, *388*, 2519–2531. [CrossRef] [PubMed]
2. Shteinberg, M.; Haq, I.J.; Polineni, D.; Davies, J.C. Cystic fibrosis. *Lancet* **2021**, *397*, 2195–2211. [CrossRef]
3. Abrami, M.; Maschio, M.; Conese, M.; Confalonieri, M.; Gerin, F.; Dapas, B.; Farra, R.; Adrover, A.; Torelli, L.; Ruaro, B.; et al. Combined use of rheology and portable low-field NMR in cystic fibrosis patients. *Respir. Med.* **2021**, *189*, 106623. [CrossRef] [PubMed]
4. McBennett, K.A.; Davis, P.B.; Konstan, M.W. Increasing life expectancy in cystic fibrosis: Advances and challenges. *Pediatr. Pulmonol.* **2022**, *57* (Suppl. 1), S5–S12. [CrossRef] [PubMed]
5. Scott, P.; Wang, S.; Onyeaghala, G.; Pankratz, N.; Starr, T.; Prizment, A.E. Lower Expression of CFTR Is Associated with Higher Mortality in a Meta-Analysis of Individuals with Colorectal Cancer. *Cancers* **2023**, *15*, 989. [CrossRef] [PubMed]
6. Bhattacharya, R.; Blankenheim, Z.; Scott, P.M.; Cormier, R.T. CFTR and Gastrointestinal Cancers: An Update. *J. Pers. Med.* **2022**, *12*, 868. [CrossRef]
7. Scott, P.; Anderson, K.; Singhania, M.; Cormier, R. Cystic Fibrosis, CFTR, and Colorectal Cancer. *Int. J. Mol. Sci.* **2020**, *21*, 2891. [CrossRef] [PubMed]
8. Carlos Dos Reis, D.; Dastoor, P.; Santos, A.K.; Sumigray, K.; Ameen, N.A. CFTR High Expresser Cells in cystic fibrosis and intestinal diseases. *Heliyon* **2023**, *9*, e14568. [CrossRef]
9. Stastna, N.; Brat, K.; Homola, L.; Os, A.; Brancikova, D. Increasing incidence rate of breast cancer in cystic fibrosis—Relationship between pathogenesis, oncogenesis and prediction of the treatment effect in the context of worse clinical outcome and prognosis of cystic fibrosis due to estrogens. *Orphanet J. Rare Dis.* **2023**, *18*, 62. [CrossRef]
10. Parisi, G.F.; Mòllica, F.; Giallongo, A.; Papale, M.; Manti, S.; Leonardi, S. Cystic fibrosis transmembrane conductance regulator (CFTR): Beyond cystic fibrosis. *Egypt. J. Med. Hum. Genet* **2022**, *23*, 94. [CrossRef]
11. Moliteo, E.; Sciacca, M.; Palmeri, A.; Papale, M.; Manti, S.; Parisi, G.F.; Leonardi, S. Cystic Fibrosis and Oxidative Stress: The Role of CFTR. *Molecules* **2022**, *27*, 5324. [CrossRef] [PubMed]
12. Cutting, G.R. Cystic fibrosis genetics: From molecular understanding to clinical application. *Nat. Rev. Genet.* **2015**, *16*, 45–56. [CrossRef] [PubMed]
13. Yu, C.; Kotsimbos, T. Respiratory Infection and Inflammation in Cystic Fibrosis: A Dynamic Interplay among the Host, Microbes, and Environment for the Ages. *Int. J. Mol. Sci.* **2023**, *24*, 4052. [CrossRef] [PubMed]
14. Zhao, H.; Wu, L.; Yan, G.; Chen, Y.; Zhou, M.; Wu, Y.; Li, Y. Inflammation and tumor progression: Signaling pathways and targeted intervention. *Signal Transduct. Target. Ther.* **2021**, *6*, 263. [CrossRef] [PubMed]
15. Murphy, S.V.; Ribeiro, C.M.P. Cystic Fibrosis Inflammation: Hyperinflammatory, Hypoinflammatory, or Both? *Am. J. Respir. Cell Mol. Biol.* **2019**, *61*, 273–274. [CrossRef] [PubMed]
16. Wu, B.; Sodji, Q.H.; Oyelere, A.K. Inflammation, Fibrosis and Cancer: Mechanisms, Therapeutic Options and Challenges. *Cancers* **2022**, *14*, 552. [CrossRef] [PubMed]
17. Appelt, D.; Fuchs, T.; Steinkamp, G.; Ellemunter, H. Malignancies in patients with cystic fibrosis: A case series. *J. Med. Case Rep.* **2022**, *16*, 27. [CrossRef] [PubMed]
18. Tam, R.Y.; van Dorst, J.M.; McKay, I.; Coffey, M.; Ooi, C.Y. Intestinal Inflammation and Alterations in the Gut Microbiota in Cystic Fibrosis: A Review of the Current Evidence, Pathophysiology and Future Directions. *J. Clin. Med.* **2022**, *11*, 649. [CrossRef]
19. Maisonneuve, P.; Lowenfels, A.B. Cancer in Cystic Fibrosis: A Narrative Review of Prevalence, Risk Factors, Screening, and Treatment Challenges: Adult Cystic Fibrosis Series. *Chest* **2022**, *161*, 356–364. [CrossRef]
20. Hanssens, L.S.; Duchateau, J.; Casimir, G.J. CFTR Protein: Not Just a Chloride Channel? *Cells* **2021**, *10*, 2844. [CrossRef]
21. Farinha, C.M.; Gentzsch, M. Revisiting CFTR Interactions: Old Partners and New Players. *Int. J. Mol. Sci.* **2021**, *22*, 13196. [CrossRef] [PubMed]
22. Lu, Y.C.; Chen, H.; Fok, K.L.; Tsang, L.L.; Yu, M.K.; Zhang, X.H.; Chen, J.; Jiang, X.; Chung, Y.W.; Ma, A.C.H.; et al. CFTR mediates bicarbonate-dependent activation of miR-125b in preimplantation embryo development. *Cell Res.* **2012**, *22*, 1453–1466. [CrossRef] [PubMed]

23. Zhang, J.; Wang, Y.; Jiang, X.; Chan, H.C. Cystic fibrosis transmembrane conductance regulator-emerging regulator of cancer. *Cell Mol. Life Sci.* **2018**, *75*, 1737–1756. [CrossRef] [PubMed]
24. Kay, J.; Thadhani, E.; Samson, L.; Engelward, B. Inflammation-induced DNA damage, mutations and cancer. *DNA Repair* **2019**, *83*, 102673. [CrossRef] [PubMed]
25. Ghigo, A.; De Santi, C.; Hart, M.; Mitash, N.; Swiatecka-Urban, A. Cell signaling and regulation of CFTR expression in cystic fibrosis cells in the era of high efficiency modulator therapy. *J. Cyst. Fibros.* **2023**, *22* (Suppl. 1), S12–S16. [CrossRef]
26. Lukasiak, A.; Zajac, M. The Distribution and Role of the CFTR Protein in the Intracellular Compartments. *Membranes* **2021**, *11*, 804. [CrossRef] [PubMed]
27. Liou, T.G. The Clinical Biology of Cystic Fibrosis Transmembrane Regulator Protein: Its Role and Function in Extrapulmonary Disease. *Chest* **2019**, *155*, 605–616. [CrossRef] [PubMed]
28. Zhu, Q.; Li, H.; Liu, Y.; Jiang, L. Knockdown of CFTR enhances sensitivity of prostate cancer cells to cisplatin via inhibition of autophagy. *Neoplasma* **2017**, *64*, 709–717. [CrossRef]
29. Wong, M.; Ziring, D.; Korin, Y.; Desai, S.; Kim, S.; Lin, J.; Gjertson, D.; Braun, J.; Reed, E.; Singh, R.R. TNFalpha blockade in human diseases: Mechanisms and future directions. *Clin. Immunol.* **2008**, *126*, 121–136. [CrossRef]
30. Yang, L.; Lu, X.; Nossa, C.W.; Francois, F.; Peek, R.M.; Pei, Z. Inflammation and intestinal metaplasia of the distal esophagus are associated with alterations in the microbiome. *Gastroenterology* **2009**, *137*, 588–597. [CrossRef]
31. Strandvik, B. Nutrition in Cystic Fibrosis-Some Notes on the Fat Recommendations. *Nutrients* **2022**, *14*, 853. [CrossRef] [PubMed]
32. Jouret, F.C.; Bernard, A.; Hermans, C.; Dom, G.; Terryn, S.; Leal, T.; Lebecque, P.; Cassiman, J.-J.; Scholte, B.J.; de Jonge, H.R.; et al. Cystic fibrosis is associated with a defect in apical receptor-mediated endocytosis in mouse and human kidney. *J. Am. Soc. Nephrol.* **2007**, *18*, 707–718. [CrossRef] [PubMed]
33. Matsumoto, Y.; Shiozaki, A.; Kosuga, T.; Kudou, M.; Shimizu, H.; Arita, T.; Konishi, H.; Komatsu, S.; Kubota, T.; Fujiwara, H.; et al. Expression and Role of CFTR in Human Esophageal Squamous Cell Carcinoma. *Ann. Surg. Oncol.* **2021**, *28*, 6424–6436. [CrossRef]
34. Shi, X.; Li, Y.; Pan, S.; Liu, X.; Ke, Y.; Guo, W.; Wang, Y.; Ruan, Q.; Zhang, X.; Ma, H. Identification and validation of an autophagy-related gene signature for predicting prognosis in patients with esophageal squamous cell carcinoma. *Sci. Rep.* **2022**, *12*, 1960. [CrossRef] [PubMed]
35. Knotts, R.M.; Solfisburg, Q.S.; Keating, C.; DiMango, E.; Lightdale, C.J.; Abrams, J.A. Cystic fibrosis is associated with an increased risk of Barrett's esophagus. *J. Cyst. Fibros.* **2019**, *18*, 425–429. [CrossRef] [PubMed]
36. Liu, H.; Wu, W.; Liu, Y.; Zhang, C.; Zhou, Z. Predictive value of cystic fibrosis transmembrane conductance regulator (CFTR) in the diagnosis of gastric cancer. *Clin. Investig. Med.* **2014**, *37*, E226–E232. [CrossRef] [PubMed]
37. Yamada, A.; Komaki, Y.; Komaki, F.; Micic, D.; Zullow, S.; Sakuraba, A. Risk of gastrointestinal cancers in patients with cystic fibrosis: A systematic review and meta-analysis. *Lancet Oncol.* **2018**, *19*, 758–767. [CrossRef] [PubMed]
38. Lim, M.C.C.; Jantaree, P.; Naumann, M. The conundrum of Helicobacter pylori-associated apoptosis in gastric cancer. *Trends Cancer* **2023**, *9*, 679–690. [CrossRef]
39. Alzahrani, S.; Lina, T.T.; Gonzalez, J.; Pinchuk, I.V.; Beswick, E.J.; Reyes, V.E. Effect of Helicobacter pylori on gastric epithelial cells. *World J. Gastroenterol.* **2014**, *20*, 12767–12780. [CrossRef] [PubMed]
40. Hou, Y.; Guan, X.; Yang, Z.; Li, C. Emerging role of cystic fibrosis transmembrane conductance regulator—An epithelial chloride channel in gastrointestinal cancers. *World J. Gastrointest. Oncol.* **2016**, *8*, 282–288. [CrossRef]
41. Anderson, K.J.; Cormier, R.T.; Scott, P.M. Role of ion channels in gastrointestinal cancer. *World J. Gastroenterol.* **2019**, *25*, 5732–5772. [CrossRef] [PubMed]
42. Patergnani, S.; Danese, A.; Bouhamida, E.; Aguiari, G.; Previati, M.; Pinton, P.; Giorgi, C. Various Aspects of Calcium Signaling in the Regulation of Apoptosis, Autophagy, Cell Proliferation, and Cancer. *Int. J. Mol. Sci.* **2020**, *21*, 8323. [CrossRef] [PubMed]
43. Rock, J.R.; O'Neal, W.K.; Gabriel, S.E.; Randell, S.H.; Harfe, B.D.; Boucher, R.C.; Grubb, B.R. Transmembrane protein 16A (TMEM16A) is a Ca2+-regulated Cl- secretory channel in mouse airways. *J. Biol. Chem.* **2009**, *284*, 14875–14880. [CrossRef] [PubMed]
44. Maisonneuve, P.; Marshall, B.C.; Lowenfels, A.B. Risk of pancreatic cancer in patients with cystic fibrosis. *Gut* **2007**, *56*, 1327–1328. [CrossRef] [PubMed]
45. McWilliams, R.R.; Petersen, G.M.; Rabe, K.G.; Holtegaard, L.M.; Lynch, P.J.; Bishop, M.D.; Highsmith, W.E. Cystic fibrosis transmembrane conductance regulator (CFTR) gene mutations and risk for pancreatic adenocarcinoma. *Cancer* **2010**, *116*, 203–209. [CrossRef] [PubMed]
46. Guerra, C.; Schuhmacher, A.J.; Cañamero, M.; Grippo, P.J.; Verdaguer, L.; Pérez-Gallego, L.; Dubus, P.; Sandgren, E.P.; Barbacid, M. Chronic pancreatitis is essential for induction of pancreatic ductal adenocarcinoma by K-Ras oncogenes in adult mice. *Cancer Cell* **2007**, *11*, 291–302. [CrossRef] [PubMed]
47. Pandol, S.J.; Apte, M.V.; Wilson, J.S.; Gukovskaya, A.S.; Edderkaoui, M. The burning question: Why is smoking a risk factor for pancreatic cancer? *Pancreatology* **2012**, *12*, 344–349. [CrossRef]
48. Cazacu, I.M.; Farkas, N.; Garami, A.; Balaskó, M.; Mosdósi, B.; Alizadeh, H.; Gyöngyi, Z.; Rakonczay, Z.; Vigh, É.; Habon, T.; et al. Pancreatitis-Associated Genes and Pancreatic Cancer Risk: A Systematic Review and Meta-analysis. *Pancreas* **2018**, *47*, 1078–1086. [CrossRef]

49. Witt, H.; Beer, S.; Rosendahl, J.; Chen, J.-M.; Chandak, G.R.; Masamune, A.; Bence, M.; Szmola, R.; Oracz, G.; Macek, M.; et al. Variants in CPA1 are strongly associated with early onset chronic pancreatitis. *Nat. Genet.* **2013**, *45*, 1216–1220. [CrossRef]
50. Earl, J.; Galindo-Pumariño, C.; Encinas, J.; Barreto, E.; Castillo, M.E.; Pachón, V.; Ferreiro, R.; Rodríguez-Garrote, M.; González-Martínez, S.; Ramon, Y.C.T.; et al. A comprehensive analysis of candidate genes in familial pancreatic cancer families reveals a high frequency of potentially pathogenic germline variants. *EBioMedicine* **2020**, *53*, 102675. [CrossRef]
51. Luu, M.; Visekruna, A. Short-chain fatty acids: Bacterial messengers modulating the immunometabolism of T cells. *Eur. J. Immunol.* **2019**, *49*, 842–848. [CrossRef]
52. Liu, T.; Sun, Z.; Yang, Z.; Qiao, X. Microbiota-derived short-chain fatty acids and modulation of host-derived peptides formation: Focused on host defense peptides. *Biomed. Pharmacother.* **2023**, *162*, 114586. [CrossRef] [PubMed]
53. Parisi, G.F.; Di Dio, G.; Franzonello, C.; Gennaro, A.; Rotolo, N.; Lionetti, E.; Leonardi, S. Liver disease in cystic fibrosis: An update. *Hepat. Mon.* **2013**, *13*, e11215. [CrossRef] [PubMed]
54. Debray, D.; Lykavieris, P.; Gauthier, F.; Dousset, B.; Sardet, A.; Munck, A.; Laselve, H.; Bernard, O. Outcome of cystic fibrosis-associated liver cirrhosis: Management of portal hypertension. *J. Hepatol.* **1999**, *31*, 77–83. [CrossRef] [PubMed]
55. Olivier, A.K.; Gibson-Corley, K.N.; Meyerholz, D.K. Animal models of gastrointestinal and liver diseases. Animal models of cystic fibrosis: Gastrointestinal, pancreatic, and hepatobiliary disease and pathophysiology. *Am. J. Physiol. Gastrointest. Liver Physiol.* **2015**, *308*, G459–G471. [CrossRef]
56. Kelleher, T.; Staunton, M.; O'Mahony, S.; McCormick, P.A. Advanced hepatocellular carcinoma associated with cystic fibrosis. *Eur. J. Gastroenterol. Hepatol.* **2005**, *17*, 1123–1124. [CrossRef]
57. McKeon, D.; Day, A.; Parmar, J.; Alexander, G.; Bilton, D. Hepatocellular carcinoma in association with cirrhosis in a patient with cystic fibrosis. *J. Cyst. Fibros.* **2004**, *3*, 193–195. [CrossRef]
58. Kinnman, N.; Lindblad, A.; Housset, C.; Buentke, E.; Scheynius, A.; Strandvik, B.; Hultcrantz, R. Expression of cystic fibrosis transmembrane conductance regulator in liver tissue from patients with cystic fibrosis. *Hepatology* **2000**, *32*, 334–340. [CrossRef]
59. Moribe, T.; Iizuka, N.; Miura, T.; Kimura, N.; Tamatsukuri, S.; Ishitsuka, H.; Hamamoto, Y.; Sakamoto, K.; Tamesa, T.; Oka, M. Methylation of multiple genes as molecular markers for diagnosis of a small, well-differentiated hepatocellular carcinoma. *Int. J. Cancer.* **2009**, *125*, 388–397. [CrossRef]
60. Paranjapye, A.; Ruffin, M.; Harris, A.; Corvol, H. Genetic variation in CFTR and modifier loci may modulate cystic fibrosis disease severity. *J. Cyst. Fibros.* **2020**, *19* (Suppl. 1), S10–S14. [CrossRef]
61. Namgoong, S.; Cheong, H.S.; Kim, J.O.; Kim, L.H.; Na, H.S.; Koh, I.S.; Chung, M.W.; Shin, H.D. Comparison of genetic variations of the SLCO1B1, SLCO1B3, and SLCO2B1 genes among five ethnic groups. *Environ. Toxicol. Pharmacol.* **2015**, *40*, 692–697. [CrossRef] [PubMed]
62. Maisonneuve, P.; Marshall, B.C.; Knapp, E.A.; Lowenfels, A.B. Cancer risk in cystic fibrosis: A 20-year nationwide study from the United States. *J. Natl. Cancer Inst.* **2013**, *105*, 122–129. [CrossRef] [PubMed]
63. Birch, R.J.; Peckham, D.; Wood, H.M.; Quirke, P.; Konstant-Hambling, R.; Brownlee, K.; Cosgriff, R.; Genomics England Research Consortium; Burr, N.; Downing, A. The risk of colorectal cancer in individuals with mutations of the cystic fibrosis transmembrane conductance regulator (CFTR) gene: An English population-based study. *J. Cyst. Fibros.* **2023**, *22*, 499–504. [CrossRef] [PubMed]
64. Miller, A.C.; Comellas, A.P.; Hornick, D.B.; Stoltz, D.A.; Cavanaugh, J.E.; Gerke, A.K.; Welsh, M.J.; Zabner, J.; Polgreen, P.M. Cystic fibrosis carriers are at increased risk for a wide range of cystic fibrosis-related conditions. *Proc. Natl. Acad. Sci. USA* **2020**, *117*, 1621–1627. [CrossRef] [PubMed]
65. Federico, A.; Morgillo, F.; Tuccillo, C.; Ciardiello, F.; Loguercio, C. Chronic inflammation and oxidative stress in human carcinogenesis. *Int. J. Cancer.* **2007**, *121*, 2381–2386. [CrossRef] [PubMed]
66. Zhao, H.; Ming, T.; Tang, S.; Ren, S.; Yang, H.; Liu, M.; Tao, Q.; Xu, H. Wnt signaling in colorectal cancer: Pathogenic role and therapeutic target. *Mol. Cancer.* **2022**, *21*, 144. [CrossRef] [PubMed]
67. Zhu, G.X.; Gao, D.; Shao, Z.Z.; Chen, L.; Ding, W.J.; Yu, Q.F. Wnt/β-catenin signaling: Causes and treatment targets of drug resistance in colorectal cancer (Review). *Mol. Med. Rep.* **2021**, *23*, 105. [CrossRef]
68. Perše, M. Oxidative stress in the pathogenesis of colorectal cancer: Cause or consequence? *Biomed. Res. Int.* **2013**, *2013*, 725710. [CrossRef]
69. Gilbert, B.; Kaiko, G.; Smith, S.; Wark, P. A systematic review of the colorectal microbiome in adult cystic fibrosis patients. *Colorectal Dis.* **2023**, *25*, 843–852. [CrossRef]
70. Karb, D.B.; Cummings, L.C. The Intestinal Microbiome and Cystic Fibrosis Transmembrane Conductance Regulator Modulators: Emerging Themes in the Management of Gastrointestinal Manifestations of Cystic Fibrosis. *Curr. Gastroenterol. Rep.* **2021**, *23*, 17. [CrossRef]
71. Amaral, M.D.; Quaresma, M.C.; Pankonien, I. What Role Does CFTR Play in Development, Differentiation, Regeneration and Cancer? *Int. J. Mol. Sci.* **2020**, *21*, 3133. [CrossRef]
72. Kim, J.; Lee, H.K. Potential Role of the Gut Microbiome In Colorectal Cancer Progression. *Front. Immunol.* **2022**, *12*, 807648. [CrossRef] [PubMed]
73. Abraham, J.M.; Taylor, C.J. Cystic Fibrosis & disorders of the large intestine: DIOS, constipation, and colorectal cancer. *J. Cyst. Fibros.* **2017**, *16* (Suppl. 2), S40–S49. [CrossRef] [PubMed]
74. Liu, C.; Song, C.; Li, J.; Sun, Q. CFTR Functions as a Tumor Suppressor and Is Regulated by DNA Methylation in Colorectal Cancer. *Cancer Manag. Res.* **2020**, *12*, 4261–4270. [CrossRef]

75. Mandal, R.K.; Khan, M.A.; Hussain, A.; Akhter, N.; Jawed, A.; Dar, S.A.; Wahid, M.; Panda, A.K.; Lohani, M.; Mishra, B.N.; et al. A trial sequential meta-analysis of TNF-α -308G>A (rs800629) gene polymorphism and susceptibility to colorectal cancer. *Biosci. Rep.* **2019**, *39*, BSR20181052. [CrossRef]
76. Smyth, A.R.; Bell, S.C.; Bojcin, S.; Bryon, M.; Duff, A.; Flume, P.; Kashirskaya, N.; Munck, A.; Ratjen, F.; Schwarzenberg, S.J.; et al. European Cystic Fibrosis Society Standards of Care: Best Practice guidelines. *J. Cyst. Fibros.* **2014**, *13* (Suppl. 1), S23–S42. [CrossRef] [PubMed]
77. Ingravalle, F.; Casella, G.; Ingravalle, A.; Monti, C.; De Salvatore, F.; Stillitano, D.; Villanacci, V. Surveillance of Colorectal Cancer (CRC) in Cystic Fibrosis (CF) Patients. *Gastrointest. Disorders.* **2021**, *3*, 84–95. [CrossRef]
78. Than, B.L.N.; Linnekamp, J.F.; Starr, T.K.; Largaespada, A.D.; Rod, A.; Zhang, Y.; Bruner, V.; Abrahante, J.; Schumann, A.; Luczak, T.; et al. CFTR is a tumor suppressor gene in murine and human intestinal cancer. *Oncogene* **2016**, *35*, 4179–4187. [CrossRef]
79. Gelsomino, F.; Balsano, R.; De Lorenzo, S.; Garajová, I. Small Bowel Adenocarcinoma: From Molecular Insights to Clinical Management. *Curr. Oncol.* **2022**, *29*, 1223–1236. [CrossRef]
80. Lam, G.Y.; Goodwin, J.; Wilcox, P.G.; Quon, B.S. Sex disparities in cystic fibrosis: Review on the effect of female sex hormones on lung pathophysiology and outcomes. *ERJ Open Res.* **2021**, *7*, 000475–2020. [CrossRef]
81. Garcia, F.U.; Galindo, L.M.; Holsclaw, D.S. Breast abnormalities in patients with cystic fibrosis: Previously unrecognized changes. *Ann. Diagn. Pathol.* **1998**, *2*, 281–285. [CrossRef] [PubMed]
82. Kelly, M.; Trudel, S.; Brouillard, F.; Bouillaud, F.; Colas, J.; Nguyen-Khoa, T.; Ollero, M.; Edelman, A.; Fritsch, J. Cystic fibrosis transmembrane regulator inhibitors CFTR(inh)-172 and GlyH-101 target mitochondrial functions, independently of chloride channel inhibition. *J. Pharmacol. Exp. Ther.* **2010**, *333*, 60–69. [CrossRef] [PubMed]
83. Chen, G.G.; Zeng, Q.; Tse, G.M. Estrogen and its receptors in cancer. *Med. Res. Rev.* **2008**, *28*, 954–974. [CrossRef] [PubMed]
84. Chotirmall, S.H.; Greene, C.M.; Oglesby, I.K.; Thomas, W.; O'Neill, S.J.; Harvey, B.J.; McElvaney, N.G. 17Beta-estradiol inhibits IL-8 in cystic fibrosis by up-regulating secretory leucoprotease inhibitor. *Am. J. Respir. Crit. Care Med.* **2010**, *182*, 62–72. [CrossRef]
85. Zhang, J.T.; Jiang, X.H.; Xie, C.; Cheng, H.; Dong, J.D.; Wang, Y.; Fok, K.L.; Zhang, X.H.; Sun, T.T.; Tsang, L.L.; et al. Downregulation of CFTR promotes epithelial-to-mesenchymal transition and is associated with poor prognosis of breast cancer. *Biochim. Biophys. Acta Mol. Cell Res.* **2013**, *1833*, 2961–2969. [CrossRef] [PubMed]
86. Hughan, K.S.; Daley, T.; Rayas, M.S.; Kelly, A.; Roe, A. Female reproductive health in cystic fibrosis. *J. Cyst. Fibros.* **2019**, *18* (Suppl. 2), S95–S104. [CrossRef] [PubMed]
87. Archangelidi, O.; Cullinan, P.; Simmonds, N.J.; Mentzakis, E.; Peckham, D.; Bilton, D.; Carr, S.B. Incidence and risk factors of cancer in individuals with cystic fibrosis in the UK; a case-control study. *J. Cyst. Fibros.* **2022**, *21*, 302–308. [CrossRef] [PubMed]
88. Iima, M.; Le Bihan, D. The road to breast cancer screening with diffusion MRI. *Front. Oncol.* **2023**, *13*, 993540. [CrossRef]
89. Vekens, K.; Vincken, S.; Hanon, S.; Demuynck, K.; Stylemans, D.; Vanderhelst, E. Lung cancer in a CF patient: Combination of bad luck or is there more to say? *Acta Clin. Belg.* **2021**, *76*, 379–380. [CrossRef]
90. Rousset-Jablonski, C.; Dalon, F.; Reynaud, Q.; Lemonnier, L.; Dehillotte, C.; Jacoud, F.; Berard, M.; Viprey, M.; Van Ganse, E.; Durieu, I.; et al. Cancer incidence and prevalence in cystic fibrosis patients with and without a lung transplant in France. *Front. Public Health* **2022**, *10*, 1043691. [CrossRef]
91. Cabrini, G.; Rimessi, A.; Borgatti, M.; Lampronti, I.; Finotti, A.; Pinton, P.; Gambari, R. Role of Cystic Fibrosis Bronchial Epithelium in Neutrophil Chemotaxis. *Front. Immunol.* **2020**, *11*, 1438. [CrossRef] [PubMed]
92. Jeffery, P.K.; Brain, A.P. Surface morphology of human airway mucosa: Normal, carcinoma or cystic fibrosis. *Scanning Microsc.* **1988**, *2*, 553–560. [PubMed]
93. Patel, V.; Majumdar, T.; Samreen, I.; Grewal, H.; Kaleekal, T. Primary lung carcinoma in cystic fibrosis: A case report and literature review. *Respir. Med. Case Rep.* **2020**, *31*, 101242. [CrossRef] [PubMed]
94. Raju, S.V.; Jackson, P.L.; Courville, C.A.; McNicholas, C.M.; Sloane, P.A.; Sabbatini, G.; Tidwell, S.; Tang, L.P.; Liu, B.; Fortenberry, J.A.; et al. Cigarette smoke induces systemic defects in cystic fibrosis transmembrane conductance regulator function. *Am. J. Respir. Crit. Care Med.* **2013**, *188*, 1321–1330. [CrossRef] [PubMed]
95. Verma, A.; Clough, D.; McKenna, D.; Dodd, M.; Webb, A.K. Smoking and cystic fibrosis. *J. R. Soc. Med.* **2001**, *94* (Suppl. 40), 29–34. [CrossRef]
96. Oh, I.-H.; Oh, C.; Yoon, T.-Y.; Choi, J.-M.; Kim, S.K.; Park, H.J.; Eun, Y.G.; Chung, D.H.; Kwon, K.H.; Choe, B.-K. Association of CFTR gene polymorphisms with papillary thyroid cancer. *Oncol. Lett.* **2012**, *3*, 455–461. [CrossRef] [PubMed]
97. Bell, S.C.; Mall, M.A.; Gutierrez, H.; Macek, M.; Madge, S.; Davies, J.C.; Burgel, P.-R.; Tullis, E.; Castaños, C.; Castellani, C.; et al. The future of cystic fibrosis care: A global perspective. *Lancet Respir. Med.* **2020**, *8*, 65–124, Erratum in *Lancet Respir. Med.* **2019**, *7*, e40. [CrossRef]
98. Jia, S.; Taylor-Cousar, J.L. Cystic Fibrosis Modulator Therapies. *Annu. Rev. Med.* **2023**, *74*, 413–426. [CrossRef]
99. Giallongo, A.; Parisi, G.F.; Papale, M.; Manti, S.; Mulé, E.; Aloisio, D.; Terlizzi, V.; Rotolo, N.; Leonardi, S. Effects of Elexacaftor/Tezacaftor/Ivacaftor on Cardiorespiratory Polygraphy Parameters and Respiratory Muscle Strength in Cystic Fibrosis Patients with Severe Lung Disease. *Genes* **2023**, *14*, 449. [CrossRef]
100. Balfour-Lynn, I.M.; King, J.A. CFTR modulator therapies-Effect on life expectancy in people with cystic fibrosis. *Paediatr. Respir. Rev.* **2022**, *42*, 3–8. [CrossRef]

101. Dagenais, R.V.E.; Su, V.C.H.; Quon, B.S. Real-World Safety of CFTR Modulators in the Treatment of Cystic Fibrosis: A Systematic Review. *J. Clin. Med.* **2020**, *10*, 23. [CrossRef]
102. Higgins, M.; Volkova, N.; Moy, K.; Marshall, B.C.; Bilton, D. Real-World Outcomes Among Patients with Cystic Fibrosis Treated with Ivacaftor: 2012-2016 Experience. *Pulm. Ther.* **2020**, *6*, 141–149. [CrossRef]
103. Bai, Y.; Higgins, M.; Volkova, N.; Bengtsson, L.; Tian, S.; Sewall, A.; Nyangoma, S.; Elbert, A.; Bilton, D. Real-world outcomes in patients (PTS) with cystic fibrosis (CF) treated with ivacaftor (IVA): Analysis of 2014 US and UK CF registries. *J. Cyst. Fibros.* **2016**, *15*, S41. [CrossRef]
104. Chilvers, M.A.; Davies, J.C.; Milla, C.; Tian, S.; Han, Z.; Cornell, A.G.; Owen, A.C.; Ratjen, F. Long-term safety and efficacy of lumacaftor-ivacaftor therapy in children aged 6-11 years with cystic fibrosis homozygous for the F508del-CFTR mutation: A phase 3, open-label, extension. *Lancet Respir. Med.* **2021**, *9*, 721–732. [CrossRef]

Disclaimer/Publisher's Note: The statements, opinions and data contained in all publications are solely those of the individual author(s) and contributor(s) and not of MDPI and/or the editor(s). MDPI and/or the editor(s) disclaim responsibility for any injury to people or property resulting from any ideas, methods, instructions or products referred to in the content.

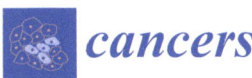

Review

PIWI-RNAs Small Noncoding RNAs with Smart Functions: Potential Theranostic Applications in Cancer

Simona Taverna [1,*], Anna Masucci [2] and Giuseppe Cammarata [1,*]

1. Institute of Translational Pharmacology (IFT), National Research Council (CNR), 90146 Palermo, Italy
2. Department of Biomedicine, Neurosciences and Advanced Diagnostics, Institute of Clinical Biochemistry, Clinical Molecular Medicine, Laboratory Medicine, University of Palermo, 90127 Palermo, Italy; anna.masucci@community.unipa.it
* Correspondence: simona.taverna@cnr.it (S.T.); giuseppe.cammarata@ift.cnr.it (G.C.)

Simple Summary: P-element-induced wimpy testis-interacting RNAs (piRNAs) are a novel class of small regulatory RNAs that often bind to PIWI proteins. First identified in animal germ line cells, piRNAs have key roles in germ line development. New insights into the functions of PIWI-piRNA complexes demonstrate that they regulate protein-coding genes. Aberrant piRNA expression has been also associated with different diseases, including cancer. Recently, piRNAs have been described in extracellular vesicles. EVs are one of the components of liquid biopsy, a revolutionary technique for detecting specific molecular biomarkers. This review focuses on piRNAs as potential biomarkers in different cancer types. Furthermore, piRNAs contained in extracellular vesicles could represent a new route for early diagnosis and therapies in a personalized medicine approach.

Abstract: P-element-induced wimpy testis (PIWI)-interacting RNAs (piRNAs) are a new class of small noncoding RNAs (ncRNAs) that bind components of the PIWI protein family. piRNAs are specifically expressed in different human tissues and regulate important signaling pathways. Aberrant expressions of piRNAs and PIWI proteins have been associated with tumorigenesis and cancer progression. Recent studies reported that piRNAs are contained in extracellular vesicles (EVs), nanosized lipid particles, with key roles in cell–cell communication. EVs contain several bioactive molecules, such as proteins, lipids, and nucleic acids, including emerging ncRNAs. EVs are one of the components of liquid biopsy (LB) a non-invasive method for detecting specific molecular biomarkers in liquid samples. LB could become a crucial tool for cancer diagnosis with piRNAs as biomarkers in a precision oncology approach. This review summarizes the current findings on the roles of piRNAs in different cancer types, focusing on potential theranostic applications of piRNAs contained in EVs (EV-piRNAs). Their roles as non-invasive diagnostic and prognostic biomarkers and as new therapeutic options have been also discussed.

Keywords: piRNAs; PIWI proteins; ncRNAs; extracellular vesicles; biomarkers; epidrugs

1. Introduction

Only 1–2% of transcriptomes are protein encoding. The latest evidence proved that a large scale of mammal genomes is transcribed to noncoding RNAs (ncRNAs). ncRNAs have emerged as an important class of genetic regulators, and their value in human diseases is becoming progressively more evident [1]. These molecules are often dysregulated in human cancers and can affect cancer progression via different mechanisms such as transcriptional and post-transcriptional modifications, epigenetics, and signal transduction [2]. The pivotal role of many ncRNAs in cancer is widely demonstrated, and they can be functionally classified into oncogenes or tumor suppressors [3–5]. ncRNAs are a heterogeneous family characterized by different lengths, biogenesis, and biological function, including (i) short ncRNAs as microRNAs (miRNAs), piwi-interacting RNAs (piRNAs), small nuclear-RNAs (snRNAs), and small nucleolar-RNAs (snoRNAs), and (ii) long ncRNAs, including circular RNAs (circRNAs) and long noncoding RNAs (lncRNAs) [4,6,7]. Among the short ncRNAs, piRNAs have emerged as the newest members of this family that are being recognized as important mediators of cell biology [8]. Several studies report that extracellular vesicles (EVs) deliver several biologically active molecules with a key role in cell–cell communication. EVs carry a wide range of cargo, such as ncRNAs, including piRNAs, which are selectively loaded into the vesicles [9]. Thus, strategies to specifically target ncRNAs contained in EVs (EV-ncRNAs) are an attractive therapeutic option [10]. This review focuses on piRNA functions in cancers and their potential clinical implications. Moreover, we discuss the potential of EV-ncRNAs as non-invasive diagnostic and prognostic biomarkers and as new therapeutic options.

2. Biogenesis of piRNAs

piRNAs were first found in germline cells and are considered critical regulators of germline maintenance. These animal-specific short-chain RNAs have a size of 24–32 nucleotides and a 2′-O-methylation at the 3′ end, a distinctive and exclusive feature of all piRNAs, and are associated with PIWI proteins. These proteins belong to the Argonaute protein family [9], which were discovered, for the first time, in *Drosophila melanogaster* ovarian germ cells and follicular cells [10]. piRNAs can bind DNA sequences of specific genes via complementary base pairing to silence transposons and regulate gene expression. The human genome contains over 30,000 piRNA genes that are mainly derived from intergenic regions. According to multiple origins, piRNAs are divided into three subclasses: mRNA-derived, lncRNA-derived, and transposon-derived piRNAs [11]. piRNAs transcribed from transposons are known as "piRNA clusters". These clusters are mainly located in the pericentromeric and sub-telomeric parts of the chromosomes. piRNA clusters are transcribed to form piRNA precursors via bidirectional or unidirectional transcription. Moreover, piRNAs can be generated from mRNA 3′ untranslated region (3′ UTR) and some long non-coding regions in the genome [12]. The mechanism of piRNA production includes two steps: a primary and a secondary amplification cycle described as the "ping-pong cycle", in which piRNAs are bound to PIWI proteins [13]. In primary amplification, newly transcribed piRNAs are exported through the nuclear envelope, processed, and matured. In the cytoplasm, the secondary structures are resolved via RNA helicase Armitage (Armi). After, piRNA precursors are cleaved by mitochondria-associated endonuclease Zucchini (Zuc) and transformed into pre-piRNAs with a 5′ monophosphate. Then, pre-piRNAs are loaded onto PIWI proteins and cut at the 3′ ends by a 3′ to 5′ exonuclease, Nibbler (Nbr) [12]. After, 3′ terminal ends are methylated at 2′ oxygen by RNA2′-O-methyltransferase Hen1 [13]. piRNAs produced in this way are named primary piRNAs. In secondary amplification, piRNAs' generation is increased with the involvement of Argonauta 3 (Ago 3) and Aubergine (Aub) proteins. Aub binds to antisense strand piRNAs and cleaves sense piRNA precursors, giving rise to sense piRNAs bound by Ago3. In contrast, Ago3 binds to sense-strand piRNAs and cleaves antisense piRNA precursors, producing antisense piRNAs that load onto Aub [14]. The round of cleavage repeats and produces several piRNA molecules. These piRNAs are then bound by PIWI proteins and transported back to the nucleus to silence target genes. Two Tudor-domain containing piRNA factors, Krimper (Krimp) and Qin/Kumo, play crucial roles in making Aub-AGO3 heterotypic ping-pong robust. This maintains the levels of piRNAs loaded onto Piwi and Aub to efficiently repress transposons at transcriptional and post-transcriptional levels, respectively [15].

To summarize, in the primary pathway, piRNA forms a complex with PIWI proteins to mediate transposon silencing. In the secondary pathway, piRNA binds to Aub protein to produce secondary piRNA, while secondary piRNA binds to Ago3 to produce primary piRNA, and the cycle continues [9] (Figure 1). Although with some differences, the piRNA ping-pong mechanism exists not only in germ cells but also in somatic cells [14]. Despite increasing interest in the role of piRNAs in human diseases, their homeostasis in cells is still a poorly understood process. RNAs' cellular concentration is maintained by a balance of biogenesis and degradation. PIWI proteins protect piRNAs from this degradation. However, when piRNAs are released from the PIWI complex, their 5′ end and 3′ end become unprotected and can easily be accessed by exoribonucleases. The degradation of human piRNAs is mainly dependent on the 5′-3′ exoribonuclease pathway mediated by XRN1 and XRN2, the two major 5′-3′ exoribonucleases involved in piRNA degradation in human somatic cells (Figure 2). It was also reported that the presence of 3′-end 2′-O-methylation in piRNAs reduced their degradation through an exosome-mediated decay pathway [16].

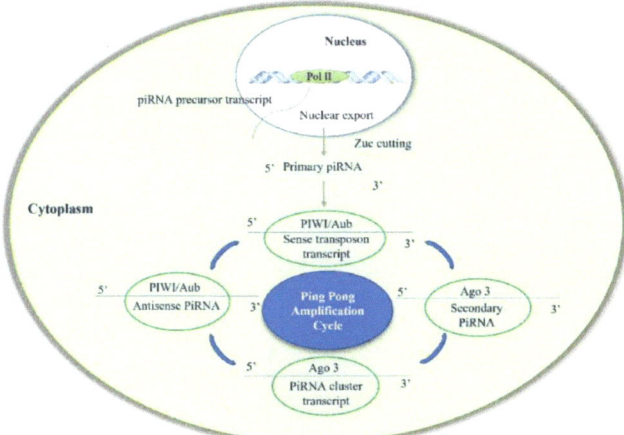

Figure 1. Simplified representation of the currently proposed model of piRNA biogenesis. Two steps of piRNA biogenesis: (1) primary amplification cycle in nucleus and (2) secondary amplification cycle described as "ping-pong cycle" in cytoplasm. Abbreviations: Pol II: polymerase II; Zuc: endonuclease Zucchini; Aub: Aubergine protein; Ago 3: Argonauta 3 protein.

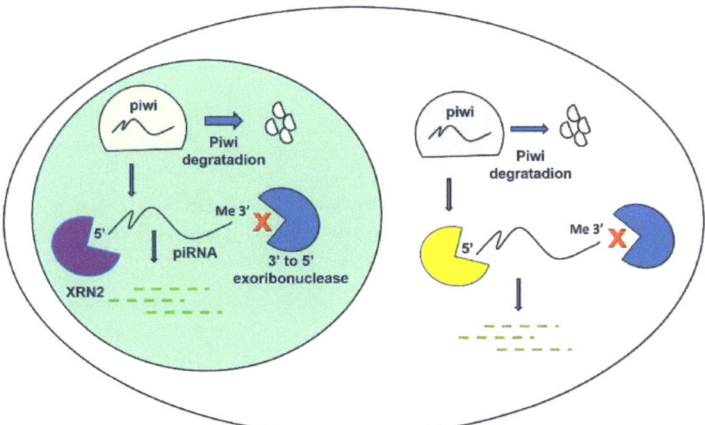

Figure 2. Homeostasis of piRNA in human cells. The degradation of human piRNAs depends on 5′-3′ exoribonuclease.

3. Function of piRNAs and PIWI Proteins

Depending on the context, piRNAs can act in the following different ways: transposon silencing, epigenetic regulation, germ stem cell maintenance, and genome rearrangement. Recently, piRNAs have been described in tumorigenesis and in various steps of cancer progression, such as proliferation, invasion, metastasis, apoptosis, and drug resistance [17] (Figure 3). piRNAs act in reproduction, in a PIWI-dependent manner, and in fertility regulation by attaching to PIWI proteins and forming a silencing ribonucleoprotein complex [9]. It seems likely their ancestral function was an adaptive mechanism to silence active transposable elements (TEs). Through complementary sequences, piRNA cluster transcripts recognize TEs, avoiding their expression, which might lead to a loss of genome integrity. piRNAs can regulate cellular processes with different mechanisms, also independently of PIWI proteins, such as increasing translation or stabilizing mRNA [18]. Recent findings on piRNAs' biological significance suggest that they can somatically regulate gene expression also via epigenetic alterations [19]. Epigenetic global changes in cancer include DNA methylation, DNA hypomethylation, CpG island methylation, and gene-specific DNA hypermethylation, leading to oncogene activation (Ras, cyclin D2) [20] and tumor suppressor silencing (RB1, p16) [21]. It was demonstrated that aberrant DNA methylation in tumor cells is linked to PIWI/piRNA disorders. Therefore, piRNA deregulation may influence the expression and stability of the genome, causing cell signaling alteration, which, in turn, may induce disease onset and progression [22–28].

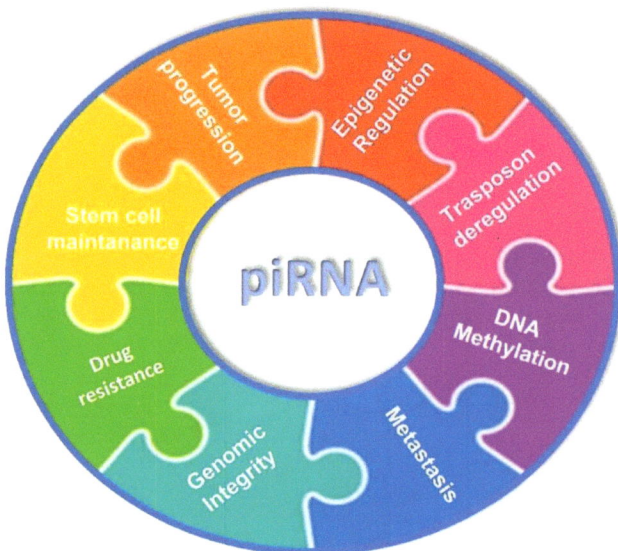

Figure 3. piRNA involvement in different biological processes, hallmarks of cancer, such as tumor progression, epigenetic regulation, transposon deregulation, DNA methylation, metastasis, genomic integrity, drug resistance, and stem cell maintenance.

PIWI family proteins consist of four members crucial for the biogenesis and function of small ncRNAs: PIWIL1, PIWIL2, PIWIL3, and PIWIL4. PIWIL proteins bind piRNAs, as a unique type of small ncRNA, forming a PIWI/piRNA complex. This complex exerts the gene regulation function, playing an important role in the stability and integrity maintenance of the germ cell genome [8]. PIWI/piRNA acts as an epigenetic modulator recruiting other epigenetic regulatory factors, such as DNA methylase, beyond its function of directly cutting and degrading target RNA, acting like an Ago protein/miRNA complex. PIWI family proteins have been considered prognostic markers for various malignancies [29]. Although specific mechanisms need further investigation, various studies have demonstrated that PIWI proteins, expressed in many cancers, affect multiple biological processes, also without interacting with piRNAs, including different steps of cancer progression such as cell proliferation, apoptosis, migration, invasion, cell cycle regulation, and self-renewal [30] (Figure 4). Specific examples of PIWIL proteins involved in cancer are described below.

PIWIL1 is the most studied PIWI protein that regulates gene expression, apoptosis, cell cycle, and proliferation. PIWIL1 is a coactivator of adenomatous polyposis coli C-terminal domain C complex that targets cell adhesion protein, Pinin, for proteolytic ubiquitination, thus promoting metastasis in pancreatic cancer (PC) [31]. PIWIL2 overexpression functions as an oncogene; its deregulation plays an important role in cancer progression and is associated with poor survival and aggressive clinicopathological properties of patients [32]. The deregulation of PIWIL3 is reported in many cancer types; it is highly expressed in both primary ovarian cancer (OC) and metastatic tissues [33]. PIWIL3 plays an important role in melanoma, and its expression correlates with the tumor stage [34]. In gastric cancer (GC), PIWIL3 upregulation increases cell proliferation, migration, and invasion [35]. Conversely, PIWIL3 overexpression seems to have a protective effect in glioma cell lines and decreased tumor size in vivo [36]. Moreover, PIWIL3 is considered a prognostic biomarker of breast cancer (BC) since its upregulation is significantly associated with poor overall survival [37].

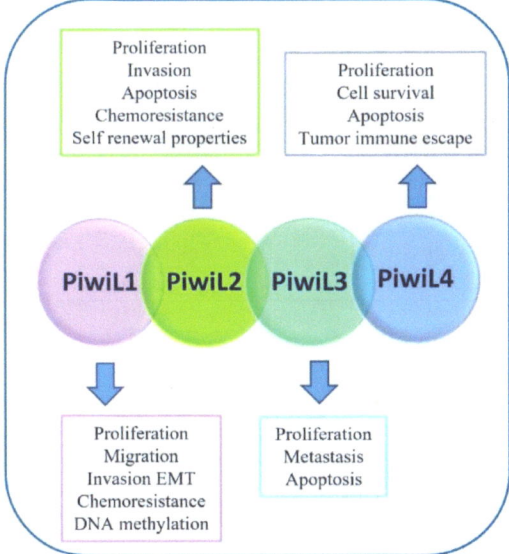

Figure 4. Roles of the four members of PIWI protein family. PIWI1, PIWI2, PIWI3, and PIWI4 have several roles in the steps of cancer progression (such as proliferation, migration, invasion, cell survival, tumor escape, chemoresistance, self-renewal properties, metastasis, apoptosis, EMT: epithelial–mesenchymal transition) and epigenetic regulation (DNA methylation).

PIWIL4 is involved in chromatin modifications in human somatic cells [38], and it can process precursor hairpins generating miRNAs in DICER independent manner [39]. PIWIL4 role in tumorigenesis is controversial; high expressions of PIWIL4 are found in colorectal, cervical, gastric, and ovarian cancer [40,41]. However, other studies reported that low PIWIL4 expression is associated with a poor prognosis in different cancer types [37]. Furthermore, the lack of PIWIL4 expression triggered by CpG island hypermethylation has been found in testicular tumors [42] (Table 1).

Table 1. PIWI protein expression and function in different cancers.

Piwi Protein	Cancer type	Expression	Function	References
PIWIL1	Gasric	Upregulated	Migration proliferation invasion	[32]
	Mieloma Multiple	Upregulated	Chemoresistance	[30]
	Lung	Upregulated	proliferation migration	[31]
	Breast	Upregulated	DNA methylation	[33]
PIWIL2	Colon Rectal	Uperegulation	Chemoresistance Proliferation	[19,22]
	Gastric	Downregulated	Self renewal properties	[19]
	Ovarian	Upregulated	Apoptosis	[20]
	Breast	Upregulated	Chemoresistance	[19]
PIWIL3	Breast	Upregulated	Proliferation Cell survival	[24]
	Ovarian	Metastasis	Metastasis	[20]
	Mieloma Multiple	Upregulated	Apoptosis	[21]
	Gastric	Upregulated	proliferation migration invasion	[22]
	Glioma	Downregulated	Tumor immune escape	[23]
PIWIL4	Lung	Upregulated	Proliferation	[39]
	Liver	Upregulated	Metastasis	[27]
	Gastric	Upregulated	Apoptosis	[28]
	Testicular	Downpregulated	Proliferation	[29]
	Ovarian	Upregulated	Metastasis	[20]

4. piRNAs in Cancer

Cancer and germ cells share important biological characteristics such as rapid proliferation and the ability for self-renewal. Recently, a growing number of studies have revealed the role of piRNAs in cancers, launching a new biological concept in which piRNAs mediate a gene regulation mechanism typical of germline cells in somatic cells [43]. It is plausible that cancer cells with a high proliferation rate can adopt and utilize self-renewal machinery like germ cells. In malignant cells, piRNAs are involved in epigenetic regulation and may be crucial to sustaining cancer stemness [30].

4.1. Role of piRNAs in Cancer Initiation and Progression

Several piRNAs affect cancer stem cells (CSCs) and somatic cells by regulating gene expression via epigenetic processes. CSCs are a small population of cancer cells with high heterogeneity and a great capacity to renew tumors. Aberrant expressions of piRNAs and PIWI proteins also in CSCs can regulate tumor initiation and progression. Examples of specific piRNAs involved in cancer are described below. In non-small cell lung cancer (NSCLC), piR-651 upregulation correlates with a significant increase in tumor growth and metastasis, affecting cell cycle arrest and inducing cyclin D1 and CDK4 and suggesting piR-651 as a potential oncogene. piR-651 overexpression promotes proliferation and invasion and reduces cell apoptosis by inducing different oncogene (CDK4, Cyclin D1, and MDM2) expressions [44]. In addition, piR-651 can increase phosphatase and tensin homolog (PTEN) methylation via DNA (cytosine-5)-methyltransferase 1 (DNMT1) [45]. It was also demonstrated that piR-651 is down-regulated in patients with Hodgkin lymphoma (HL) with respect to healthy controls; low levels of piR-651 correlate with poor prognosis in HL patients [46]. High expressions of piR-30473 support the aggressive phenotype of diffuse large B-cell lymphoma, exerting its oncogenic role through a mechanism involving the upregulation of Wilms Tumor-1 Associated Protein (WTAP), an m6A mRNA methylase, that enhances the global m6A level. WTAP induces the expression of its critical target gene, hexokinase 2 (HK2), by enhancing HK2 m6A level, thereby promoting lymphoma progression [47]. An imbalance in piRNA regulatory processes modifies several levels of gene regulation that control DNA damage repair, chromatin organization, and mitogenic signals, inducing uncontrolled cell proliferation [48]. piR-55490 expression is downregulated in lung cancer (LC), restoring piR-55490 can reduce LC cell proliferation rates, whereas suppressing piR-55490 increases cell proliferation rates. piR-55490 acts by inhibiting the serine/threonine kinase 1 (AKT)/mTOR pathway, thereby suppressing cell growth [49]. piR-211106 binding to pyruvate carboxylase can inhibit the progression of LC-enhancing chemotherapy sensitivity, suggesting that it is a potential therapeutic target [50]. In BC has been described an aberrant expression of various piRNAs. piR-36712 is lowly expressed in this cancer type compared with non-tumor tissues and acts as a possible tumor suppressor. It was also reported that piR-36712 upregulation has a synergistic anticancer effect with chemotherapy on BC cells via the Interaction with SEPW1 pseudogene SEPW1P RNA [51]. piR-36712 can be considered a novel tumor suppressor and a prognostic predictor of BC. Moreover, piR-36712 modulates the expression levels of tumor suppressor genes p53 and P21; its increase leads to cell cycle arrest in the G0/G1 phase of cancer cells [52]. piR-021285 induces methylation at cancer-relevant genes, and it is considered a potential modulator of BC invasiveness by remodeling the cancer epigenome. The exogenous expression of piR-021285 induces significant methylation differences at BC-related genes, including the attenuated methylation of 5' UTR first exon at the pro-invasive ARHGAP11A gene. There is an increased ARHGAP11A mRNA expression and enhanced invasiveness in variant versus WT piR-021285 mimic-transfected BC cell lines, supporting the role of this piRNA in tumorigenesis via a piRNA-mediated epigenetic mechanism [53]. In clear cells renal carcinoma (ccRC), by using piRNA microarray in a large cohort study, three piRNAs (piR-30924, piR-57125, and piR-38756) have been identified as piRNAs significantly associated with tumor recurrence and overall survival [54]. In cells and plasma of various cancer patients, an altered expression of piR-823 has been observed, with a role in regulating tumor cell growth. In GC, piR-823 acts as a tumor suppressor, and its expression is dramatically decreased in GC tissues. The restoration of piR-823 in GC cells inhibits cancer cell growth both in vitro and in vivo [55]. Also, in colorectal cancer (CRC), piR-823 downregulation inhibits cell proliferation and increases cell apoptosis by inducing an apoptosis activator gene, the transcription factor HSF1 [56]. Moreover, in CRC tissue and serum, piR-54265 is upregulated and induces cancer progression activating STAT3 signaling [57]. Furthermore, it was reported that piR-18 is involved and contributed to the tumorigenesis and progression of CRC. The overexpression of piR-18 inhibits the cell proliferation, migration, and invasion of CRC; thus, it could potentially be used as a new biomarker for diagnosis and therapy [52]. In hepatocellular carcinoma (HCC), a new piRNA, piR-Hep1 has been identified; it is upregulated in HCC with respect to non-tumoral liver cells. The silencing of piR-Hep1 inhibits cell viability, migration, and invasion, with a concomitant decrease in AKT phosphorylation [58,59] (Figure 5).

In BC, piR-2158 is downregulated in CSCs; it was demonstrated that the overexpression of piR-2158 prevents mammary gland tumorigenesis via regulating CSCs and tumor angiogenesis. piR-2158 acts as a transcriptional repressor of Interleukin 11 (IL11) by competing with AP-1 transcription factor subunit FOSL1 to bind the promoter of IL11. piR-2158 can also provide a potential therapeutic strategy in BC treatment [60]. Moreover, the piRNA/PIWI complex can selectively control the phosphorylation of target proteins. It was reported that piR-54265-binding PIWIL2 promotes the formation of PIWIL2/STAT3/phosphorylated SRC complex, inducing phosphorylated SRC-mediated STAT3 phosphorylation that, in turn, causes the proliferation, metastasis, and chemotherapy resistance of CRC cells [19]. The piR-823/PIWIL2 complex mediates STAT3 phosphorylation and the activation of the STAT3/BCL-xl/cyclin D1 pathway, inducing the expression of cyclin-dependent kinase inhibitors and controlling G1 phase regulators Cyclin D1 and CDK4, thus promoting CRC progression [39]. piRNA/PIWI complex can interact with other ncRNAs, including miRNAs and lncRNAs, to regulate cancer progression. piR-30188/PIWIL3 binds to OIP5-AS1, a cancer-associated lncRNA, a target of miR-367-3p in gliomas. miR-367-3p negatively regulates CEBPA mRNA expression and increases TRAF4 expression [36]. The combination of OIP5-AS1 knockdown with the over-expression of PIWIL3 and miR-367-3p leads to tumor regression, identifying a novel molecular pathway in glioma cells that may provide a potential innovative approach for cancer therapy [23]. Overall, these findings indicate that piRNAs can have several potential clinical applications in diagnosis, prognosis, and therapy (Table 2).

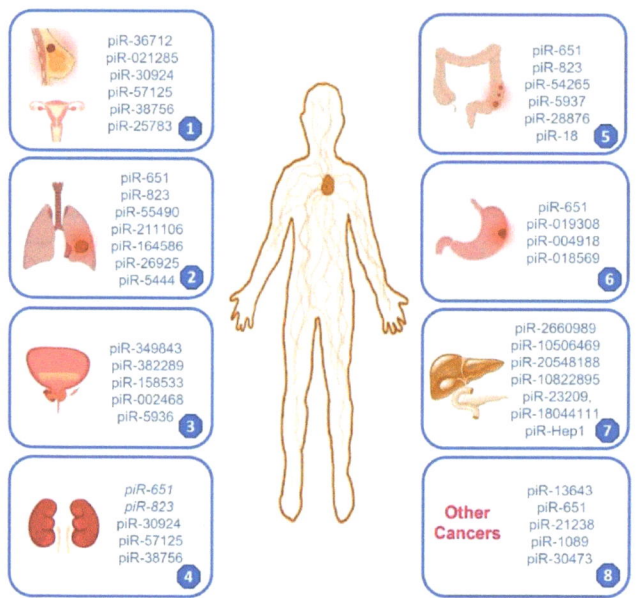

Figure 5. Schematic representation of the piRNAs localization in various cancer types. 1: Breast and ovarian cancer; 2: lung cancer; 3: prostate cancer; 4: renal cancer; 5: colon rectal cancer; 6: gastric cancer; 7: pancreatic and biliary cancer; 8: other cancer type.

Table 2. piRNA localization and their potential clinical applications in different cancers.

Cancer Type	piRNA	Expression	Sample Type	Target	Potential Clinical Application	References
Lung	piR-651	Upregulation	Cell	CDK4 Cyclin D1 MDM2 PTEN DNMT1	Diagnosis	[34,51]
	piR-211106	Upregulation	Cell	Pyruvate carboxylase	Therapy	[56]
	piR-55490	Downregulation	Cell	AKT mTOR	Therapy	[55]
	piR-5444	Upregulation	EV		Diagnosis Prognosis Therapy	[61]
	piR-26925	Upregulation	EV		Diagnosis Prognosis Therapy	[61]
	piR-164586	Upregulation	EV		Diagnosis	[62]

Table 2. Cont.

Cancer Type	piRNA	Expression	Sample Type	Target	Potential Clinical Application	References
Gastric	piR-823	Downregulation	Cell Plasma		Diagnosis	[63]
	piR-019308	Upregulation	EV		Diagnosis	[64]
	piR-004918	Upregulation	EV		Diagnosis	[64]
	piR-018569	Upregulation	EV		Diagnosis	[64]
Breast	piR-2158	Downregulation	Stem cell	IL11	Therapy	[65]
	piR-823	Upregulation	Stem cell	DNMT	Therapy	[66]
	piR-36712	Upregulation	Cell	SEPW1 p53 p21	Prognosis	[57,58]
	piR-021285	Upregulation	Cell	ARHGAP11A	Therapy	[53,61]
Colon Rectal	piR-823	Downregulation	Cell	HSF1		[67]
	piR-54265	Upregulation	Tissue Serum	STAT3	Prognosis	[35]
	piR-5937	Upregulation	Serum		Diagnosis	[68]
	piR-28876	Upregulation	Serum		Diagnosis	[68]
	piR-18	Upregulation	Tissue Cell		Diagnosis Therapy	[58]
Liver	piR-Hep1	Upregulation	Tissue Cell	AKT	Diagnosis	[69,70]
Neuroblastoma	piR-1089	Upregulation	EV	KEAP1	Prognosis	[71]
Lymphoma	piR-651	Downregulation	Serum		Prognosis	[52]
Renal	piR-38756	Upregulation	Tissue		Prognosis	[60]
	piR-57125	Upregulation	Tissue		Prognosis	[60]
	piR-30924	Upregulation	Tissue		Prognosis	[60]
B-cell lymphoma	piR-30473	Upregulation	Serum	WTAP HK2	Prognosis	[53]
Bladder	piR-5936	Upregulation	Plasma EV		Diagnosis	[72,73]
Ovarian	piR-25783	Upregulation	Plasma EV		Diagnosis Prognosis	[74]
Thyroid	piR-13643	Upregulation	Tissue		Diagnosis	[75]
	piR-21238	Upregulation	Tissue		Diagnosis	[75]
Cholangio Gallbladder	piR-2660989	Upregulation	EV		Diagnosis Prognosis	[76]
	piR-10506469	Upregulation	EV		Diagnosis Prognosis	[76]
	piR-20548188	Upregulation	EV		Diagnosis Prognosis	[76]
	piR-10822895	Upregulation	EV		Diagnosis Prognosis	[76]
	piR-23209	Upregulation	EV		Diagnosis Prognosis	[76]
	piR-18044111	Upregulation	EV		Diagnosis Prognosis	[76]

4.2. piRNAs as Cancer Biomarkers

ncRNAs have received a lot of attention as one factor contributing to genetic and epigenetic instability. Clinically, ncRNA alterations have a relevant diagnostic and prognostic significance [26]. Epigenetic biomarkers can be useful in predicting therapeutic drug responses, and piRNAs are considered emerging biomarkers for therapy monitoring. A biomarker is a significant indicator that can be used to assess a target's diagnostic potential, risk of recurrence, and clinical prognosis [63]. Aberrant expressions of piRNAs and their correlation with cancer patient features suggest that these may have an important clinical impact, not only as diagnostic biomarkers but also as druggable targets [67]. Altered piRNA levels may be considered good cancer biomarkers, with higher sensitivity and specificity than miRNAs [69]. Nowadays, few studies investigate the role of piRNAs as cancer biomarkers, but the field is in progress and updated [70]. Some studies indicate that piRNAs have a better diagnostic ability than traditional biomarkers. It was reported that piR-13643 and piR-21238 performed better than conventional biomarkers, such as hector battifora mesothelial antigen-1 (HBME1), conventionally used to discriminate malignant nodules from benign ones in papillary thyroid carcinoma [65]. Moreover, serum piR-5937 and piR-28876 were able to distinguish CRC from healthy controls with higher sensitivity and specificity than traditional markers such as Carcinoembryonic Antigen (CEA) and Carbohydrate antigen 19-9 (CA199) [61]. It was also suggested that piR-54265 can be used as a biomarker for the early detection and clinical monitoring of CRC [77].

5. piRNAs and Liquid Biopsy

Liquid biopsy is considered an ideal tool for discovering new cancer biomarkers, and in the current era of personalized medicine, LB has acquired high relevance in cancer patient management [66]. LB serves as a safe alternative to solid biopsies; its main components are circulating tumor cells (CTCs), circulating tumor DNA (ctDNA), circulating tumor RNA (ctRNA), tumor-associated platelets, and EVs [78]. Nowadays, clinical oncology adopts next-generation sequencing (NGS)-based diagnostics; these high throughput technologies allow for the identification of ncRNA profiles and significant genetic mutations across the human genome. LB is increasingly being used for early diagnosis and to determine the best therapeutic option for cancer patients [79].

5.1. piRNAs in Extracellular Vesicles

Extracellular vesicles (EVs) are nanoscale membrane particles released by all cytotypes in physiological and pathological conditions. EVs are internalized by target cells through a different mechanism and transport a plethora of bioactive molecules, including proteins, lipids, and nucleic acids [68,75,80–82]. EVs have a key role in several steps of cancer progression; they are involved in proliferation, migration, premetastatic niche formation, and immune response [62,76]. EVs have been reported to contain an abundance of RNAs, such as ncRNAs, including miRNAs, lncRNAs, circRNAs, and piRNAs [74]. The packaging of different ncRNAs into EVs is selective and mirrors the status of parental cells. EV-RNAs, with regulatory effects, have been implicated in many EV-mediated biological functions [64,75]. EVs are widely present in biofluids, such as blood, urine, saliva, and malignant effusions. Moreover, piRNAs can cross the plasma membrane, and EVs released by cancer cells contained piRNAs that remain stable in body fluids. This feature suggests that piRNAs can easily be detected in body fluids as accurate biomarkers [44]. Several studies have focused on plasma EV's role as an early and non-invasive diagnostic biomarker for cancers. EV-cargo represents a valuable source of genetic materials, mainly ncRNA biomarkers [83]. These findings indicate that LB can allow for the detection of piRNAs that may become therapeutic and diagnostic tools for various cancer types. Differentially expressed EV-piRNAs have been identified in patients with specific disease conditions compared to healthy controls, suggesting an association between piRNA and progression in various diseases [72]. Although we are currently lacking guidelines on piRNA bioinformatic analysis, EV-piRNA can be considered a new research niche in human cancer pathology.

piRNAs encapsulated in EVs are stable in body fluids and have the potential to be promising markers for cancer diagnosis and prognosis and new tools for innovative therapies [73]. Examples of specific piRNAs shuttled by EVs are described below and summarized in Table 3.

It was reported that piR-26925 and piR-5444 are upregulated In EVs isolated from the serum of LC patients [84]. A high-throughput sequencing of small ncRNAs from EVs, cancerous and adjacent noncancerous tissues in patients with NSCLC, was applied to recognize candidate piRNAs as diagnostic biomarkers. This study reveals that piR-164586 was significantly upregulated in paracancerous tissues and EVs from serum samples of healthy individuals [85].

Recently, it was demonstrated that EVs isolated from the plasma of neuroblastoma (NB) patients contain high levels of piR-1089. In vitro, studies indicated that EV-piR-1089 promoted NB cell proliferation and migration by inhibiting Kelch-like ECH-associated protein 1 (*KEAP1*) expression. Low *KEAP1* expressions were associated with NB progression in clinical samples [86]. piRNAs are also involved in the crosstalk between multiple myeloma (MM) cells and bone marrow microenvironment. In MM, piR-823 silencing causes cell cycle dysregulation, reduction of apoptosis-related proteins, and de novo DNA methyltransferases, thus inhibiting the tumorigenicity of MM in vitro and in vivo [87]. piR-823 contained in EVs from peripheral blood of MM patients and cell lines plays an important role in cell–cell communication between endothelial and myeloma cells in the tumor microenvironment. EV-piR-823 from MM cells can be effectively transferred to endothelial cells and alter their biological characteristics, promoting anti-apoptotic and pro-angiogenic activity and creating a favorable microenvironment for MM cell survival. The upregulation of piR-823 can increase the expressions of IL-6, VEGF, and ICAM-1, promoting endothelial cell proliferation, invasion, and tube formation [88]. Granulocytic myeloid-derived suppressor cells (MDSCs) can trigger piR-823 expression, and silencing piR-823 can decrease the stemness of MM stem cells maintained by granulocytic MDSCs [89]. Moreover, piR-823 expression has been correlated with the stage and prognosis of MM, indicating its potential as a therapeutic target and prognostic stratification biomarker [88,90]. Gu et al. reported that the EV-piRNA population is altered in the plasma of cholangiocarcinoma (CCA) and gallbladder carcinoma (GBC) patients compared to healthy individuals. EV-piRNA profiling revealed unique piRNA signatures of CCA and GBC. Small RNA sequencing data, obtained by the NGS system, showed piR-2660989, piR-10506469, piR-20548188, piR-10822895, piR-23209, and piR-18044111 in EVs isolated from CCA and GBC plasma. Interestingly, expression level analyses of EV-piRNAs in plasma of CCA and GBC patients, before and after surgeries, have demonstrated that piR-10506469 and piR-20548188 were significantly decreased in patients who underwent surgeries [91]. In OC, EVs drive the crosstalk between cancer cells and omental fibroblasts. EV-piR-25783 activates TGF-β/SMAD2/SMAD3 pathway in fibroblasts and promotes the fibroblast-to-myofibroblast transition in the omentum, secretion of various cytokines, proliferation, migration, and invasion, contributing to the premetastatic niche formation. piR-25783-induced myofibroblasts improve tumor implantation and growth in the omentum. EV-piR-25783 upregulation is thus associated with adverse clinicopathological characteristics and shorter survival [92]. Moreover, EV-piRNAs can be considered promising non-invasive diagnostic biomarkers for GC, piR-019308, piR-004918, and piR-018569 contained in serum EVs were significantly increased in GC patients compared to healthy controls [93].

In prostate cancer (PCa), piRNAs were involved in the proliferation, migration, and invasion of PCa cells by activating different signal pathways, which may represent a new marker of PCa diagnosis. It was reported that piRNAs contained in urinary EVs, isolated from patients with PCa and detected using NGS technology, are useful for diagnosis. The fraction of PCa-derived EVs in urine is larger than in plasma and allows for a better detection and tracking of PCa-derived RNAs [94]. The expressions of piR-349843, piR-382289, piR-158533, and piR-002468 in urinary EVs were significantly increased in PCa patients compared with healthy controls [95]. Interestingly, it was also indicated that in plasma EVs of patients with bladder cancer (BCa), two small ncRNAs, miR-4508 and piR-5936, were associated with the risk class: miR-4508 with a descendant trend going from controls to high-risk BCa; piR-5936 with an ascending trend [96]. Taken together, these reports indicate that EV-piRNAs have an important role in tumor–host crosstalk, contributing to cancer progression and showing a great potential as theranostic biomarkers.

5.2. piRNA-Based Therapeutic Approaches in Cancer

On-target specificity is a significant difficulty to overcome for an RNA-based therapeutic strategy that involves gene silencing. Moreover, RNAs are unstable molecules, and the development of ways to enhance RNA stability and its uptake are crucial points. Although siRNA molecules are structurally susceptible to RNases and degradation, some advances to overcome these limits are ongoing, employing various chemical and structural modifications that make RNAi delivery more physiologically amenable. Synthetic lipid nanoparticles have been developed and have enabled successful systemic delivery of RNAi. Each of these RNA components can be modified to overcome their susceptibility to degradation [94]. Stability and barriers to delivery were overcome thanks to the success of the mRNA vaccine for COVID-19 in early 2021, opening new routes for targeted RNA therapies [95]. siRNAs are double-stranded ncRNAs with similar biological functions to miRNAs but are synthetically derived (exogenously) via the process of RNA interference (RNAi). siRNAs, like miRNAs, degrade target mRNAs in a sequence-specific manner, leading to gene silencing. RNAi machinery targets and can silence pathologic mRNA sequences [94].

Some typical limitations of siRNAs and miRNAs can be overcome using piRNAs and EVs as their shuttles. Nowadays, the potential role of piRNAs as therapeutic tools has been reported; piRNA treatment is performed via the correction of pathological alteration of piRNA expression, including the reactivation of endogenous piRNA as a pathological inhibitor and functional blocking or reduction in piRNA expression as a pathological driver [30]. Synthetic piRNAs are very intriguing as they could block the synthesis of cancer-related proteins by binding to mRNAs. Different from miRNAs, which need to be processed by enzymes and regulate several mRNAs, piRNAs have the advantage of not requiring enzyme processing and better specificity than other ncRNAs to targets [97]. Since epigenetic regulatory mechanisms are closely related to cancer progression, the epigenetic reprogramming of cancer cells can be a potentially powerful therapeutic approach [43]. Epigenetic drugs (epidrugs) consist of small molecules targeting epigenetic key signaling pathways, promoting transcriptional and post-transcriptional modifications and acting mainly on tumor suppressor and DNA repair gene activation [44]. Since piRNAs regulate protein-coding genes involved in the development of various diseases, they can be considered molecules useful as innovative epidrugs [45]. Although the studies on piRNAs as new therapeutic methods are still in the early stage, understanding the mechanisms and functions of piRNAs could enhance therapeutic alternatives in cancer. Recently, EV-mediated ncRNA delivery systems have attracted tremendous attention in the research of next-generation therapeutics for the treatment of several pathologies, including cancer [98]. EVs, thanks to their small size, low immunogenicity, and high biocompatibility due to their natural origin [99,100], are more attractive than synthetic vehicles. Moreover, EV cargos are protected from degradation in the bloodstream by a lipid bilayer membrane; they have the potential to escape from immune system clearance and cross the physiological barriers [101]. Despite these advantages, natural EVs show some pitfalls. The procedures for EV isolation are time consuming, monitoring methods for cargo dosage are insufficient, and EV stability after storage is not easy to monitor [102]. Currently, the yield of EVs isolated from body fluids or culture media is insufficient to supply clinical demands, and EV-quality control is a challenge that limits their clinical application [103]. To overcome this limit, EVs collected from non-human sources such as plants, bacteria, and milk are considered a potential alternative for cancer therapy. Since EV-mediated communication is involved in all the domains of life and in several cellular physiological and pathological processes,

EVs are involved in a universal, evolutionarily conserved mechanism for inter-kingdom and intra-kingdom communication [104]. It was reported that plant EVs can be used as nanoplatforms to transfer ncRNAs in inter-kingdom communication [28,71]. ncRNAs contained in plant EVs are considered a new class of cross-kingdom modulators, capable of mediating animal-plant interactions at the molecular level [105]. Applications of plant EVs in nanomedicine and nutraceutics are based on their intrinsic biological properties, such as anti-cancer, anti-inflammatory, and anti-aging, and on their use as shuttles of therapeutic biomolecules [106]. It was also reported that bacterial EVs isolated from the host gut microbiome can enter the circulatory system to disseminate to distant organs and tissues and be detected in human biofluids. Bacterial EVs in microbiome-based liquid biopsies might be useful for cancer diagnostics and bioengineering strategies for cancer therapy [107]. Moreover, bovine milk-derived EVs have been shown to increase the oral bioavailability of drugs and are optimal vehicles to transport bioactive compounds for nutritional and therapeutic purposes [108]. In cancer therapy, milk EVs can be functionalized with ligands such as folic acid to achieve cancer targeting [109]. In addition, milk-derived EVs have shown several therapeutic effects, such as a selective interaction with macrophages and an increase in intestinal stem cell proliferation as potential adjuvant therapy to standard clinical management of malnourished children [110].

Table 3. piRNAs content in EVs collected from different cancer types.

Cancer Type	piRNA	EV Origin	Target/Role	References
Lung	piR-26925 piR-5444 piR-164586	Serum	Biomarker	[61,62]
Ovarian	piR-25783	CM	TGF-β/SMAD2/SMAD3 pathway	[74]
Gastric	piR-019308 piR-004918 piR-018569	Serum	Biomarker	[64]
Prostate	piR-349843 piR-382289 piR-158533 piR-002468	Urine	Biomarker	[72]
Neuroblastoma	piR-1089	Plasma	KEAP1	[71]
Multiple Mieloma	piR-823	CM, Plasma	IL-6, VEGF ICAM-1	[105]
Cholangio Gallbladder carcinoma	piR-2660989 piR-10506469 piR-20548188 piR-10822895 piR23209 piR-18044111	Plasma	Biomarker	[76]
Bladder	piR-5936	Plasma	Biomarker	[73]

6. Conclusions and Outlook

Recently, significant advances in the piRNA field have been made, providing mechanistic insights into the transcription of piRNA clusters, piRNA biogenesis, and piRNA function. Although the knowledge of piRNAs in cancers remains in its infancy, a growing number of studies have shown that piRNAs can be considered good diagnostic and prognostic markers and new therapeutic tools. However, it needs to report a few studies indicating that piRNAs could be fragments of other ncRNAs and could correspond to false positives due to the use of noncurated piRNA databases [111,112]. Many studies have found aberrant piRNAs in biofluids of cancer patients; thus, LB is considered an ideal tool for developing cancer biomarkers. Even if a single piRNA can be sufficient to distinguish cancer patients from healthy controls, combined biomarkers may be more diagnostically accurate than one. EVs can have a dual role in cancer management as a source of diagnostic biomarkers with the identification of specific piRNAs and as a therapeutic tool consisting of engineered EVs with piRNAs useful as potential and breakthrough epidrugs (Figure 6). Future research efforts should concentrate on wide studies on piRNA profiles in different cancer types and stages. This effort can allow for the identification of comprehensive diagnostic panels able to compliant the heterogeneous landscape of cancer. Preclinical studies show how smart EVs have the potential to expand into next-generation drugs to address the current demand for precision cancer therapies. However, numerous milestones on piRNAs contained in EVs are yet to be achieved. To date, the clinical trials with piRNAs and EV-piRNAs are still a hard challenge, and only a few clinical studies on these emerging ncRNAs are ongoing (www.clinical.trials.org, accessed on 20 April 2023). Further clinical studies are needed to demonstrate that EV-piRNAs are smart tools useful for theranostic applications in precision oncology.

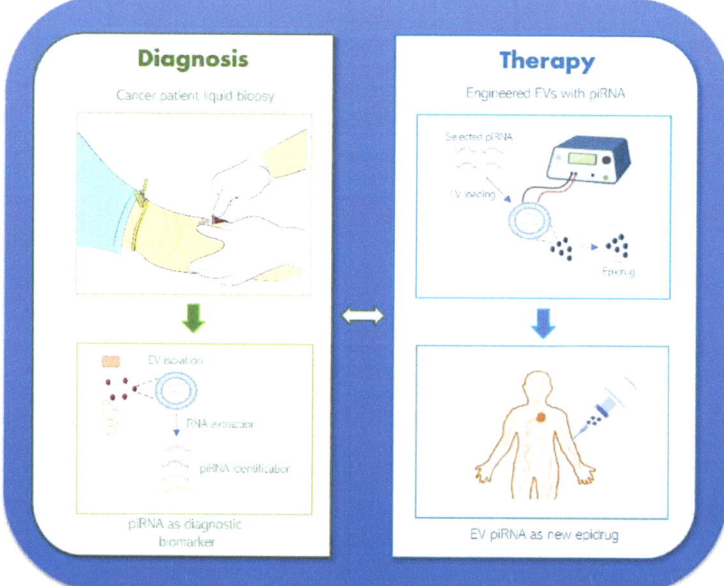

Figure 6. Working hypothesis of piRNA use in diagnosis and therapies. The identification of EV-piRNAs collected by the blood of cancer patients can be useful as diagnostic biomarkers. The engineering of EVs, loading ectopic piRNA, may allow shuttling piRNA useful as new epidrugs.

Author Contributions: Conceptualization: S.T. and G.C.; methodology, data curation; writing—original draft preparation: S.T., A.M. and G.C.; writing—review and editing: S.T. and G.C.; visualization: S.T., A.M. and G.C.; supervision: S.T. and G.C. All authors have read and agreed to the published version of the manuscript.

Funding: This research received no external funding.

Institutional Review Board Statement: Not applicable.

Informed Consent Statement: Not applicable.

Data Availability Statement: Not applicable.

Conflicts of Interest: The authors declare no conflict of interest.

References

1. Dhamija, S.; Menon, M.B. Non-Coding Transcript Variants of Protein-Coding Genes-What Are They Good For? *RNA Biol.* **2018**, *15*, 1025–1031. [CrossRef] [PubMed]
2. Kumar, S.; Gonzalez, E.A.; Rameshwar, P.; Etchegaray, J.-P. Non-Coding RNAs as Mediators of Epigenetic Changes in Malignancies. *Cancers* **2020**, *12*, 3657. [CrossRef] [PubMed]
3. Ye, J.; Li, J.; Zhao, P. Roles of NcRNAs as CeRNAs in Gastric Cancer. *Genes* **2021**, *12*, 1036. [CrossRef]
4. Cammarata, G.; Barraco, N.; Giusti, I.; Gristina, V.; Dolo, V.; Taverna, S. Extracellular Vesicles-CeRNAs as Ovarian Cancer Biomarkers: Looking into CircRNA-MiRNA-MRNA Code. *Cancers* **2022**, *14*, 3404. [CrossRef] [PubMed]
5. Pucci, M.; Reclusa Asiain, P.; Durendez Saez, E.; Jantus-Lewintre, E.; Malarani, M.; Khan, S.; Fontana, S.; Naing, A.; Passiglia, F.; Raez, L.E.; et al. Extracellular Vesicles As MiRNA Nano-Shuttles: Dual Role in Tumor Progression. *Target. Oncol.* **2018**, *13*, 175–187. [CrossRef] [PubMed]
6. Ameli Mojarad, M.; Ameli Mojarad, M.; Shojaee, B.; Nazemalhosseini-Mojarad, E. PiRNA: A Promising Biomarker in Early Detection of Gastrointestinal Cancer. *Pathol. Res. Pract.* **2022**, *230*, 153757. [CrossRef] [PubMed]
7. Cammarata, G.; de Miguel-Perez, D.; Russo, A.; Peleg, A.; Dolo, V.; Rolfo, C.; Taverna, S. Emerging Noncoding RNAs Contained in Extracellular Vesicles: Rising Stars as Biomarkers in Lung Cancer Liquid Biopsy. *Ther. Adv. Med. Oncol.* **2022**, *14*, 17588359221131228. [CrossRef]
8. Weng, W.; Li, H.; Goel, A. Piwi-Interacting RNAs (PiRNAs) and Cancer: Emerging Biological Concepts and Potential Clinical Implications. *Biochim. Biophys. Acta Rev. Cancer* **2019**, *1871*, 160–169. [CrossRef]
9. Koch, B.; Geßner, A.; Farmand, S.; Fuhrmann, D.C.; Chiocchetti, A.G.; Schubert, R.; Baer, P.C. Effects of Hypoxia on RNA Cargo in Extracellular Vesicles from Human Adipose-Derived Stromal/Stem Cells. *Int. J. Mol. Sci.* **2022**, *23*, 7384. [CrossRef]
10. Huang, M.; Peng, X.; Yang, L.; Yang, S.; Li, X.; Tang, S.; Li, B.; Jin, H.; Wu, B.; Liu, J.; et al. Non-Coding RNA Derived from Extracellular Vesicles in Cancer Immune Escape: Biological Functions and Potential Clinical Applications. *Cancer Lett.* **2021**, *501*, 234–246. [CrossRef]
11. Sadoughi, F.; Mirhashemi, S.M.; Asemi, Z. Epigenetic Roles of PIWI Proteins and PiRNAs in Colorectal Cancer. *Cancer Cell Int.* **2021**, *21*, 328. [CrossRef] [PubMed]
12. Houwing, S.; Kamminga, L.M.; Berezikov, E.; Cronembold, D.; Girard, A.; van den Elst, H.; Filippov, D.V.; Blaser, H.; Raz, E.; Moens, C.B.; et al. A Role for Piwi and PiRNAs in Germ Cell Maintenance and Transposon Silencing in Zebrafish. *Cell* **2007**, *129*, 69–82. [CrossRef] [PubMed]
13. Billi, A.C.; Alessi, A.F.; Khivansara, V.; Han, T.; Freeberg, M.; Mitani, S.; Kim, J.K. The Caenorhabditis Elegans HEN1 Ortholog, HENN-1, Methylates and Stabilizes Select Subclasses of Germline Small RNAs. *PLoS Genet.* **2012**, *8*, e1002617. [CrossRef] [PubMed]
14. Zhang, Z.; Xu, J.; Koppetsch, B.S.; Wang, J.; Tipping, C.; Ma, S.; Weng, Z.; Theurkauf, W.E.; Zamore, P.D. Heterotypic PiRNA Ping-Pong Requires Qin, a Protein with Both E3 Ligase and Tudor Domains. *Mol. Cell* **2011**, *44*, 572–584. [CrossRef]
15. Sato, K.; Iwasaki, Y.W.; Siomi, H.; Siomi, M.C. Tudor-Domain Containing Proteins Act to Make the PiRNA Pathways More Robust in Drosophila. *Fly* **2015**, *9*, 86–90. [CrossRef]
16. Balaratnam, S.; Hoque, M.E.; West, N.; Basu, S. Decay of Piwi-Interacting RNAs in Human Cells Is Primarily Mediated by 5′ to 3′ Exoribonucleases. *ACS Chem. Biol.* **2022**, *17*, 1723–1732. [CrossRef]
17. Fonseca Cabral, G.; Azevedo Dos Santos Pinheiro, J.; Vidal, A.F.; Santos, S.; Ribeiro-Dos-Santos, Â. PiRNAs in Gastric Cancer: A New Approach Towards Translational Research. *Int. J. Mol. Sci.* **2020**, *21*, 2126. [CrossRef]
18. Tóth, K.F.; Pezic, D.; Stuwe, E.; Webster, A. The PiRNA Pathway Guards the Germline Genome Against Transposable Elements. *Adv. Exp. Med. Biol.* **2016**, *886*, 51–77. [CrossRef]
19. Li, Z.; Tang, X.; Shen, E.-Z. How Mammalian PiRNAs Instruct de Novo DNA Methylation of Transposons. *Signal Transduct. Target. Ther.* **2020**, *5*, 190. [CrossRef]
20. Wilson, A.S.; Power, B.E.; Molloy, P.L. DNA Hypomethylation and Human Diseases. *Biochim. Biophys. Acta-Rev. Cancer* **2007**, *1775*, 138–162. [CrossRef]
21. Baylin, S.B. DNA Methylation and Gene Silencing in Cancer. *Nat. Clin. Pract. Oncol.* **2005**, *2*, S4–S11. [CrossRef] [PubMed]
22. Yao, J.; Xie, M.; Ma, X.; Song, J.; Wang, Y.; Xue, X. PIWI-Interacting RNAs in Cancer: Biogenesis, Function, and Clinical Significance. *Front. Oncol.* **2022**, *12*, 965684. [CrossRef] [PubMed]
23. Chénais, B. Transposable Elements and Human Cancer: A Causal Relationship? *Biochim. Biophys. Acta-Rev. Cancer* **2013**, *1835*, 28–35. [CrossRef] [PubMed]
24. Fabry, M.H.; Ciabrelli, F.; Munafò, M.; Eastwood, E.L.; Kneuss, E.; Falciatori, I.; Falconio, F.A.; Hannon, G.J.; Czech, B. PiRNA-Guided Co-Transcriptional Silencing Coopts Nuclear Export Factors. *Elife* **2019**, *8*, e47999. [CrossRef]
25. Jia, D.-D.; Jiang, H.; Zhang, Y.-F.; Zhang, Y.; Qian, L.-L.; Zhang, Y.-F. The Regulatory Function of PiRNA/PIWI Complex in Cancer and Other Human Diseases: The Role of DNA Methylation. *Int. J. Biol. Sci.* **2022**, *18*, 3358–3373. [CrossRef]
26. Ali, R.; Laskar, S.A.; Khan, N.J.; Wahab, S.; Khalid, M. Non-Coding RNA's Prevalence as Biomarkers for Prognostic, Diagnostic, and Clinical Utility in Breast Cancer. *Funct. Integr. Genomics* **2023**, *23*, 195. [CrossRef]
27. Baylin, S.B.; Jones, P.A. A Decade of Exploring the Cancer Epigenome—Biological and Translational Implications. *Nat. Rev. Cancer* **2011**, *11*, 726–734. [CrossRef]

28. Siddiqi, S.; Matushansky, I. Piwis and Piwi-Interacting RNAs in the Epigenetics of Cancer. *J. Cell. Biochem.* **2012**, *113*, 373–380. [CrossRef]
29. Mentis, A.-F.A.; Dardiotis, E.; Romas, N.A.; Papavassiliou, A.G. PIWI Family Proteins as Prognostic Markers in Cancer: A Systematic Review and Meta-Analysis. *Cell. Mol. Life Sci.* **2020**, *77*, 2289–2314. [CrossRef]
30. Zhou, J.; Xie, H.; Liu, J.; Huang, R.; Xiang, Y.; Tian, D.; Bian, E. PIWI-Interacting RNAs: Critical Roles and Therapeutic Targets in Cancer. *Cancer Lett.* **2023**, *562*, 216189. [CrossRef]
31. Li, F.; Yuan, P.; Rao, M.; Jin, C.-H.; Tang, W.; Rong, Y.-F.; Hu, Y.-P.; Zhang, F.; Wei, T.; Yin, Q.; et al. PiRNA-Independent Function of PIWIL1 as a Co-Activator for Anaphase Promoting Complex/Cyclosome to Drive Pancreatic Cancer Metastasis. *Nat. Cell Biol.* **2020**, *22*, 425–438. [CrossRef] [PubMed]
32. Zhao, X.; Huang, L.; Lu, Y.; Jiang, W.; Song, Y.; Qiu, B.; Tao, D.; Liu, Y.; Ma, Y. PIWIL2 Interacting with IKK to Regulate Autophagy and Apoptosis in Esophageal Squamous Cell Carcinoma. *Cell Death Differ.* **2021**, *28*, 1941–1954. [CrossRef]
33. Chen, C.; Liu, J.; Xu, G. Overexpression of PIWI Proteins in Human Stage III Epithelial Ovarian Cancer with Lymph Node Metastasis. *Cancer Biomark.* **2013**, *13*, 315–321. [CrossRef] [PubMed]
34. Gambichler, T.; Kohsik, C.; Höh, A.-K.; Lang, K.; Käfferlein, H.U.; Brüning, T.; Stockfleth, E.; Stücker, M.; Dreißigacker, M.; Sand, M. Expression of PIWIL3 in Primary and Metastatic Melanoma. *J. Cancer Res. Clin. Oncol.* **2017**, *143*, 433–437. [CrossRef]
35. Jiang, L.; Wang, W.-J.; Li, Z.-W.; Wang, X.-Z. Downregulation of Piwil3 Suppresses Cell Proliferation, Migration and Invasion in Gastric Cancer. *Cancer Biomark.* **2017**, *20*, 499–509. [CrossRef]
36. Liu, X.; Zheng, J.; Xue, Y.; Yu, H.; Gong, W.; Wang, P.; Li, Z.; Liu, Y. PIWIL3/OIP5-AS1/MiR-367-3p/CEBPA Feedback Loop Regulates the Biological Behavior of Glioma Cells. *Theranostics* **2018**, *8*, 1084–1105. [CrossRef]
37. Li, W.; Martinez-Useros, J.; Garcia-Carbonero, N.; Fernandez-Aceñero, M.J.; Orta, A.; Ortega-Medina, L.; Garcia-Botella, S.; Perez-Aguirre, E.; Diez-Valladares, L.; Celdran, A.; et al. The Clinical Significance of PIWIL3 and PIWIL4 Expression in Pancreatic Cancer. *J. Clin. Med.* **2020**, *9*, 1252. [CrossRef] [PubMed]
38. Sugimoto, K.; Kage, H.; Aki, N.; Sano, A.; Kitagawa, H.; Nagase, T.; Yatomi, Y.; Ohishi, N.; Takai, D. The Induction of H3K9 Methylation by PIWIL4 at the P16Ink4a Locus. *Biochem. Biophys. Res. Commun.* **2007**, *359*, 497–502. [CrossRef] [PubMed]
39. Coley, W.; Van Duyne, R.; Carpio, L.; Guendel, I.; Kehn-Hall, K.; Chevalier, S.; Narayanan, A.; Luu, T.; Lee, N.; Klase, Z.; et al. Absence of DICER in Monocytes and Its Regulation by HIV-1. *J. Biol. Chem.* **2010**, *285*, 31930–31943. [CrossRef] [PubMed]
40. Zoch, A.; Auchynnikava, T.; Berrens, R.V.; Kabayama, Y.; Schöpp, T.; Heep, M.; Vasiliauskaitė, L.; Pérez-Rico, Y.A.; Cook, A.G.; Shkumatava, A.; et al. SPOCD1 Is an Essential Executor of PiRNA-Directed de Novo DNA Methylation. *Nature* **2020**, *584*, 635–639. [CrossRef]
41. Sohn, E.J.; Oh, S.-O. P-Element-Induced Wimpy Testis Proteins and P-Element-Induced Wimpy Testis-Interacting RNAs Expression in Ovarian Cancer Stem Cells. *Genet. Test. Mol. Biomark.* **2023**, *27*, 56–64. [CrossRef] [PubMed]
42. Ferreira, H.J.; Heyn, H.; Garcia del Muro, X.; Vidal, A.; Larriba, S.; Muñoz, C.; Villanueva, A.; Esteller, M. Epigenetic Loss of the PIWI/PiRNA Machinery in Human Testicular Tumorigenesis. *Epigenetics* **2014**, *9*, 113–118. [CrossRef] [PubMed]
43. Cheng, Y.; Wang, Q.; Jiang, W.; Bian, Y.; Zhou, Y.; Gou, A.; Zhang, W.; Fu, K.; Shi, W. Emerging Roles of PiRNAs in Cancer: Challenges and Prospects. *Aging* **2019**, *11*, 9932–9946. [CrossRef]
44. Li, D.; Luo, Y.; Gao, Y.; Yang, Y.; Wang, Y.; Xu, Y.; Tan, S.; Zhang, Y.; Duan, J.; Yang, Y. PiR-651 Promotes Tumor Formation in Non-Small Cell Lung Carcinoma through the Upregulation of Cyclin D1 and CDK4. *Int. J. Mol. Med.* **2016**, *38*, 927–936. [CrossRef] [PubMed]
45. Liu, T.; Wang, J.; Sun, L.; Li, M.; He, X.; Jiang, J.; Zhou, Q. Piwi-Interacting RNA-651 Promotes Cell Proliferation and Migration and Inhibits Apoptosis in Breast Cancer by Facilitating DNMT1-Mediated PTEN Promoter Methylation. *Cell Cycle* **2021**, *20*, 1603–1616. [CrossRef]
46. Cordeiro, A.; Navarro, A.; Gaya, A.; Díaz-Beyá, M.; Gonzalez-Farré, B.; Castellano, J.J.; Fuster, D.; Martínez, C.; Martínez, A.; Monzó, M. PiwiRNA-651 as Marker of Treatment Response and Survival in Classical Hodgkin Lymphoma. *Oncotarget* **2016**, *7*, 46002–46013. [CrossRef]
47. Han, F.; Fan, G.; Song, S.; Jiang, Y.; Qian, C.; Zhang, W.; Su, Q.; Xue, X.; Zhuang, W.; Li, B. PiRNA-30473 Contributes to Tumorigenesis and Poor Prognosis by Regulating M6A RNA Methylation in DLBCL. *Blood* **2021**, *137*, 1603–1614. [CrossRef]
48. Wang, X.; Ramat, A.; Simonelig, M.; Liu, M.-F. Emerging Roles and Functional Mechanisms of PIWI-Interacting RNAs. *Nat. Rev. Mol. Cell Biol.* **2022**, *24*, 123–141. [CrossRef]
49. Peng, L.; Song, L.; Liu, C.; Lv, X.; Li, X.; Jie, J.; Zhao, D.; Li, D. PiR-55490 Inhibits the Growth of Lung Carcinoma by Suppressing MTOR Signaling. *Tumour Biol.* **2016**, *37*, 2749–2756. [CrossRef]
50. Liu, Y.; Dong, Y.; He, X.; Gong, A.; Gao, J.; Hao, X.; Wang, S.; Fan, Y.; Wang, Z.; Li, M.; et al. PiR-Hsa-211106 Inhibits the Progression of Lung Adenocarcinoma Through Pyruvate Carboxylase and Enhances Chemotherapy Sensitivity. *Front. Oncol.* **2021**, *11*, 651915. [CrossRef]
51. Tan, L.; Mai, D.; Zhang, B.; Jiang, X.; Zhang, J.; Bai, R.; Ye, Y.; Li, M.; Pan, L.; Su, J.; et al. PIWI-Interacting RNA-36712 Restrains Breast Cancer Progression and Chemoresistance by Interaction with SEPW1 Pseudogene SEPW1P RNA. *Mol. Cancer* **2019**, *18*, 9. [CrossRef] [PubMed]
52. Liu, Q.; Chen, Q.; Zhou, Z.; Tian, Z.; Zheng, X.; Wang, K. PiRNA-18 Inhibition Cell Proliferation, Migration and Invasion in Colorectal Cancer. *Biochem. Genet.* **2023**. [CrossRef] [PubMed]

53. Fu, A.; Jacobs, D.I.; Hoffman, A.E.; Zheng, T.; Zhu, Y. PIWI-Interacting RNA 021285 Is Involved in Breast Tumorigenesis Possibly by Remodeling the Cancer Epigenome. *Carcinogenesis* **2015**, *36*, 1094–1102. [CrossRef] [PubMed]
54. Busch, J.; Ralla, B.; Jung, M.; Wotschofsky, Z.; Trujillo-Arribas, E.; Schwabe, P.; Kilic, E.; Fendler, A.; Jung, K. Piwi-Interacting RNAs as Novel Prognostic Markers in Clear Cell Renal Cell Carcinomas. *J. Exp. Clin. Cancer Res.* **2015**, *34*, 61. [CrossRef] [PubMed]
55. Cheng, J.; Deng, H.; Xiao, B.; Zhou, H.; Zhou, F.; Shen, Z.; Guo, J. piR-823, a Novel Non-Coding Small RNA, Demonstrates in Vitro and in Vivo Tumor Suppressive Activity in Human Gastric Cancer Cells. *Cancer Lett.* **2012**, *315*, 12–17. [CrossRef] [PubMed]
56. Yin, J.; Jiang, X.-Y.; Qi, W.; Ji, C.-G.; Xie, X.-L.; Zhang, D.-X.; Cui, Z.-J.; Wang, C.-K.; Bai, Y.; Wang, J.; et al. PiR-823 Contributes to Colorectal Tumorigenesis by Enhancing the Transcriptional Activity of HSF1. *Cancer Sci.* **2017**, *108*, 1746–1756. [CrossRef]
57. Mai, D.; Ding, P.; Tan, L.; Zhang, J.; Pan, Z.; Bai, R.; Li, C.; Li, M.; Zhou, Y.; Tan, W.; et al. PIWI-Interacting RNA-54265 Is Oncogenic and a Potential Therapeutic Target in Colorectal Adenocarcinoma. *Theranostics* **2018**, *8*, 5213–5230. [CrossRef]
58. Law, P.T.-Y.; Qin, H.; Ching, A.K.-K.; Lai, K.P.; Co, N.N.; He, M.; Lung, R.W.-M.; Chan, A.W.-H.; Chan, T.-F.; Wong, N. Deep Sequencing of Small RNA Transcriptome Reveals Novel Non-Coding RNAs in Hepatocellular Carcinoma. *J. Hepatol.* **2013**, *58*, 1165–1173. [CrossRef]
59. Yuan, C.; Qin, H.; Ponnusamy, M.; Chen, Y.; Lin, Z. PIWI-interacting RNA in Cancer: Molecular Mechanisms and Possible Clinical Implications (Review). *Oncol. Rep.* **2021**, *46*, 209. [CrossRef]
60. Zhao, Q.; Qian, L.; Guo, Y.; Lü, J.; Li, D.; Xie, H.; Wang, Q.; Ma, W.; Liu, P.; Liu, Y.; et al. IL11 Signaling Mediates PiR-2158 Suppression of Cell Stemness and Angiogenesis in Breast Cancer. *Theranostics* **2023**, *13*, 2337–2349. [CrossRef]
61. Vychytilova-Faltejskova, P.; Stitkovcova, K.; Radova, L.; Sachlova, M.; Kosarova, Z.; Slaba, K.; Kala, Z.; Svoboda, M.; Kiss, I.; Vyzula, R.; et al. Circulating PIWI-Interacting RNAs PiR-5937 and PiR-28876 Are Promising Diagnostic Biomarkers of Colon Cancer. *Cancer Epidemiol. Biomark. Prev.* **2018**, *27*, 1019–1028. [CrossRef] [PubMed]
62. de Miguel-Perez, D.; Russo, A.; Arrieta, O.; Ak, M.; Barron, F.; Gunasekaran, M.; Mamindla, P.; Lara-Mejia, L.; Peterson, C.B.; Er, M.E.; et al. Extracellular Vesicle PD-L1 Dynamics Predict Durable Response to Immune-Checkpoint Inhibitors and Survival in Patients with Non-Small Cell Lung Cancer. *J. Exp. Clin. Cancer Res.* **2022**, *41*, 186. [CrossRef] [PubMed]
63. Califf, R.M. Biomarker Definitions and Their Applications. *Exp. Biol. Med.* **2018**, *243*, 213–221. [CrossRef] [PubMed]
64. Rigogliuso, S.; Donati, C.; Cassarà, D.; Taverna, S.; Salamone, M.; Bruni, P.; Vittorelli, M.L. An Active Form of Sphingosine Kinase-1 Is Released in the Extracellular Medium as Component of Membrane Vesicles Shed by Two Human Tumor Cell Lines. *J. Oncol.* **2010**, *2010*, 509329. [CrossRef] [PubMed]
65. Chen, Y.-J.; Zhao, R.-M.; Zhao, Q.; Li, B.-Y.; Ma, Q.-Y.; Li, X.; Chen, X. Diagnostic Significance of Elevated Expression of HBME-1 in Papillary Thyroid Carcinoma. *Tumour Biol.* **2016**, *37*, 8715–8720. [CrossRef] [PubMed]
66. Serrano, M.J.; Garrido-Navas, M.C.; Diaz Mochon, J.J.; Cristofanilli, M.; Gil-Bazo, I.; Pauwels, P.; Malapelle, U.; Russo, A.; Lorente, J.A.; Ruiz-Rodriguez, A.J.; et al. Precision Prevention and Cancer Interception: The New Challenges of Liquid Biopsy. *Cancer Discov.* **2020**, *10*, 1635–1644. [CrossRef]
67. Perera, B.P.U.; Morgan, R.K.; Polemi, K.M.; Sala-Hamrick, K.E.; Svoboda, L.K.; Dolinoy, D.C. PIWI-Interacting RNA (PiRNA) and Epigenetic Editing in Environmental Health Sciences. *Curr. Environ. Health Rep.* **2022**, *9*, 650–660. [CrossRef]
68. Galvano, A.; Taverna, S.; Badalamenti, G.; Incorvaia, L.; Castiglia, M.; Barraco, N.; Passiglia, F.; Fulfaro, F.; Beretta, G.; Duro, G.; et al. Detection of RAS Mutations in Circulating Tumor DNA: A New Weapon in an Old War against Colorectal Cancer. A Systematic Review of Literature and Meta-Analysis. *Ther. Adv. Med. Oncol.* **2019**, *11*, 1758835919874653. [CrossRef]
69. Ray, S.K.; Mukherjee, S. Piwi-Interacting RNAs (PiRNAs) and Colorectal Carcinoma: Emerging Non-Invasive Diagnostic Biomarkers with Potential Therapeutic Target Based Clinical Implications. *Curr. Mol. Med.* **2023**, *23*, 300–311. [CrossRef]
70. Pardini, B.; Sabo, A.A.; Birolo, G.; Calin, G.A. Noncoding RNAs in Extracellular Fluids as Cancer Biomarkers: The New Frontier of Liquid Biopsies. *Cancers* **2019**, *11*, 1170. [CrossRef]
71. He, B.; Cai, Q.; Qiao, L.; Huang, C.-Y.; Wang, S.; Miao, W.; Ha, T.; Wang, Y.; Jin, H. RNA-Binding Proteins Contribute to Small RNA Loading in Plant Extracellular Vesicles. *Nat. Plants* **2021**, *7*, 342–352. [CrossRef]
72. Goh, T.-X.; Tan, S.-L.; Roebuck, M.M.; Teo, S.-H.; Kamarul, T. A Systematic Review of Extracellular Vesicle-Derived Piwi-Interacting RNA in Human Body Fluid and Its Role in Disease Progression. *Tissue Eng. Part C. Methods* **2022**, *28*, 511–528. [CrossRef]
73. Mokarram, P.; Niknam, M.; Sadeghdoust, M.; Aligolighasemabadi, F.; Siri, M.; Dastghaib, S.; Brim, H.; Ashktorab, H. PIWI Interacting RNAs Perspectives: A New Avenues in Future Cancer Investigations. *Bioengineered* **2021**, *12*, 10401–10419. [CrossRef] [PubMed]
74. Zimta, A.-A.; Sigurjonsson, O.E.; Gulei, D.; Tomuleasa, C. The Malignant Role of Exosomes as Nanocarriers of Rare RNA Species. *Int. J. Mol. Sci.* **2020**, *21*, 5866. [CrossRef] [PubMed]
75. Monteleone, F.; Taverna, S.; Alessandro, R.; Fontana, S. SWATH-MS Based Quantitative Proteomics Analysis Reveals That Curcumin Alters the Metabolic Enzyme Profile of CML Cells by Affecting the Activity of MiR-22/IPO7/HIF-1alpha Axis. *J. Exp. Clin. Cancer Res.* **2018**, *37*, 170. [CrossRef]
76. Oliveres, H.; Caglevic, C.; Passiglia, F.; Taverna, S.; Smits, E.; Rolfo, C. Vaccine and Immune Cell Therapy in Non-Small Cell Lung Cancer. *J. Thorac. Dis.* **2018**, *10*, S1602–S1614. [CrossRef]

77. Mai, D.; Zheng, Y.; Guo, H.; Ding, P.; Bai, R.; Li, M.; Ye, Y.; Zhang, J.; Huang, X.; Liu, D.; et al. Serum PiRNA-54265 Is a New Biomarker for Early Detection and Clinical Surveillance of Human Colorectal Cancer. *Theranostics* **2020**, *10*, 8468–8478. [CrossRef] [PubMed]
78. Al-Obeidi, E.; Riess, J.W.; Malapelle, U.; Rolfo, C.; Gandara, D.R. Convergence of Precision Oncology and Liquid Biopsy in Non-Small Cell Lung Cancer. *Hematol. Oncol. Clin. N. Am.* **2023**, *37*, 475–487. [CrossRef]
79. Connors, D.; Allen, J.; Alvarez, J.D.; Boyle, J.; Cristofanilli, M.; Hiller, C.; Keating, S.; Kelloff, G.; Leiman, L.; McCormack, R.; et al. International Liquid Biopsy Standardization Alliance White Paper. *Crit. Rev. Oncol. Hematol.* **2020**, *156*, 103112. [CrossRef]
80. Candela, M.E.; Geraci, F.; Turturici, G.; Taverna, S.; Albanese, I.; Sconzo, G. Membrane Vesicles Containing Matrix Metalloproteinase-9 and Fibroblast Growth Factor-2 Are Released into the Extracellular Space from Mouse Mesoangioblast Stem Cells. *J. Cell. Physiol.* **2010**, *224*, 144–151. [CrossRef]
81. Taverna, S.; Giusti, I.; D'Ascenzo, S.; Pizzorno, L.; Dolo, V. Breast Cancer Derived Extracellular Vesicles in Bone Metastasis Induction and Their Clinical Implications as Biomarkers. *Int. J. Mol. Sci.* **2020**, *21*, 3573. [CrossRef] [PubMed]
82. Reclusa, P.; Verstraelen, P.; Taverna, S.; Gunasekaran, M.; Pucci, M.; Pintelon, I.; Claes, N.; de Miguel-Pérez, D.; Alessandro, R.; Bals, S.; et al. Improving Extracellular Vesicles Visualization: From Static to Motion. *Sci. Rep.* **2020**, *10*, 6494. [CrossRef] [PubMed]
83. Kalluri, R.; LeBleu, V.S. The Biology, Function, and Biomedical Applications of Exosomes. *Science* **2020**, *367*, eaau6977. [CrossRef]
84. Li, J.; Wang, N.; Zhang, F.; Jin, S.; Dong, Y.; Dong, X.; Chen, Y.; Kong, X.; Tong, Y.; Mi, Q.; et al. PIWI-Interacting RNAs Are Aberrantly Expressed and May Serve as Novel Biomarkers for Diagnosis of Lung Adenocarcinoma. *Thorac. Cancer* **2021**, *12*, 2468–2477. [CrossRef] [PubMed]
85. Li, Y.; Dong, Y.; Zhao, S.; Gao, J.; Hao, X.; Wang, Z.; Li, M.; Wang, M.; Liu, Y.; Yu, X.; et al. Serum-Derived PiR-Hsa-164586 of Extracellular Vesicles as a Novel Biomarker for Early Diagnosis of Non-Small Cell Lung Cancer. *Front. Oncol.* **2022**, *12*, 850363. [CrossRef] [PubMed]
86. Wang, H.; Shi, B.; Zhang, X.; Shen, P.; He, Q.; Yin, M.; Pan, Y.; Ma, J. Exosomal Hsa-PiR1089 Promotes Proliferation and Migration in Neuroblastoma via Targeting KEAP1. *Pathol. Res. Pract.* **2023**, *241*, 154240. [CrossRef]
87. Yan, H.; Wu, Q.-L.; Sun, C.-Y.; Ai, L.-S.; Deng, J.; Zhang, L.; Chen, L.; Chu, Z.-B.; Tang, B.; Wang, K.; et al. PiRNA-823 Contributes to Tumorigenesis by Regulating de Novo DNA Methylation and Angiogenesis in Multiple Myeloma. *Leukemia* **2015**, *29*, 196–206. [CrossRef]
88. Li, B.; Hong, J.; Hong, M.; Wang, Y.; Yu, T.; Zang, S.; Wu, Q. PiRNA-823 Delivered by Multiple Myeloma-Derived Extracellular Vesicles Promoted Tumorigenesis through Re-Educating Endothelial Cells in the Tumor Environment. *Oncogene* **2019**, *38*, 5227–5238. [CrossRef]
89. Ai, L.; Mu, S.; Sun, C.; Fan, F.; Yan, H.; Qin, Y.; Cui, G.; Wang, Y.; Guo, T.; Mei, H.; et al. Myeloid-Derived Suppressor Cells Endow Stem-like Qualities to Multiple Myeloma Cells by Inducing PiRNA-823 Expression and DNMT3B Activation. *Mol. Cancer* **2019**, *18*, 88. [CrossRef]
90. Feng, J.; Yang, M.; Wei, Q.; Song, F.; Zhang, Y.; Wang, X.; Liu, B.; Li, J. Novel Evidence for Oncogenic PiRNA-823 as a Promising Prognostic Biomarker and a Potential Therapeutic Target in Colorectal Cancer. *J. Cell. Mol. Med.* **2020**, *24*, 9028–9040. [CrossRef]
91. Gu, X.; Wang, C.; Deng, H.; Qing, C.; Liu, R.; Liu, S.; Xue, X. Exosomal PiRNA Profiling Revealed Unique Circulating PiRNA Signatures of Cholangiocarcinoma and Gallbladder Carcinoma. *Acta Biochim. Biophys. Sin.* **2020**, *52*, 475–484. [CrossRef]
92. Li, Y.; Yi, X.; Du, S.; Gong, L.; Wu, Q.; Cai, J.; Sun, S.; Cao, Y.; Chen, L.; Xu, L.; et al. Tumour-Derived Exosomal PiR-25783 Promotes Omental Metastasis of Ovarian Carcinoma by Inducing the Fibroblast to Myofibroblast Transition. *Oncogene* **2023**, *42*, 421–433. [CrossRef] [PubMed]
93. Ge, L.; Zhang, N.; Li, D.; Wu, Y.; Wang, H.; Wang, J. Circulating Exosomal Small RNAs Are Promising Non-Invasive Diagnostic Biomarkers for Gastric Cancer. *J. Cell. Mol. Med.* **2020**, *24*, 14502–14513. [CrossRef] [PubMed]
94. Bajo-Santos, C.; Brokāne, A.; Zayakin, P.; Endzeliņš, E.; Soboļevska, K.; Belovs, A.; Jansons, J.; Sperga, M.; Llorente, A.; Radoviča-Spalviņa, I.; et al. Plasma and Urinary Extracellular Vesicles as a Source of RNA Biomarkers for Prostate Cancer in Liquid Biopsies. *Front. Mol. Biosci.* **2023**, *10*, 980433. [CrossRef] [PubMed]
95. Peng, Q.; Chiu, P.K.-F.; Wong, C.Y.-P.; Cheng, C.K.-L.; Teoh, J.Y.-C.; Ng, C.-F. Identification of PiRNA Targets in Urinary Extracellular Vesicles for the Diagnosis of Prostate Cancer. *Diagnostics* **2021**, *11*, 1828. [CrossRef] [PubMed]
96. Sabo, A.A.; Birolo, G.; Naccarati, A.; Dragomir, M.P.; Aneli, S.; Allione, A.; Oderda, M.; Allasia, M.; Gontero, P.; Sacerdote, C.; et al. Small Non-Coding RNA Profiling in Plasma Extracellular Vesicles of Bladder Cancer Patients by Next-Generation Sequencing: Expression Levels of MiR-126-3p and PiR-5936 Increase with Higher Histologic Grades. *Cancers* **2020**, *12*, 1507. [CrossRef]
97. Rayford, K.J.; Cooley, A.; Rumph, J.T.; Arun, A.; Rachakonda, G.; Villalta, F.; Lima, M.F.; Pratap, S.; Misra, S.; Nde, P.N. PiRNAs as Modulators of Disease Pathogenesis. *Int. J. Mol. Sci.* **2021**, *22*, 2373. [CrossRef]
98. Bobis-Wozowicz, S.; Marbán, E. Editorial: Extracellular Vesicles as Next Generation Therapeutics. *Front. Cell Dev. Biol.* **2022**, *10*, 919426. [CrossRef]
99. Armstrong, J.P.K.; Stevens, M.M. Strategic Design of Extracellular Vesicle Drug Delivery Systems. *Adv. Drug Deliv. Rev.* **2018**, *130*, 12–16. [CrossRef]
100. Huang, J.; Xiao, K. Nanoparticles-Based Strategies to Improve the Delivery of Therapeutic Small Interfering RNA in Precision Oncology. *Pharmaceutics* **2022**, *14*, 1586. [CrossRef]

101. Liu, J.; Peng, X.; Yang, S.; Li, X.; Huang, M.; Wei, S.; Zhang, S.; He, G.; Zheng, H.; Fan, Q.; et al. Extracellular Vesicle PD-L1 in Reshaping Tumor Immune Microenvironment: Biological Function and Potential Therapy Strategies. *Cell Commun. Signal.* **2022**, *20*, 14. [CrossRef] [PubMed]
102. Taverna, S.; Pucci, M.; Alessandro, R. Extracellular Vesicles: Small Bricks for Tissue Repair/Regeneration. *Ann. Transl. Med.* **2017**, *5*, 83. [CrossRef]
103. Kadota, T.; Yoshioka, Y.; Fujita, Y.; Kuwano, K.; Ochiya, T. Extracellular Vesicles in Lung Cancer-From Bench to Bedside. *Semin. Cell Dev. Biol.* **2017**, *67*, 39–47. [CrossRef] [PubMed]
104. Giancaterino, S.; Boi, C. Alternative Biological Sources for Extracellular Vesicles Production and Purification Strategies for Process Scale-Up. *Biotechnol. Adv.* **2023**, *63*, 108092. [CrossRef]
105. Rome, S. Biological Properties of Plant-Derived Extracellular Vesicles. *Food Funct.* **2019**, *10*, 529–538. [CrossRef] [PubMed]
106. Fang, Z.; Liu, K. Plant-Derived Extracellular Vesicles as Oral Drug Delivery Carriers. *J. Control. Release* **2022**, *350*, 389–400. [CrossRef]
107. Chronopoulos, A.; Kalluri, R. Emerging Role of Bacterial Extracellular Vesicles in Cancer. *Oncogene* **2020**, *39*, 6951–6960. [CrossRef] [PubMed]
108. Carobolante, G.; Mantaj, J.; Ferrari, E.; Vllasaliu, D. Cow Milk and Intestinal Epithelial Cell-Derived Extracellular Vesicles as Systems for Enhancing Oral Drug Delivery. *Pharmaceutics* **2020**, *12*, 226. [CrossRef]
109. Munagala, R.; Aqil, F.; Jeyabalan, J.; Gupta, R.C. Bovine Milk-Derived Exosomes for Drug Delivery. *Cancer Lett.* **2016**, *371*, 48–61. [CrossRef]
110. Maghraby, M.K.; Li, B.; Chi, L.; Ling, C.; Benmoussa, A.; Provost, P.; Postmus, A.C.; Abdi, A.; Pierro, A.; Bourdon, C.; et al. Extracellular Vesicles Isolated from Milk Can Improve Gut Barrier Dysfunction Induced by Malnutrition. *Sci. Rep.* **2021**, *11*, 7635. [CrossRef]
111. Tosar, J.P.; García-Silva, M.R.; Cayota, A. Circulating SNORD57 Rather than PiR-54265 Is a Promising Biomarker for Colorectal Cancer: Common Pitfalls in the Study of Somatic PiRNAs in Cancer. *RNA* **2021**, *27*, 403–410. [CrossRef] [PubMed]
112. Tosar, J.P.; Rovira, C.; Cayota, A. Non-Coding RNA Fragments Account for the Majority of Annotated PiRNAs Expressed in Somatic Non-Gonadal Tissues. *Commun. Biol.* **2018**, *1*, 2. [CrossRef] [PubMed]

Disclaimer/Publisher's Note: The statements, opinions and data contained in all publications are solely those of the individual author(s) and contributor(s) and not of MDPI and/or the editor(s). MDPI and/or the editor(s) disclaim responsibility for any injury to people or property resulting from any ideas, methods, instructions or products referred to in the content.

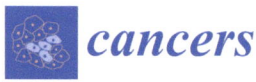 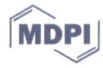

Review

Modulating Effects of Cancer-Derived Exosomal miRNAs and Exosomal Processing by Natural Products

Ya-Ting Chuang [1,†], Jen-Yang Tang [2,3,†], Jun-Ping Shiau [4], Ching-Yu Yen [5,6], Fang-Rong Chang [7], Kun-Han Yang [7], Ming-Feng Hou [4,8], Ammad Ahmad Farooqi [9,*] and Hsueh-Wei Chang [1,8,10,11,*]

[1] Graduate Institute of Medicine, College of Medicine, Kaohsiung Medical University, Kaohsiung 80708, Taiwan
[2] School of Post-Baccalaureate Medicine, Kaohsiung Medical University, Kaohsiung 80708, Taiwan
[3] Department of Radiation Oncology, Kaohsiung Medical University Hospital, Kaohsiung Medical University, Kaohsiung 80708, Taiwan
[4] Division of Breast Oncology and Surgery, Department of Surgery, Kaohsiung Medical University Hospital, Kaohsiung Medical University, Kaohsiung 80708, Taiwan
[5] School of Dentistry, Taipei Medical University, Taipei 11031, Taiwan
[6] Department of Oral and Maxillofacial Surgery, Chi-Mei Medical Center, Tainan 71004, Taiwan
[7] Graduate Institute of Natural Products, Kaohsiung Medical University, Kaohsiung 80708, Taiwan
[8] Department of Biomedical Science and Environmental Biology, College of Life Science, Kaohsiung Medical University, Kaohsiung 80708, Taiwan
[9] Institute of Biomedical and Genetic Engineering (IBGE), Islamabad 54000, Pakistan
[10] Institute of Medical Science and Technology, National Sun Yat-sen University, Kaohsiung 80424, Taiwan
[11] Center for Cancer Research, Kaohsiung Medical University, Kaohsiung 80708, Taiwan
* Correspondence: farooqiammadahmad@gmail.com (A.A.F.); changhw@kmu.edu.tw (H.-W.C.); Tel.: +92-0334-4346213 (A.A.F.); +886-7-312-1101 (ext. 2691) (H.-W.C.)
† These authors contributed equally to this work.

Simple Summary: Cancer cells generate exosomes (extracellular vesicles) to regulate many cell functions for tumor progression. Many exosome-modulating clinical drugs have been developed for effective cancer therapy, but the functions and exosome processing (secretion and assembly) modulation by natural products are not well understood. In this review, we fill the gaps between natural products-modulated miRNAs and exosome-processing by the target gene prediction of the bioinformatics database. The cancer-derived exosomal miRNAs and their exosome processing and modulated cell functions by natural products are well organized. Consequently, this review provides a comprehensive and potential modulating mechanism and targets for exosome processing and cancer cell functions for natural products.

Abstract: Cancer-derived exosomes exhibit sophisticated functions, such as proliferation, apoptosis, migration, resistance, and tumor microenvironment changes. Several clinical drugs modulate these exosome functions, but the impacts of natural products are not well understood. Exosome functions are regulated by exosome processing, such as secretion and assembly. The modulation of these exosome-processing genes can exert the anticancer and precancer effects of cancer-derived exosomes. This review focuses on the cancer-derived exosomal miRNAs that regulate exosome processing, acting on the natural-product-modulating cell functions of cancer cells. However, the role of exosomal processing has been overlooked in several studies of exosomal miRNAs and natural products. In this study, utilizing the bioinformatics database (miRDB), the exosome-processing genes of natural-product-modulated exosomal miRNAs were predicted. Consequently, several natural drugs that modulate exosome processing and exosomal miRNAs and regulate cancer cell functions are described here. This review sheds light on and improves our understanding of the modulating effects of exosomal miRNAs and their potential exosomal processing targets on anticancer treatments based on the use of natural products.

Keywords: exosome; miRNA; cell function; natural product

1. Introduction

Exosomes are extracellular vesicles of 30–100 nm in size that are secreted by both cancer and normal cells [1,2]. Cancer cells secrete more abundant and complex compositions in exosomes than normal cells. Cancer-derived exosomes exhibit diverse functions in regulating proliferation, migration, invasion, metastasis, drug resistance, inflammation, and immune responses [1,3,4].

The general structure and biogenesis of exosomes are shown in Figure 1 [5–13]. Many proteins, lipids, DNAs, mRNAs, and non-coding RNAs (circular RNAs, long-noncoding RNAs, and microRNAs (miRNAs)) exist in exosomes [1–3]. In general, the membrane proteins of exosomes include major histocompatibility complex (MHC)-I, MHC-II, flotillin, tetraspanins (CD9, CD82, CD81, and CD63), cell adhesion molecules (CAMs), integrins, and transmembrane proteins. The soluble proteins of exosomes include TSG101, heat shock protein 70 (Hsp70), Hsp90, and protein kinase B (AKT). The lipid rafts of exosomes include ceramides, sphingolipids, and cholesterol [5–13]. The process of exosome biogenesis starts with the initiation of endocytosis, early endosome, late endosome, and multivesicular body (MVB) formation, plasma membrane fusion, and release by exocytosis [5–13]. Exosome biogenesis consists of two stages, namely exosomal assembly and secretion. Many exosomal components (DNA, RNA, and proteins) are uploaded during exosome biogenesis.

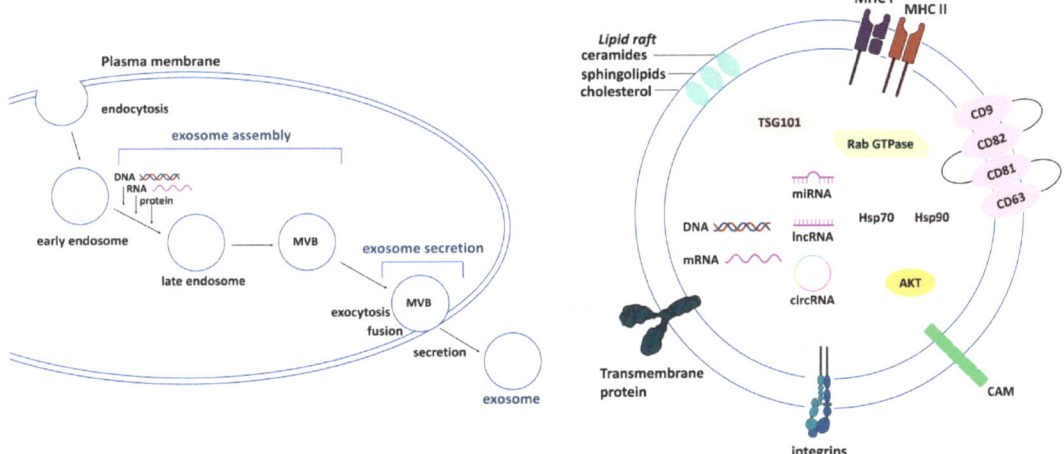

Figure 1. General structure and biogenesis of exosomes. The basic steps of exosome biogenesis, consisting of two main stages, are provided: exosome assembly and secretion. Exosomes generally contain nucleic acids, membrane and soluble proteins, and lipids. Different cells or treatments may have different compositions of exosomes. MVB, multivesicular body.

miRNAs are a group of small non-coding RNAs of 21–25 nucleotides in size. miRNAs can modulate gene expression by inhibiting mRNA translation or improving the mRNA degradation of target genes [14]. By binding to the 3′-untranslated regions (UTR) of target genes, miRNAs can knock down target gene expressions to assess their diverse functions.

Among the non-coding RNAs, this review focuses only on miRNAs, particularly exosomal miRNAs. miRNA uptake into exosomes is not a random but selective process involving secretion and transportation between exosome donors and receptors [15]. Exosomes play a vital role in regulating the development of oral [16,17], head/neck [18], breast [19], prostate [20], pancreatic [21], colon [22], gynecologic [23], liver [24], and myeloma cancer cells. In preclinical applications, exosomes are applied in diagnosis as several cancer biomarkers [25,26] and in cancer therapy using animal models [27–30]. Moreover, the exosomal miRNAs also function as modulators of drug resistance and cancer metastasis [25].

As mentioned above, exosomes and miRNAs have a close relationship in regulating cell functions. Recently, anticancer studies using natural products have shown progression in research involving exosomes and miRNAs. However, the potential impacts of exosomes and miRNAs on natural-product-regulating cancer cell functions lack systemic organization. The modulating effects of natural products on exosome biogenesis and exosomal miRNAs are discussed later, particularly in regard to their capacity for regulating exosomal processing (secretion and assembly). Moreover, some natural products and exosomal miRNAs show anticancer effects but lack investigation regarding their impacts on exosomal processing. This gap can be filled by utilizing the miRDB database [31], a bioinformatic tool which can predict the target genes of exosome processing by inputting natural-product-modulated exosomal miRNAs.

In the following review, we first explore the relationship between exosome processing (secretion and assembly) and natural products (Section 2), because the impact of exosome processing is rarely discussed in detail in the literature. Next, the prediction of the targeting of exosome-processing and AKT-signaling genes of exosome miRNAs is assessed (Section 3), because the contribution of exosome processing is rarely emphasized in the literature. The modulating effects of exosome production by natural products and their exosome delivery potential for cancer treatment (Section 4) are explored. Finally, the regulation of the cancer cell functions of natural-product-modulating miRNAs and exosomes (Section 5) is summarized (Figure 2). Consequently, this review sheds light on the organization of the relationship between exosomal processing and its related genes, exosomal miRNAs, cell functions, and natural products.

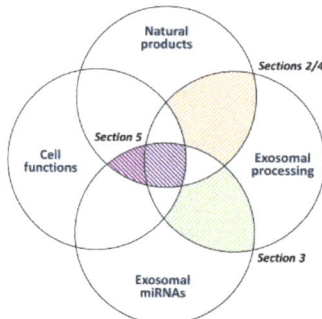

Figure 2. Connections between different sections of this review. Connections between natural products and exosomal processing are examined in Sections 2 and 4. The connection between exosomal processing and exosomal miRNAs is examined in Section 3. Finally, connections between cancer cell functions, exosomal miRNAs, and natural products are examined in Section 5.

2. Exosome Processing (Secretion and Assembly) and Natural-Product-Modulated Cell Functions

2.1. Exosome Processing (Secretion and Assembly) Genes

Several extracellular biogenesis genes, including exosomal secretion and assembly, were summarized using the Mouse Genome Database in Gene Oncology (GO) functions http://www.informatics.jax.org/vocab/gene_ontology/GO:1990182 (retrieval date: 11 November 2022) [32]. Exosomal secretion begins with the fusion of the partial endosomal membrane of a multivesicular body (MVB) with the plasma membrane, and it ends with the release of membrane-bounded vesicles into the extracellular space (Figure 1). Three main functions of exosomal secretion are classified: multiple vesicular body fusion into the apical plasma membrane, the negative regulation of exosomal secretion, and the positive regulation of exosomal secretion. Furthermore, exosomal assembly is the process in which a set of components are incorporated, aggregated, and bonded to generate an extracellular vesicular exosome. Three main functions of exosomal assembly are classified: extracellular exosome assembly, the positive regulation of extracellular exosome assembly, and the negative regulation of extracellular exosome assembly.

For exosomal secretion, "multiple vesicular body fusion into the apical plasma membrane" includes four genes, including COP9 signalosome subunit 5 (COPS5), RAB11A, a member of the RAS oncogene family (RAB11A), RAB27A, a member of the RAS oncogene family (RAB27A), and STEAP family member 3 (STEAP3). Five genes are listed as modulators of "negative regulation of exosomal secretion", including ATPase class II, type 9A (ATP9A), parkin RBR E3 ubiquitin protein ligase (PRKN), RAB7A, a member of the RAS oncogene family (RAB7A), RAB7B, a member of the RAS oncogene family (RAB7B), and vacuolar protein sorting 4B (VPS4B).

For exosomal secretion, 14 genes are listed as modulators of the "positive regulation of exosomal secretion", including ATPase type 13A2 (ATP13A2), charged multivesicular body protein 2A (CHMP2A), HGF-regulated tyrosine kinase substrate (HGS), myosin VB (MYO5B), programmed cell death 6 interacting protein (PDCD6IP), RAB7A, RAB7B, syndecan 1 (SDC1), syndecan 4 (SDC4), syndecan binding protein (SDCBP), sphingomyelin phosphodiesterase 3, neutral (SMPD3), SNF8, the endosomal sorting complexes required for transport (ESCRT)-II complex subunit, homolog (*S. cerevisiae*) (SNF8), signal-transducing adaptor molecule (SH3 domain and ITAM motif) 1 (STAM), tumor susceptibility gene 101 (TSG101), vacuolar protein sorting 4A (VPS4A), and VPS4B. RAB7A, RAB7B, and VPS4B also belong to the genes with a "negative regulation of exosomal secretion" function.

For exosomal assembly, the CD34 antigen (CD34) gene is listed among the cells that affect "extracellular exosome assembly". Four genes are listed as modulators of "positive regulation of extracellular exosome assembly", including PDCD6IP, SDC1, SDC4, and SDCBP, which also belong to the group of genes with an exosomal secretion function. Three genes are listed among the cells that affect the "regulation of extracellular exosome assembly", including PDCD6IP, STAM, and TSG101, which also belong to the group of cells with an exosomal secretion function mentioned above.

2.2. Exosomal Secretion and Assembly Effects of Natural Products in Regulating Cell Functions

Some of the exosomal secretion (Section 2.2.1) and assembly (Section 2.2.2) genes have been reported to be regulated by natural products (Table 1).

2.2.1. Exosomal Secretion Effects of Natural Products in Regulating Cell Functions

Natural-product-derived exosomes exhibit a capacity for the sophisticated regulation of cell functions in non-cancer and cancer cells. The potential roles of exosome-processing genes in natural product treatments can be predicted by target gene retrieval using the miRDB database (Table 1).

For non-cancer cells, several natural products exhibit modulating effects on cell functions in regard to exosome processing. Drug-triggered hepatic precancerous lesions upregulate exosomal RAB11A mRNA. Hesperidin downregulates exosomal RAB11A mRNA and upregulates exosomal miR-1298, resulting in hepatoprotective effects on rats (Table 1) [33]. Several natural products, such as tenuifolin, schisandrin A, celastrol, salidroside, and carnosic acid, were demonstrated to exhibit neuroprotection effects through PINK1 modulation [34]. Moreover, PINK1 and PRKN cooperate to regulate the mitophagy of renal proximal tubular cells [35]. Hence, these natural products (tenuifolin, schisandrin A, celastrol, salidroside, and carnosic acid) may modulate PRKN expression. Salvianolic acid B, a *Salvia miltiorrhiza* Bge-derived bioactive compound, suppresses renal interstitial fibrosis by inducing SDC1/E-cadherin in angiotensin II-treated proximal tubular cells [36]. Combined, *Echinacea angustifolia* DC. and *Zingiber officinale* lipophilic extracts show immunomodulatory effects by downregulating SDCBP expression based on human studies [37]. Bavachinin, a *Fructus psoraleae*-derived natural product, provides protection against the palmitic-acid-induced death of hepatocytes by upregulating VPS4B expression (Table 1) [38].

Table 1. Connecting natural products to exosomal secretion and assembly in the regulation of cell functions.

Natural Products	Genes	Cell Functions	Cancer	References
Exosomal secretion				
Methanolic extract of Moringa oleifera	↓COPS5	apoptosis	cervical	[39]
Rutin	↓COPS5	apoptosis	cervical	[40]
Hesperidin	↓RAB11A	hepatoprotective	(rat)	[33]
Heteronemin	↑STEAP3	ferroptosis	pancreatic	[41]
Dihydroartemisinin	↓STEAP3	anti-iron uptake	liver	[42]
Robustaflavone A	↓STEAP3	ferroptosis	breast	[43]
Tenuifolin, Schisandrin A, Celastrol, Salidroside, Carnosic acid	↑PRKN	mitophagy	(renal tubular cells)	[35]
Liensinine	↑RAB7A	anti-autophagy	breast	[44]
Sulfisoxazole	↓VPS4B	antimetastatic	breast	[45]
Bavachinin	↑VPS4B	pro-survival	(hepatocyte)	[38]
Squalamine	↑ATP13A2	α-synuclein aggregation	neuroblastoma	[46]
7-α-Hydroxyfrullanolide	↑PDCD6IP	apoptosis	breast	[47]
Salvianolic acid B	↓SDC1	renal interstitial fibrosis	(proximal tubular cells)	[36]
Rutaecarpine	↓SDC1	antimigration	glioblastoma	[48]
Echinacea angustifolia/ Zingiber officinale extracts	↓SDCBP	immunomodulation	(human study)	[37]
Dioscin	↑SDCBP	apoptosis, autophagy, DNA damage	liver ca	[49]
Sulforaphane	↑SDCBP	apoptosis	leukemia	[50]
Acetyl-11-keto-b-boswellic acid	↑SMPD3	antiproliferation	colon	[51]
Withanolide D	↑/↓SMPD3	apoptosis	leukemia	[52]
Resveratrol	↑TSG101	antiproliferation	intestinal tumor	[53]
Exosomal assembly				
Astragalus membranaceus extract	↑CD34	angiogenesis	(myocardial infarction)	[54]
D Rhamnose bhederin	↓STAM	chemoresistance	breast	[55]

↑, enhance or activate; ↓, inhibit or inactivate. Some are non-cancer studies, shown in parentheses. PDCD6IP, SDC1, SDC4, SDCBP, STAM, and TSG101 exhibit the regulating functions of both exosomal secretion and assembly, as described in Section 2.1.

For cancer cells, several natural products exhibit modulating effects on cell functions in regard to exosome processing. The methanolic extract of *Moringa oleifera* leaves suppresses the proliferation and causes the G1 arrest and apoptosis of cervical cancer cells by downregulating COPS5 (Table 1) [39]. Rutin, a bioflavonoid, induces the apoptosis of cervical cancer cells by downregulating COPS5 [40]. Heteronemin, a marine sesterterpenoid, induces ferroptosis by upregulating the protein expression of divalent metal transporter-1 (DMT1) and STEAP3 in pancreatic cancer cells [41]. Dihydroartemisinin, a metabolite of artemisinin, downregulates the DMT1 and STEAP3 genes controlling iron uptake in liver cancer HepG2 cells (Table 1) [42].

Selaginella trichoclada-derived robustaflavone A induces ferroptosis by downregulating the expressions of acyl-CoA synthetase long-chain family member 4 (ACSL4), ACSL5, STEAP3, lysophosphatidylcholine acyltransferase (LPCAT3), and autophagy-related 7 (ATG7) genes in breast cancer cells (Table 1) [43]. Liensinine, a *Nelumbo nucifera*-derived isoquinoline alkaloid, induces the expression of the small GTP-binding protein RAB7A and suppresses autophagosome–lysosome fusion for the degradation of breast cancer cells [44]. Squalamine inhibits the α-synuclein aggregation of neuroblastoma cells [56]. The inhibition of ATP13A2 destroys lysosomal membrane integrity and induces the α-synuclein accumulation of neuroblastoma cells (Table 1) [46]. All this warrants a detailed assessment of the role of ATP13A2 in squalamine treatment.

Sulfisoxazole shows antimetastatic effects on breast cancer cells by downregulating VPS4B mRNA expression (Table 1) [45]. 7-α-Hydroxyfrullanolide, an Asteraceae-plant-derived natural product, upregulates PDCD6IP expression in breast cancer cells [47]. Rutaecarpine downregulates the mRNA expression of the SDC1 gene to suppress glioblastoma cell migration [48]. Dioscin, a steroid saponin, causes the apoptosis, autophagy, and DNA damage of liver cancer cells by upregulating SDCBP expression [49]. Sulforaphane, a cruciferous-vegetable-derived compound, triggers apoptosis by upregulating SDCBP expression in leukemia HL-60 cells [50]. Acetyl-11-keto-b-boswellic acid (AKBA), a *Boswellia serrata*-derived natural product, inhibits the proliferation of colon cancer cells by upregulating SMPD3 [51]. Withanolide D triggers the apoptosis of leukemia MOLT-4 cells by upregulating SMPD3 expression after 15 min and downregulating after 45 min [52]. The oral administration of resveratrol suppresses intestinal tumorigenesis in mice and upregulates TSG101 mRNA expression (Table 1) [53]. All this warrants a detailed assessment exploring the roles of more natural-product-regulated cell functions in exosomal secretion in the future.

2.2.2. Exosomal Assembly Effects of Natural Products in Regulating Cell Functions

Natural products also regulate exosomal assembly. *Astragalus membranaceus* extract enhances angiogenesis in myocardial infarction rats by upregulating vascular endothelial growth factor (VEGF), CD34, and endothelial nitric oxide synthase (eNOS) expression [54]. Moreover, D Rhamnose bhederin, a *Clematis ganpiniana*-derived bioactive component, inhibits exosome secretion from docetaxel-resistant breast cancer cells and alleviates the transmission of resistance [55]. D Rhamnose bhederin downregulates several miRNAs (miR-16-5p, miR-23a-3p, miR-24-3p, miR-26a-5p, and miR-27a-3p), in which miR-24-3p is predicted to target exosomal-assembly related genes, such as STAM, according to the miRDB database [31]. This warrants a detailed assessment exploring the roles of more natural-product-regulated cell functions in exosomal assembly in the future.

3. Prediction of the Targeting of Exosome-Processing and AKT-Signaling Genes of Certain Exosome miRNAs

Several exosomal miRNAs have been reviewed previously [4,16,57]. However, their potential impacts on exosomal processing (secretion and assembly) have rarely been investigated. In this study, utilizing the miRDB database [31], these exosomal miRNAs targeting exosome-processing genes (Section 2) were retrieved (Table 2). miR-29a-3p is predicted to target SMPD3. miR-101-3p and miR-21-5p/miR-30a-5p are predicted to target RAB27A and RAB11A, respectively. miR-6887-5p is predicted to target RAB7A and RAB7B. miR-142-3p and miR-24-3p are predicted to target HGS and ATP13A2/STAM, respectively. miR-106a-5p, miR-106b-5p, miR-21-5p, miR-223-3p, miR-365a-3p, and miR-374a-5p are predicted to target MYO5B. miR-522-3p and miR-8485 are predicted to target PDCD6IP (Table 2).

Additionally, miR-8485 is also predicted to target SDC1 and SDCBP. miR-128-3p, miR-142-3p, miR-200c-3p, miR-223-3p, and miR-8485 are predicted to target STAM. miR-106a-5p and miR-106b-5p are predicted to target TSG101. Finally, miR-128-3p, miR-32-5p, and miR-92a-3p are predicted to target VPS4B (Table 2). Consequently, these examples demonstrate that many of the reported exosomal miRNAs have the potential to target exosomal processing genes. This warrants an advanced examination exploring the roles of exosomal processing genes in several reported exosomal miRNA studies in the future.

Moreover, some exosomal miRNAs are reported to regulate AKT signaling [58–61]. Among the examples of exosomal miRNAs listed in Table 2, miR-29a-3p is predicted to target AKT2 and AKT3 (Table 2). miR-374a-5p is predicted to target AKT1. miR-101-3p, miR-106a-5p, miR-106b-5p, miR-365a-3p, miR-6887-5p, and miR-30a-3p are predicted to target AKT1, ATK2, or AKT3. Those AKT1-, AKT2-, and AKT3-targeting exosomal miRNAs (miR-29a-3p, miR-374a-5p, miR-101-3p, miR-106a-5p, miR-106b-5p, miR-365a-3p, miR-6887-5p, and miR-30a-3p) also target some exosomal processing genes (Table 2).

Exosomal proteins can activate AKT signaling in the regulation of metastasis. Annexin A5, one of the exosome proteins in prostate cancer tissues, activates AKT signaling to stimulate the epithelial–mesenchymal transition (EMT) and upregulate matrix metalloproteinase-2 (MMP2) and MMP9 expression [5]. The exosomal miRNAs involved in AKT signaling have been applied in animal [59] and preclinical experiments [60]. Bone-marrow—mesenchymal-stem-cell-derived exosomes, which are rich in miR-126-3p (miR-126), enhance the migration and angiogenesis of human umbilical vein endothelial cells (HUVECs) [59]. This exosomal miR-126-3p stimulates vascularization at wound sites and improves cutaneous wound healing in mice models. Plasma exosomes isolated from Graves ophthalmopathy with an effective response to intravenous glucocorticoid therapy contain a high level of miR-885-3p, showing AKT inhibition and improving glucocorticoid sensitivity [60]. Consequently, the exosomal miRNAs with AKT modulating ability are potential tools for preclinical applications.

Table 2. Connecting some exosomal miRNAs to the predicted targets of exosome processing and AKT genes.

	ATP9A	ATP13A2	HGS	MYO5B	RAB27A	RAB11A	RAB7A	RAB7B	PDCD6IP	SDC1	SDCBP	SMPD3	STAM	TSG101	VPS4B	AKT
miR-29a-3p [4,16]												SMPD3				AKT2/3
miR-101-3p [4]					RAB27A											AKT3
miR-106a-5p [16,57]				MYO5B										TSG101		AKT3
miR-106b-3p [57]				MYO5B										TSG101		AKT3
miR-128-3p [57]																
miR-142-3p [4,16]			HGS										STAM		VPS4B	
miR-200c-3p [4,16]													STAM			
miR-21-5p [4,57]				MYO5B		RAB11A							STAM			
miR-223-3p [16]				MYO5B												
miR-24-3p [4,16]		ATP13A2											STAM			
miR-32-5p [57]													STAM		VPS4B	
miR-365a-3p [57]				MYO5B												AKT3
miR-374a-5p [57]				MYO5B												AKT1
miR-522-3p [57]									PDCD6IP							
miR-6887-5p [4]							RAB7A	RAB7B								AKT3
miR-8485 [4]	ATP9A								PDCD6IP	SDC1	SDCBP		STAM		VPS4B	
miR-92a-3p [57]																AKT3
miR-30a-3p [62]						RAB11A										

The predicted targets for exosomal processing and AKT genes of the exosomal miRNAs were retrieved from the miRDB database (retrieval date: 12 November 2022).

4. Natural Products Modulate Exosome Production and Their Exosome Delivery for the Purpose of Cancer Treatment

Many natural-product-derived exosomes have been demonstrated to exhibit theranostic effects in cancer therapy [63–66]. The modulating results of exosome biogenesis and delivery by natural products are discussed as follows below.

Some natural products improve exosome biogenesis. Sulforaphane suppresses the fusion of early and late endosomes (GFP-Rab5a and GFP-Rab7a) with the lysosome, blocks the autophagy flux, promotes exosome production, and triggers exosome-dependent paracrine senescence by downregulating mTOR and transcription factor binding to IGHM enhancer 3 (TFE3) [67]. Sulforaphane induces a high protein concentration of exosomes and causes the accumulation of exosome marker CD63 in esophageal cancer cells. Moreover, supernatants from sulforaphane-treated cancer cells show high CD63 expression [67]. Consequently, sulforaphane triggers exosome biogenesis and secretion in esophageal cancer cells.

In contrast, some natural products suppress exosome biogenesis. Autophagy and lysosome dysfunction enhance exosome secretion [68,69] and vice versa. Asteltoxin inhibits mitochondrial ATP synthase and exosome generation by upregulating AMPK-dependent mTORC1 inactivation and lysosome activation [70]. Transmission electron microscopy analysis shows that asteltoxin induces lysosome–MVB fusion, causing the downregulation of exosome generation. Berberine suppresses the proliferation of colon cancer cells by downregulating acetyl-CoA carboxylase (ACC) for fatty acid synthesis and reducing exosome biogenesis and the secretion of colon and cervical cancer cells [71], an observation which is supported by the finding that berberine downregulates syntenin and TSG101, as intracellular vesicle markers.

Some natural-product-derived exosomes exhibit modulating effects on cell functions. Exosomes used in phytoagent deoxyelephantopin treatment, a plant deoxyelephantopin derivative, suppress the ROS-mediated proliferation of breast cancer cells, reversed by *N*-acetylcysteine [72]. Phytoagent deoxyelephantopin also enhances calcium-dependent exosome secretion from breast cancer cells. *Momordica charantia*-derived exosome-like nanovesicles suppress the proliferation and migration of glioma cells by downregulating phosphorylated PI3K/AKT [73]. *Fusobacterium nucleatum* is rich in colon cancer lesions associated with colon cancer carcinogenesis and metastases. Exosomes from *Fusobacterium nucleatum* enhance the invasion of colon cancer cells. This invasion is prevented by the bioactive compounds of *Paris polyphylla*, such as pennogenin 3-O-beta-chacotrioside and polyphyllin VI, which exhibit cell-killing effects on *Fusobacterium nucleatum* [74]. All this warrants an advanced examination exploring the impacts of exosomal biogenesis by natural products and natural-product-derived exosomes on cell functions in the future.

Moreover, exosomes are naturally generated, showing lower cytotoxicity and immunogenicity and higher biocompatibility than lipid-based nanoparticles [6,65,75]. Exosomes were reported to effectively deliver several natural products that can be exploited for preclinical anticancer therapy in vitro and in vivo [65]. The oral delivery of paclitaxel using milk-derived exosomes results in less side effects of immunologic toxicity and higher antitumor effects than i.v. in lung-tumor-xenograft nude mice [76]. Exosome-delivered curcumin exhibits a high in vitro stability and in vivo bioavailability [77]. Celastrol-loaded milk exosomes show a high degree of anti-lung tumor growth with in vivo biosafety [78]. This warrants the advanced testing of more natural products based on exosome delivery strategies in the future.

5. The Role of Natural-Product-Modulating miRNAs and Exosomes in Regulating Cancer Cell Functions

A mounting array of literature reports that natural products modulate many miRNAs that regulate their target genes to affect several of the cell functions of cancer cells [79]. However, most of these studies did not investigate the impacts of exosomal miRNAs on anticancer effects using natural products.

Recently, several natural-product-induced exosomal miRNA studies have been reported. *Aurea helianthus* extract inhibits the migration and induces the senescence and autophagy of endometrial cancer cells [80]. Several miRNAs derived from the induced exosomes in these extract-treated endometrial cancer cells were upregulated or downregulated. However, there is a lack of systemic information on the modulating effects of drug-induced exosomal miRNAs based on natural products. Most natural-product-modulating miRNA studies have focused on impacts on cancer cell functions without considering the contribution of exosomes. Consequently, there are gaps between exosomal miRNAs and natural products in terms of their anticancer effects.

A total of 26 natural-product-modulated exosomal miRNAs that regulate cancer cell functions, such as antiproliferation (Section 5.1), apoptosis (Section 5.2), antimigration/anti-invasion/anti-EMT/anti-angiogenesis (Section 5.3), the modulation of chemo- and radioresistance (Section 5.4), and others (Section 5.5), are summarized in Table 3. Many non-exosomal miRNA studies have assessed the impacts of the anticancer effects of natural products. In the future, a detailed examination of the roles of exosomes and investigations of their anticancer effects related to miRNAs and natural products should be carried out.

Table 3. Connecting natural products to exosomal miRNA-regulated cell functions.

Natural Products	miRNAs	Cell Functions	Cancer	References
Ursolic acid	↓miR-21-5p	apoptosis	glioblastoma	[81]
	↑miR-200c-3p	apoptosis, anti-invasion	colon	[82]
Resveratrol	↓miR-21-5p	apoptosis	bladder	[83]
	↓miR-31-5p	anticolitis	(T cells)	[84]
	↑miR-424-5p	antiproliferation	breast	[85]
Berberine	↓miR-21-5p	antiproliferation	myeloma	[86]
	↑miR-144-3p	apoptosis, autophagy	lung	[87]
	↑miR-101-3p	antiproliferation, antimigration	endometrial	[88]
Butylcycloheptyl prodiginine	↓miR-21-5p	antiproliferation	colon	[89]
Honokiol	↓miR-21-5p	apoptosis	osteosarcoma	[90]
	↑miR-34a-5p	anti-EMT	breast	[91]
Sophocarpine	↓miR-21-5p	antiproliferation, anti-EMT	head/neck	[92]
Tricin	↓miR-21-5p	chemosensitization	prostate	[93]
Dihydromyricetin	↓miR-21-5p	antiproliferation, antimigration	cholangiocarcinoma	[94]
Curcumin	↓miR-21-5p	antiproliferation, antimigration	liver	[95]
	↑miR-200c-3p	anti-EMT	colon	[96]
	↑miR-142-3p	20S proteasome suppression	breast	[97]
	↓miR-1246	antiproliferation	bladder	[98]
Curcumol	↓miR-21-5p	antiproliferation	colon	[99]
PRP1	↓miR-21-5p	apoptosis	liver	[100]
Sinomenine	↓miR-21-5p	antimigration	lung	[101]
Psoralen	↑miR-196a-5p	apoptosis	gastric	[102]
Pinolenic acid	↑miR-3188	anti-inflammation	(rheumatoid arthritis)	[103]
Pachymic acid	↓miR-24-3p	anti-heart failure	(left ventricle)	[104]
Genistein	↓miR-155-5p	antiproliferation	(cardiac)	[105]
(−)-Epigallocatechin gallate	↓miR-155-5p	chemosensitization	colon	[106]
	↑miR-34a-5p	radiosensitization	liver	[107]
Enoxolone, Magnolol, Palmatine chloride	↑miR-200c-3p	anti-invasion	breast	[108]
(−)-Sativan	↑miR-200c-3p	apoptosis, antimigration	breast	[109]
Isoliquiritigenin	↑miR-200c-3p	antimigration	breast	[110]
Thymoquinone	↑miR-30a-5p	anti-liver fibrosis	(liver)	[111]
Nicotine	↑miR-30a-5p	G1 arrest	(periodontal ligament)	[112]
Norcantharidin	↑miR-30a-5p	antiproliferation, antimigration	giant cell tumor of bone	[62]
1′S-1′-acetoxychavicol acetate	↓miR-210-3p	apoptosis	cervical	[113]
Crocin	↓miR-365a-3p	apoptosis	cervical	[114]
	↓miR-34a-5p	apoptosis	papillary thyroid	[115]
Isoliquiritigenin	↓miR-421	apoptosis, DNA damage	oral	[116]
Anisomycin	↑miR-421	anti-angiogenesis	ovarian	[117]
Asparanin A	↓miR-421	antimigration	endometrial	[118]
Rhamnetin, Cirsiliol	↑miR-34a-5p	radiosensitization, anti-EMT	lung	[119]
Dihydroartemisinin	↑miR-34a-5p	apoptosis, antimigration	prostate	[120]
Isovitexin	↑miR-34a-5p	apoptosis	osteosarcoma	[121]
Emodin	↑miR-34a-5p	antiproliferation	liver	[122]
Kaempferol	↑miR-130a-3p	cytokine reduction	(chondrocyte)	[123]
Chicoric acid	↓miR-130a-3p	anti-inflammation	lung	[124]
Mitomycin C	↑miR-31-5p	chemosensitization	bladder	[125]
Licochalcone A	↑miR-144-3p	ER stress, apoptosis	lung	[126]
10-Hydroxycamptothecin	↑miR-23b-3p	apoptosis	(fibroblast)	[127]
Astaxanthin	↓miR-382-5p	anti-liver fibrosis	(liver)	[128]
Polydatin	↑miR-382-5p	apoptosis	colon	[129]
Piperlongumine	↓miR-30d-5p	antiproliferation	osteosarcoma	[130]

↑, enhance or activate; ↓, inhibit or inactivate. Non-cancer studies are shown in parentheses.

5.1. Antiproliferation by Natural-Product-Modulated Exosomal miRNAs

Natural products may regulate cell proliferation by modulating miR-424-5p, miR-21-5p (miR-21), miR-101-3p, miR-1246, miR-155-5p (miR-155), miR-30a-5p, miR-34a-5p, and miR-30d-5p (Table 3), as described in the following section.

miR-424-5p is downregulated in breast cancer tissues. Resveratrol inhibits the proliferation of breast cancer cells by upregulating miR-424-5p and downregulating heterogeneous nuclear ribonucleoprotein A1 (HNRNPA1) [85] (Table 3).

Berberine, a natural alkaloid, inhibits the proliferation of multiple myeloma cells by downregulating miR-21-5p and upregulating its target, programmed cell death 4 (*PDCD4*) [86] (Table 3). The natural product butylcycloheptyl prodiginine promotes the antiproliferation of colon cancer cells by binding pre-miR-21-5p to inhibit the function of miR-21-5p [89]. Honokiol, a *Magnolia officinalis*-derived natural product, promotes the antiproliferation of osteosarcoma cells by downregulating miR-21-5p/AKT signaling [90]. Sophocarpine, a *Sophora flavescens*-derived bioactive compound, suppresses the proliferation of head and neck cancer cells by targeting miR-21-5p [92]. Dihydromyricetin, a natural flavonoid, suppresses the proliferation of cholangiocarcinoma cells by downregulating miR-21-5p [94]. Curcumin decreases the proliferation of liver cancer cells by downregulating miR-21-5p and upregulating its target, SRY-box transcription factor 6 (*SOX6*) [95] (Table 3).

Exosomal miR-101-3p displays tumor-suppressive and oncogenic functions. Oral cancer cells express low levels of miR-101-3p by targeting the collagen type X alpha 1 chain (*COL10A1*). In contrast, exosomes derived from bone marrow mesenchymal stem cells overexpress miR-101-3p to suppress oral cancer proliferation and migration [131]. miR-101-3p mimics suppress the proliferation and migration and trigger the apoptosis of medulloblastoma cells by targeting the enhancer of zeste homolog 2 (*EZH2*), a histone methyltransferase [132]. In contrast, exosomal miR-101-3p exhibits an oncogenic function to improve the proliferation and migration of colon cancer cells by downregulating its target, the homeodomain-interacting protein kinase (*HIPK3*) [133]. Berberine, a plant-bark-derived alkaloid, suppresses the proliferation of endometrial cancer cells by upregulating miR-101-3p to downregulate cyclo-oxygenase-2 (COX-2) [88] (Table 3).

Exosomal miR-1246 is reported to regulate cell migration. Exosomal miR-1246 from highly metastatic oral cancer cells promotes the migration and invasion of poorly metastatic oral cancer cells by downregulating the DENN/MADD-domain-containing 2D (DENND2D) [134]. In addition to antimigration, miR-1246 was reported to modulate proliferation (Table 3). Bladder cancer T24 cells highly express miR-1246. Curcumin inhibits the proliferation of bladder cancer cells by downregulating miR-1246 [98]. Combined treatment (curcumin and X-ray) synergistically suppresses its proliferation to a greater extent than individual treatments by decreasing miR-1246 expression [98].

Moreover, natural products were reported to modulate miR-155-5p, miR-30a-5p, and miR-34a-5p expression, regulating cancer cell proliferation (Table 3). Genistein, a soy isoflavone phytoestrogen, suppresses the proliferation of breast cancer cells by downregulating miR-155-5p [105]. Thymoquinone, a black-seed-oil-derived compound, suppresses liver fibrosis by upregulating miR-30a-5p to inhibit its target, such as snail family transcriptional repressor 1 (*SNAI1*), inhibiting EMT [111]. Norcantharidin, a cantharidin derivative, inhibits the proliferation of giant-cell tumors of the bone by upregulating miR-30a-5p and downregulating AKT, reversed by inhibiting miR-30a-5p [62]. Emodin, a natural anthraquinone derivative, suppresses liver cancer cell proliferation by upregulating miR-34a-5p [122].

Exosomal miR-30d-5p appears in higher levels in cervical cancer tissues than in normal controls [135]. However, the miR-30d-5p-modulating cell function has rarely been reported, particularly in regard to the antiproliferation of cancer cells. A recent study of natural products reported the antiproliferation effect achieved by the modulation of miR-30d-5p (Table 3). Piperlongumine, a long-pepper-derived amide alkaloid, suppresses the proliferation of osteosarcoma cells by downregulating miR-30d-5p and upregulating its target, the suppressor of cytokine signaling 3 (*SOCS3*) [130].

Furthermore, natural products may regulate cancer cell proliferation by modulating miR-200c-3p (Table 3). (−)-Sativan, a *Spatholobus suberectus*-derived isoflavane, suppresses the proliferation of breast cancer cells by upregulating miR-200c-3p to downregulate its direct target, such as prickle planar cell polarity protein 2 (*PRICKLE2*; *EPM5*) [109].

5.2. Apoptosis by Natural-Product-Modulated Exosomal miRNAs

Several natural products modulate apoptosis in cancer cells by downregulating miR-21-5p, miR-196a-5p (miR-196a), miR-210-3p, miR-365a-3p (miR-365), miR-34a-5p (miR-34a), miR-144-3p (miR-144), miR-23b-3p, and miR-382-5p (Table 3), as described in the following section.

Several natural products promote apoptosis through miR-21-5p in cancer cells. Ursolic acid triggers the apoptosis of glioblastoma cells by downregulating miR-21-5p [81] (Table 3). Resveratrol triggers the apoptosis of bladder cancer cells by downregulating miR-21-5p and AKT phosphorylation, reversed by miR-21-5p overexpression [83]. The downregulation of miR-196a-5p enhances cisplatin resistance [102]. Psoralen, a natural photosensitizing drug, triggers the apoptosis of gastric cancer cells to alleviate cisplatin resistance by upregulating miR-196a-5p and downregulating homeobox B7 (HOXB7) and HER2 expression [102]. Honokiol enhances the apoptosis of osteosarcoma cells by downregulating miR-21-5p/AKT signaling [90]. Dihydromyricetin triggers the apoptosis of cholangiocarcinoma cells by downregulating miR-21-5p [94]. PRP1, a *Platycodonis*-radix-derived polysaccharide, promotes the apoptosis of liver cancer cells by reducing miR-21-5p expression and inactivating AKT [100].

Exosomal miR-210-3p promotes the angiogenesis and tubulogenesis of endothelial cells [136] and enhances the metastasis of lung cancer cells [137]. A recent study demonstrated the novel function of the apoptosis-modulating effect of miR-210-3p, regulated by natural products. In hypoxic conditions, colon cancer cells enhance tumor progression. The transmission of hypoxic colon-cancer-cell-derived exosomal miR-210-3p to normoxic tumor cells prevents apoptosis and induces a protumoral effect [138]. 1′S-1′-Acetoxychavicol acetate (ACA), a wild ginger *Alpinia conchigera*-derived natural product, triggers the apoptosis of cervical cancer cells by downregulating miR-210-3p to upregulate its target, SMAD family member 4 (*SMAD4*) [113] (Table 3).

Exosomal miR-365a-3p regulates the chemoresistance of cancer cells involved in apoptosis. Exosomal miR-365a-3p derived from imatinib-resistant chronic myeloid leukemia (CML) cells provides drug resistance to, and prevents apoptosis in, sensitive CML cells [139]. Natural product studies showed that miR-365a-3p exhibits an apoptosis-modulating effect (Table 3). Crocin, a carotenoid pigment of saffron, induces cervical cancer cell apoptosis by upregulating Bax and downregulating BCL2 and miR-365a-3p [114]. The combination treatment of cervical cancer cells with crocin and cisplatin promotes antiproliferation and apoptosis by downregulating miR-365a-3p, an upregulator of BAX and BCL2 [140].

Exosomal miR-421 regulates the chemoresistance of cancer cells. Exosomes from cisplatin-resistant oral cancer patients enhance the proliferation and reduce the cisplatin sensitivity of cisplatin-resistant cells by downregulating miR-421 expression [141]. The hypermethylation of transcription-factor-activating-enhancer-binding protein 2e (TFAP2E) enhances 5-fluorouracil chemoresistance in gastric cancer cells by upregulating exosomal miR-421 [142]. However, the impact of apoptosis by exosomal miR-421 is unclear. A recent natural product study reported the apoptosis function through the modulation of miR-421 (Table 3). Isoliquiritigenin induces the apoptosis and DNA damage of oral cancer cells by downregulating miR-421 expression [116].

Exosomal miR-34a-5p regulates the proliferation of cancer cells. Normal fibroblasts exhibit higher miR-34a-5p levels than cancer-associated fibroblasts from oral cancer patients. miR-34a-5p overexpression in cancer-associated fibroblasts suppresses cancer cell proliferation and migration [143]. Exosomal miR-34a-5p induces the antiproliferation and apoptosis of pancreatic cancer cells [144]. Several natural product studies have demonstrated the apoptosis function of cancer cells through the modulation of miR-34a-5p (Table 3). Dihydroartemisinin triggers the apoptosis of prostate cancer cells by upregulating miR-34a-5p [120]. Isovitexin, a flavonoid, triggers the apoptosis of osteosarcoma cells by upregulating miR-34a-5p and downregulating BCL2 [121]. Crocin, a saffron-derived pigment, triggers the ROS-dependent apoptosis of papillary thyroid cancer cells by downregulating the miR-34a-5p and upregulating its target, protein tyrosine phosphatase non-receptor type 4 (*PTPN4*) [115].

miR-144-3p exhibits differential expressions in different cancer cells. miR-144-3p is downregulated in lung cancer cells. Exosomal miR-144-3p from bone marrow-derived mesenchymal stem cells suppresses the proliferation of lung cancer cells by downregulating cyclin E1 (CCNE1) and CCNE2 [145]. In contrast, miR-144-3p is upregulated in nasopharyngeal cancer cells. Exosomal miR-144-3p from nasopharyngeal cancer cells promotes angiogenesis [146]. However, the apoptosis-inducing effect of exosomal miR-421 has rarely been examined. Recent natural product studies demonstrated apoptosis induction through the modulation of miR-144-3p (Table 3). Berberine induces the apoptosis of lung cancer cells by upregulating miR-144-3p [87]. Licochalcone A, a *Glycyrrhiza inflata*-derived natural product, induces ER stress and the apoptosis of lung cancer cells by upregulating miR-144-3p [126].

miR-23b-3p suppresses the proliferation and migration of prostate [147] cancer cells, while it enhances pancreatic cell migration [148] and salivary cancer cell angiogenesis and metastasis [149]. However, the apoptosis function of exosomal miR-421 has rarely been reported. A natural product investigation validated the fact that apoptosis induction results from the modulation of miR-23b-3p (Table 3). 10-Hydroxycamptothecin, a *Nothapodytes nimmoniana*-derived natural product, causes the apoptosis of fibroblasts by upregulating miR-23b-3p [127].

Exosomal miR-382-5p from cancer-associated fibroblasts enhances the migration of oral cancer cells [150]. A recent natural product study demonstrated the novel function of apoptosis induction through the modulation of miR-382-5p (Table 3). Polydatin, a metabolite of trans-resveratrol, inhibits the proliferation and causes the apoptosis of colon cancer cells by upregulating miR-382-5p and downregulating its target, programmed cell death ligand 1 (*PD-L1*) [129].

5.3. Antimigration/Anti-Invasion/Anti-EMT/Anti-Angiogenesis by Natural-Product-Modulated Exosomal miRNAs

Several natural products regulate the migration, invasion, and angiogenesis of cancer cells by modulating miR-101-3p, miR-30a-5p, miR-34a-5p, miR-200c-3p, miR-21-5p, and miR-421 (Table 3), as described in the following section.

Some miRNAs showing migration-suppressing effects are upregulated by several natural products. Berberine suppresses the migration of endometrial cancer cells by upregulating miR-101-3p to downregulate cyclo-oxygenase-2 (COX-2) [88] (Table 3). Norcantharidin inhibits the migration of giant-cell tumors of the bone by upregulating miR-30a-5p and downregulating AKT, reversed by inhibiting miR-30a-5p [62]. Dihydroartemisinin suppresses the migration of prostate cancer cells by upregulating miR-34a-5p [120]. Honokiol, a *Magnolia grandiflora*-derived polyphenol, suppresses the leptin-promoted EMT of breast cancer cells by upregulating miR-34a-5p [91]. Anisomycin suppresses angiogenesis in ovarian cancer stem cells by upregulating miR-421 [117].

Similarly, exosomal miR-200c-3p suppresses the migration and invasion of lipopolysaccharide (LPS)-treated colon cancer cells by targeting zinc finger E-box-binding homeobox-1 (*ZEB-1*) [151]. The natural compounds enoxolone, magnolol, and palmatine chloride suppress the invasion of breast cancer cells by upregulating miR-200c-3p [108]. (−)-Sativan inhibits the migration of breast cancer cells by upregulating miR-200c-3p [109]. Similarly, curcumin, acting on colon cancer cells, exhibits the downregulation of EMT-related gene expression by upregulating miR-200c-3p and downregulating its target, *PRICKLE2* [96]. Isoliquiritigenin, a Glycyrrhizae Rhizoma-derived bioactive component, inhibits migration, metastasis, and breast tumor growth by inhibiting EMT and upregulating miR-200c-3p, which is downregulated in breast cancer tissues [110]. Ursolic acid, a pentacyclic triterpenoid, induces the apoptosis and inhibits the invasive ability of colon cancer cells by upregulating miR-200c-3p [82].

In contrast, some miRNAs showing migration-promoting effects are suppressed by natural product treatments. The transfer of hypoxic oral cancer exosomes containing miR-21-5p to normal cells improves their pro-metastatic effects [152]. Sophocarpine suppresses the epithelial–mesenchymal transition (EMT) of head and neck cancer cells by targeting miR-21-5p [92]. Dihydromyricetin inhibits the migration of cholangiocarcinoma cells by downregulating miR-21-5p [94]. Curcumin decreases the migration of liver cancer cells by downregulating miR-21-5p [95]. Sinomenine, a *Sinomenium acutum*-derived alkaloid, shows antimigration effects on lung cancer cells by suppressing miR-21-5p and MMP2/9 [101]. Asparanin A, a vegetable- and *Asparagus officinalis-derived natural product*, suppresses the migration of endometrial cancer cells by downregulating miR-421 [118].

5.4. Modulation of Chemo- and Radio-Resistance by Natural-Product-Modulated Exosomal miRNAs

Several natural products regulate migration, invasion, and angiogenesis in cancer cells by modulating miR-21-5p, miR-155-5p, miR-34a-5p, and miR-31-5p, as described in the following section.

Some miRNAs showing resistance-promoting effects are downregulated by several natural products. miR-21-5p has been identified in exosomes from hypoxic oral cancer cells. miR-21-5p-containing hypoxic oral cancer exosomes also exhibit cisplatin resistance in oral cancer cells, as evidenced by exosome transfer experiments [153]. Natural products may inhibit drug resistance in cancer cells by downregulating miR-21-5p. Tricin, an *Allium atroviolaceum*-derived compound, sensitizes the docetaxel response to prostate cancer cells by downregulating miR-21-5p [93] (Table 3).

Similarly, exosomal miR-155-5p enhances the migration or metastasis of gastric [154], lung [155], renal [156], and colon [157] cancer cells. Recently, a resistance-modulating function of exosome miR-155-5p was reported. Exosome miR-155-5p from oral cancer cells improves cisplatin resistance to cisplatin-sensitive cells by upregulating EMT [158]. A natural product study showed the resistance-modulating function of miR-155-5p (Table 3). (−)-Epigallocatechin gallate (EGCG), a green- or red-tea-derived bioactive compound, improves 5-fluorouracil (5-FU) sensitivity in colon cancer cells by suppressing miR-155-5p expression [106].

In contrast, some miRNAs showing resistance-suppressing effects are upregulated by several natural products. Rhamnetin and cirsiliol, the quercetin and flavonoid derivatives, enhance radiosensitization and suppress lung cancer cell EMT by upregulating miR-34a-5p [119]. miR-34a-5p is downregulated in liver cancer tissues. EGCG improves the radiosensitization of liver cancer cells by upregulating miR-34a-5p [107]. Similarly, bladder cancer tissues exhibit a low level of miR-31-5p. Mitomycin C sensitivity is enhanced in bladder cancer cells by upregulating miR-31-5p to target integrin α5 (*ITGA5*) [125].

5.5. Potential Modulation Effects of Target Immunotherapy of Cancer by Natural-Product-Modulated Exosomal miRNAs

The tumor immune microenvironment (TIME) comprises several types of immune cells. Some miRNAs were identified in the tumor-associated macrophages (TAM), natural killer (NK) cells, and myeloid-derived suppressor cells (MDSC) of TIME [159]. A comparison illustrated that some of them overlapped with the exosomal miRNAs modulated by natural products (Table 3). Upon inspection, some of the exosomal miRNAs (miR-21-5p, miR-200c-3p, miR-155-5p, miR-30a-5p, miR-34a-5p, miR-130a-3p, miR-101-3p, miR-142-3p, and miR-24-3p) listed in Table 3 were reported in certain immune cells of TIME [159], such as TAM, NK, and MDSC. However, the review in question [159] rarely mentioned the impacts of natural products.

Here, we discuss the indirect connections of these exosomal miRNAs to natural products (Table 4). TAM upregulates several exosomal miRNAs (miR-21-5p, miR-155-5p, miR-30a-5p, miR-101-3p, and miR-142-3p) but downregulates miR-34a-5p [159]. NK upregulates miR-155-5p, miR-130a-3p, miR-101-3p, and miR-24-3p. MDSC upregulates miR-21-5p, miR-200c-3p, miR-155-5p, and miR-30a-5p. Since some of the miRNAs listed in Table 4 are downregulated or upregulated by several natural products, their potential impacts in modulating the expressions of the TAM, NK, and MDSC of TIME are worthy of attention. Notably, TIME miRNAs that are not included in Tables 3 and 4 may be modulated by natural products and, thus, require detailed investigation.

Table 4. Connecting natural-product-modulated exosomal miRNAs to TIME.

miRNAs	miRNAs Status in TIME	miRNA Effects of Natural Products *
miR-21-5p	↑TAM [159] ↑MDSC [159]	↓ miR-21-5p (Ursolic acid [81], Resveratrol [83], Berberine [86], Butylcycloheptyl prodiginine [89], Honokiol [90], Sophocarpine [92], Tricin [93], Dihydromyricetin [94], Curcumin [95], Curcumol [99], PRP1 [100], Sinomenine [101])
miR-200c-3p	↑MDSC [159]	↑ miR-200c-3p (Urolic acid [82], Curcumin [96], Enoxolone, Magnolol, Palmatine chloride [108], (−)-Sativan [109], Isoliquiritigenin [110])
miR-155-5p	↑TAM,↑MDSC,↑NK [159]	↓ miR-155-5p (Genistein [105], (−)-Epigallocatechin gallate [106])
miR-30a-5p	↑TAM,↑MDSC [159]	↑ miR-30a-5p (Thymoquinone [111], Nicotine [112], Norcantharidin [62])
miR-34a-5p	↓TAM [159]	↑ miR-34a-5p (Honokiol [91], (−)-Epigallocatechin gallate [107], Rhamnetin, Cirsiliol [119], Dihydroartemisinin [120], Isovitexin [121], Emodin [122]) ↓ miR-34a-5p (Crocin [115])
miR-130a-3p	↑NK [159]	↑ miR-130a-3p (Kaempferol [123]) ↓ miR-130a-3p (Chicoric acid [124])
miR-101-3p	↑TAM [159]	↑ miR-101-3p (Berberine [88])
miR-142-3p	↑TAM [159]	↑ miR-142-3p (Curcumin [97])
miR-24-3p	↑NK [159]	↓ miR-24-3p (Pachymic acid [104])

* These natural products and their modulated exosomal miRNAs were collected from Table 3. The literature [159] did not provide information on natural products. ↑, enhance; ↓, inhibit. Tumor immune microenvironment (TIME); tumor-associated macrophages (TAM); natural killer (NK); myeloid-derived suppressor cells (MDSC).

All this warrants a detailed assessment of all the miRNA-modulating effects of these natural products that are employed in cancer studies in the future.

5.6. Other Cell Functions Influenced by Natural-Product-Modulated Exosomal miRNAs

Several miRNAs, such as miR-31-5p, miR-3188, miR-24-3p, miR-30a-5p, miR-130a-3p, miR-142-3p, miR-30a-5p, and miR-382-5p, exhibit diverse effects other than the modulation of proliferation, apoptosis, migration, and resistance. Although these miRNAs modulate many functions, only a few natural products were retrieved from Pubmed and Google scholar.

Exosomal miR-31-5p regulates the proliferation and drug resistance of cancer cells. Macrophage-derived exosomal miR-31-5p enhances oral cancer cell proliferation by downregulating large tumor suppressor 2 (LATS2) [160]. Exosomal miR-31-5p from hypoxic lung cancer cells promotes metastasis [161]. Moreover, exosomal miR-31-5p is also involved in the regulation of drug resistance. Exosomal miR-31-5p enhances sorafenib resistance in renal cancer cells by targeting mutL homolog 1 (*MLH1*) [162]. Forkhead box C1 (FOXC1) functions as a transcriptional factor to promote the transcription of miR-31-5p and downregulate LATS2, leading to oxaliplatin resistance in colon cancer cells [163]. A natural product study showed that resveratrol alleviates 2,4,6-trinitrobenzenesulfonic-acid-solution (TNBS)-induced colitis by suppressing miR-31-5p expression to increase the number of regulatory T-cells [84] (Table 3).

Cancer-associated fibroblasts enhance the progression of head and neck cancer cells by downregulating exosomal miR-3188 [164]. Without considering exosomes, other cancer studies also reported the tumor suppressive function of miR-3188. miR-3188 inhibits the proliferation of nasopharyngeal [165] and lung [166] cancer cells by targeting *mTOR*. A natural product study showed that pinolenic acid, a *Pinus*-species-derived natural product, upregulates miR-3188 to target the pyruvate dehydrogenase Kinase 4 (*PDK4*) and the mitochondrially encoded ATP synthase membrane subunit 6 (*MT-ATP6*) genes, showing anti-inflammatory effects in rheumatoid arthritis patients [103] (Table 3).

Exosomal miR-24-3p modulates proliferation and drug resistance in cancer cells. Salivary exosomal miR-24-3p promotes the proliferation of oral cancer cells by targeting period circadian regulator 1 (*PER1*) [167]. Exosomal miR-24-3p from cancer-associated fibroblasts enhances methotrexate resistance and inhibits the apoptosis of colon cancer cells by suppressing caudal type homeobox 2 (CDX2) or hephaestin (HEPH) expression [168]. A natural product study showed that doxorubicin causes the miR-24-3p overexpression of the left ventricle [104]. Pachymic acid, a *Poria cocos*-derived natural product, alleviates doxorubicin-induced heart failure in rats by downregulating miR-24-3p [104] (Table 3).

Exosomal miR-30a-5p (miR-30a) regulates several cell functions, such as chemoresistance and migration. Cisplatin-sensitive oral cancer cells exhibit higher miR-30a and lower Beclin 1 (BECN1) expression levels than cisplatin-resistant cells [169]. Exosomes from miR-30a-mimic-transfected cisplatin-resistant cells downregulate BECN1 and BCL2 expression to sensitize the cells to cisplatin. Vascular endothelial cells express exosomes containing higher miR-30a-5p levels than lung cancer cells. Exosomal miR-30a-5p derived from vascular endothelial cells suppresses the proliferation and migration of lung cancer cells by targeting cyclin E2 (*CCNE2*) [170]. Colon cancer mesenchymal stem cells are abundant in exosomal miR-30a-5p. This stem cell exosomal miR-30a-5p improves the proliferation and migration of colon cancer cells by targeting the MIA SH3 domain ER export factor 3 (*MIA3*) [171]. A natural product study showed that Nicotine causes the G1 arrest of periodontal ligament cells by upregulating miR-30a-5p to target *CCNE2* [95] (Table 3).

Exosomal miR-130a-3p (miR-130a) regulates the proliferation and migration of cancer cells. Breast cancer tissues and plasma exosomes exhibit low miR-130a-3p levels. The overexpression of miR-130a-3p in breast cancer stem-cell-like cells suppresses proliferation and migration by targeting *RAB5B*, member of the RAS oncogene family (RAB5B) [172]. The serum of differentiated thyroid cancer patients shows low levels of exosomal miR-130a-3p, which upregulates its target, insulin-like growth factor 1 (*IGF-1*) [173]. Some natural product studies showed that miR-130a-3p possessed inflammation-related functions (Table 3). Kaempferol, a dietary flavonoid, suppresses the cytokine production of chondrocytes by upregulating miR-130a-3p and downregulating its targets, such as the signal transducer and activator of transcription 3 (*STAT3*) [123]. Chicoric acid, an Echinacea-derived natural product, reduces the LPS-induced inflammation of lung cancer cells by downregulating miR-130a-3p and upregulating IGF-1 [124] (Table 3).

miR-142-3p exhibits differential patterns in regulating proliferation in different cancer cells. An increase in miR-142-3p in oral cancer cells suppresses tumor-promoting changes in the recipient endothelial cells [174]. Exosomal miR-142-3p from monocytes can be transferred to retinoblastoma cells, inhibiting their proliferation [175]. In contrast, exosomal miR-142-3p may exhibit a proliferation-promoting effect. Exosomal miR-142-3p from HBV-infected liver cancer cells induces the ferroptosis of M1 macrophages to improve the proliferation of liver cancer cells [176]. Some natural product studies showed that miR-144-3p can modulate several cell functions, such as the regulation of proteasome, ER stress, and autophagy. Curcumin suppresses 20S proteasome activity in breast cancer cells by upregulating miR-142-3p and downregulating its target, such as the proteasome 20S subunit beta 5 (*PSMB5*) [97]. Licochalcone A, a *Glycyrrhiza inflata*-derived natural product, induces ER stress in lung cancer cells by upregulating miR-144-3p [126]. Berberine induces the autophagy of lung cancer cells by upregulating miR-144-3p [87] (Table 3).

Some natural product studies showed that miRNAs can modulate liver fibrosis. Thymoquinone, a black-seed-oil-derived compound, suppresses liver fibrosis by upregulating miR-30a-5p to inhibit its target, such as snail family transcriptional repressor 1 (*SNAI1*), suppressing EMT [111]. Astaxanthin, a xanthophyll carotenoid, inactivates liver-fibrosis-associated hepatic stellate cells by downregulating miR-382-5p [128]. This warrants a detailed evaluation of all the miRNA-modulating effects of the aforementioned natural products employed in cancer studies.

Furthermore, several exosomal miRNAs have been identified in a number of cancer cells, but no natural product studies have been reported to date. Some exosomal miRNAs show proliferation-/invasion-promoting effects. Exosomal miR-626 enhances the proliferation and migration of oral cancer cells by targeting nuclear factor I/B (*NFIB*) [177]. miR-10b-5p shows a higher expression in metastatic breast cancer cells than in non-metastatic breast cancer or normal cells. Exosomal miR-10b-5p transmission enhances the invasion capacity of normal breast cancer [178]. The delivery of exosomal miR-10b-5p from gastric cancer cells also improves the proliferation of fibroblasts [179].

In contrast, some exosomal miRNAs show proliferation-/invasion-suppressing effects. A vitamin D analog, eldecalcitol (ED-71)-induced exosomal miR-6887-5p, suppresses oral cancer cell proliferation by targeting the 3′-UTR of heparin-binding protein 17/fibroblast growth-factor-binding protein-1 (*HBp17/FGFBP-1*) [180]. Exosomal miR-3180-3p suppresses lung cancer proliferation and metastasis by targeting forkhead box P4 (*FOXP4*) [181].

5.7. Overview of the Natural Products and Their Modulating Exosomal miRNAs That Regulate Exosomal Processing

The connections of natural products with their exosomal miRNA-regulated cell functions are summarized in Table 3. However, the impacts of exosomal processing, their genes related to these natural products, and their modulated exosomal miRNAs remain unclear. Utilizing the miRDB database [31], the target prediction of the exosome-processing genes for these natural-product-modulated exosomal miRNAs (Table 3) was performed. From exosomal assembly to secretion, the exosomal processing genes targeted by natural-product-modulated exosomal miRNAs were plotted (Figure 3). This warrants a careful investigation of the predicted targets of these natural-product-modulated exosomal miRNAs based on experiments in the future.

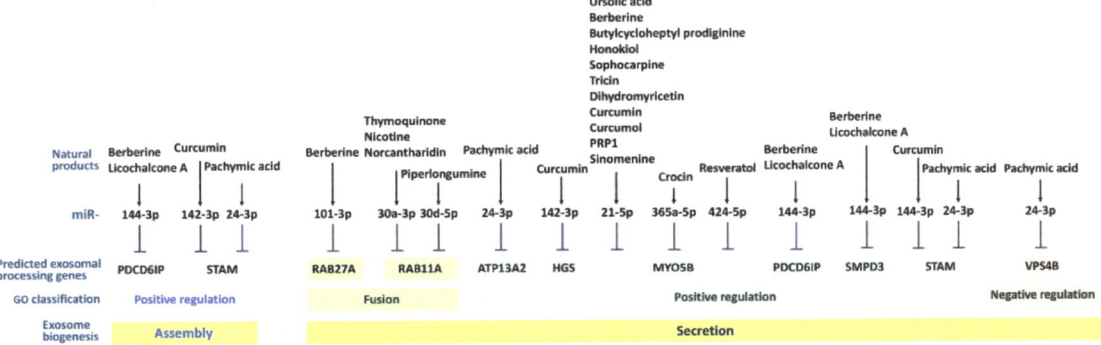

Figure 3. Overview of natural products modulating exosomal miRNAs through exosomal processing genes and exosomal assembly and secretion. The targets of exosomal processing genes with respect to natural-product-modulated miRNAs (Table 3) were predicted using the miRDB database. Some natural products (Table 3) are not shown here because the exosomal processing gene targets of their modulated miRNAs could not be identified in miRDB.

6. Conclusions

Tumor-derived exosomes containing many biomolecules can regulate sophisticated cell functions. This review focused on our understanding of the roles of exosomal miRNAs in controlling cancer cell functions. The impacts of the modulating effects of natural products in regulating exosome processing and exosomal miRNAs were also summarized.

Many natural products exhibit diverse functions and affect the expression of many genes, but they the impacts of natural products on exosome biogenesis have been overlooked. By examining exosomal processing information derived from the GO database and PubMed/Google scholar searches, we noted that some of the altered genes belong to the classification of exosomal processing. Accordingly, this work represents a novel contribution to the study of the exosomal processing of natural products.

Similarly, many exosomal miRNAs have been reported but lack detailed investigations of their regulation of exosomal processing. By utilizing the miRDB database, the potential impacts of exosomal processing genes were predicted to be targeted by exosomal miRNAs. This prediction further provides a direction for future research, which should aim to assess the detailed mechanisms of exosomal miRNAs, although further experiments are still required to confirm them.

Finally, we collected and organized several natural products and their associated modulations of exosomal miRNAs and cell functions, such as proliferation, apoptosis, migration, the tumor immune microenvironment, and other diverse effects. The potential roles of exosomal processing in these natural product investigations were further assessed using information retrieved from the miRDB database. Similarly, we demonstrated that some natural-product-modulated exosomal miRNAs overlap with tumor-immune-microenvironment-associated miRNAs. Although they are indirectly connected, this information provides a future direction for research, which should aim to validate whether these natural products can modulate exosomal miRNAs to regulate the tumor immune microenvironment.

Consequently, we offer a clear conclusion that several exosome-processing genes involved in exosomal secretion and assembly are organized in connection to natural products based on our utilization of the miRDB database to retrieve the target predictions of exosomal miRNAs. Accordingly, we filled the gaps in current knowledge between the exosomal processing of exosomal miRNAs and natural products.

Notably, the miRDB-database-predicted targets of exosomal processing genes were collected based on different cell types. Different cell types may show various miRNAs and targeting responses. This warrants careful examination based on wet experiments to validate the relationship between exosomal miRNAs and natural products in order to explore their impacts on the modulation of cancer cell functions.

This review sheds light on the connections between exosomes, exosomal miRNAs, natural products, and cancer cell functions, providing a clear direction for future research on the modulation of exosomal miRNAs by natural products.

Author Contributions: Conceptualization, Y.-T.C., J.-Y.T., A.A.F. and H.-W.C.; methodology, Y.-T.C., J.-P.S., C.-Y.Y., F.-R.C., K.-H.Y. and M.-F.H.; supervision, A.A.F. and H.-W.C.; writing—original draft, Y.-T.C., J.-Y.T. and H.-W.C.; writing—review and editing, A.A.F. and H.-W.C. All authors have read and agreed to the published version of the manuscript.

Funding: This study was partly supported by funds from the Ministry of Science and Technology (MOST 111-2320-B-037-015-MY3 and MOST 110-2314-B-037-074-MY3), the Kaohsiung Medical University (KMU-DK(A)111008), and the Kaohsiung Medical University Research Center (KMU-TC108A04).

Acknowledgments: We: the authors, thank our colleague Hans-Uwe Dahms for editing the manuscript.

Conflicts of Interest: The authors declare that there are no conflict of interest.

References

1. Zhang, C.; Ji, Q.; Yang, Y.; Li, Q.; Wang, Z. Exosome: Function and role in cancer metastasis and drug resistance. *Technol. Cancer Res. Treat.* **2018**, *17*, 1533033818763450. [CrossRef] [PubMed]
2. Dilsiz, N. Role of exosomes and exosomal microRNAs in cancer. *Future Sci. OA* **2020**, *6*, FSO465. [CrossRef] [PubMed]

3. Thery, C.; Zitvogel, L.; Amigorena, S. Exosomes: Composition, biogenesis and function. *Nat. Rev. Immunol.* **2002**, *2*, 569–579. [CrossRef] [PubMed]
4. Zhao, C.; Zhang, G.; Liu, J.; Zhang, C.; Yao, Y.; Liao, W. Exosomal cargoes in OSCC: Current findings and potential functions. *PeerJ* **2020**, *8*, e10062. [CrossRef] [PubMed]
5. Feng, S.; Lou, K.; Zou, X.; Zou, J.; Zhang, G. The potential role of exosomal proteins in prostate cancer. *Front. Oncol.* **2022**, *12*, 873296. [CrossRef] [PubMed]
6. Liang, Y.; Duan, L.; Lu, J.; Xia, J. Engineering exosomes for targeted drug delivery. *Theranostics* **2021**, *11*, 3183–3195. [CrossRef]
7. Jan, A.T.; Rahman, S.; Badierah, R.; Lee, E.J.; Mattar, E.H.; Redwan, E.M.; Choi, I. Expedition into exosome biology: A perspective of progress from discovery to therapeutic development. *Cancers* **2021**, *13*, 1157. [CrossRef]
8. Kalluri, R.; LeBleu, V.S. The biology, function, and biomedical applications of exosomes. *Science* **2020**, *367*, eaau6977. [CrossRef]
9. Gurunathan, S.; Kang, M.H.; Jeyaraj, M.; Qasim, M.; Kim, J.H. Review of the isolation, characterization, biological function, and multifarious therapeutic approaches of exosomes. *Cells* **2019**, *8*, 307. [CrossRef]
10. Pegtel, D.M.; Gould, S.J. Exosomes. *Annu. Rev. Biochem.* **2019**, *88*, 487–514. [CrossRef]
11. Farooqi, A.A.; Desai, N.N.; Qureshi, M.Z.; Librelotto, D.R.N.; Gasparri, M.L.; Bishayee, A.; Nabavi, S.M.; Curti, V.; Daglia, M. Exosome biogenesis, bioactivities and functions as new delivery systems of natural compounds. *Biotechnol. Adv.* **2018**, *36*, 328–334. [CrossRef] [PubMed]
12. Teng, F.; Fussenegger, M. Shedding light on extracellular vesicle biogenesis and bioengineering. *Adv. Sci.* **2020**, *8*, 2003505. [CrossRef] [PubMed]
13. Hu, S.; Liu, Y.; Guan, S.; Qiu, Z.; Liu, D. Natural products exert anti-tumor effects by regulating exosomal ncRNA. *Front. Oncol.* **2022**, *12*, 1006114. [CrossRef] [PubMed]
14. Cai, Y.; Yu, X.; Hu, S.; Yu, J. A brief review on the mechanisms of miRNA regulation. *Genom. Proteom. Bioinform.* **2009**, *7*, 147–154. [CrossRef] [PubMed]
15. Bhome, R.; Del Vecchio, F.; Lee, G.H.; Bullock, M.D.; Primrose, J.N.; Sayan, A.E.; Mirnezami, A.H. Exosomal microRNAs (exomiRs): Small molecules with a big role in cancer. *Cancer Lett.* **2018**, *420*, 228–235. [CrossRef]
16. Lu, Y.; Zheng, Z.; Yuan, Y.; Pathak, J.L.; Yang, X.; Wang, L.; Ye, Z.; Cho, W.C.; Zeng, M.; Wu, L. The emerging role of exosomes in oral squamous cell carcinoma. *Front. Cell Dev. Biol.* **2021**, *9*, 628103. [CrossRef]
17. Dhar, R.; Mallik, S.; Devi, A. Exosomal microRNAs (exoMIRs): Micromolecules with macro impact in oral cancer. *3 Biotech* **2022**, *12*, 155. [CrossRef]
18. Li, Y.; Gao, S.; Hu, Q.; Wu, F. Functional properties of cancer epithelium and stroma-derived exosomes in head and neck squamous cell carcinoma. *Life* **2022**, *12*, 757. [CrossRef]
19. St-Denis-Bissonnette, F.; Khoury, R.; Mediratta, K.; El-Sahli, S.; Wang, L.; Lavoie, J.R. Applications of extracellular vesicles in triple-negative breast cancer. *Cancers* **2022**, *14*, 451. [CrossRef]
20. Lorenc, T.; Klimczyk, K.; Michalczewska, I.; Slomka, M.; Kubiak-Tomaszewska, G.; Olejarz, W. Exosomes in prostate cancer diagnosis, prognosis and therapy. *Int. J. Mol. Sci.* **2020**, *21*, 2118. [CrossRef]
21. Li, X.; Jiang, W.; Gan, Y.; Zhou, W. The application of exosomal microRNAs in the treatment of pancreatic cancer and its research progress. *Pancreas* **2021**, *50*, 12–16. [CrossRef] [PubMed]
22. Babaker, M.A.; Aljoud, F.A.; Alkhilaiwi, F.; Algarni, A.; Ahmed, A.; Khan, M.I.; Saadeldin, I.M.; Alzahrani, F.A. The Therapeutic Potential of Milk Extracellular Vesicles on Colorectal Cancer. *Int. J. Mol. Sci.* **2022**, *23*, 6812. [CrossRef] [PubMed]
23. Hashemipour, M.; Boroumand, H.; Mollazadeh, S.; Tajiknia, V.; Nourollahzadeh, Z.; Rohani Borj, M.; Pourghadamyari, H.; Rahimian, N.; Hamblin, M.R.; Mirzaei, H. Exosomal microRNAs and exosomal long non-coding RNAs in gynecologic cancers. *Gynecol. Oncol.* **2021**, *161*, 314–327. [CrossRef] [PubMed]
24. Sun, W.; Fu, S.; Wu, S.; Tu, R. Growing evidence of exosomal microRNA-related metastasis of hepatocellular carcinoma. *BioMed Res. Int.* **2020**, *2020*, 4501454. [CrossRef] [PubMed]
25. Bhattacharjee, R.; Mitra, P.; Gupta, N.; Sharma, S.; Singh, V.K.; Mukerjee, N.; Dhasmana, A.; Gundamaraju, R. Cellular landscaping of exosomal miRNAs in cancer metastasis: From chemoresistance to prognostic markers. *Adv. Cancer Biol.-Metastasis* **2022**, *5*, 100050. [CrossRef]
26. Sorop, A.; Constantinescu, D.; Cojocaru, F.; Dinischiotu, A.; Cucu, D.; Dima, S.O. Exosomal microRNAs as biomarkers and therapeutic targets for hepatocellular carcinoma. *Int. J. Mol. Sci.* **2021**, *22*, 4997. [CrossRef] [PubMed]
27. Hu, M.; Cao, Z.; Jiang, D. The effect of miRNA-modified exosomes in animal models of spinal cord injury: A meta-analysis. *Front. Bioeng Biotechnol* **2021**, *9*, 819651. [CrossRef]
28. Cetin, Z.; Saygili, E.I.; Gorgisen, G.; Sokullu, E. Preclinical experimental applications of miRNA loaded BMSC extracellular vesicles. *Stem Cell Rev. Rep.* **2021**, *17*, 471–501. [CrossRef]
29. Rezaei, R.; Baghaei, K.; Hashemi, S.M.; Zali, M.R.; Ghanbarian, H.; Amani, D. Tumor-derived exosomes enriched by miRNA-124 promote anti-tumor immune response in CT-26 tumor-bearing mice. *Front. Med.* **2021**, *8*, 619939. [CrossRef]
30. Guglielmi, L.; Nardella, M.; Musa, C.; Cifola, I.; Porru, M.; Cardinali, B.; Iannetti, I.; Di Pietro, C.; Bolasco, G.; Palmieri, V.; et al. Circulating miRNAs in small extracellular vesicles secreted by a human melanoma xenograft in mouse brains. *Cancers* **2020**, *12*, 1635. [CrossRef]
31. Chen, Y.; Wang, X. miRDB: An online database for prediction of functional microRNA targets. *Nucleic Acids Res.* **2020**, *48*, D127–D131. [CrossRef] [PubMed]

32. Bult, C.J.; Blake, J.A.; Smith, C.L.; Kadin, J.A.; Richardson, J.E.; Mouse Genome Database, G. Mouse Genome Database (MGD) 2019. *Nucleic Acids Res.* **2019**, *47*, D801–D806. [CrossRef] [PubMed]
33. Hasanin, A.H.; Matboli, M.; Seleem, H.S. Hesperidin suppressed hepatic precancerous lesions via modulation of exophagy in rats. *J. Cell. Biochem.* **2020**, *121*, 1295–1306. [CrossRef] [PubMed]
34. Li, Y.Q.; Zhang, F.; Yu, L.P.; Mu, J.K.; Yang, Y.Q.; Yu, J.; Yang, X.X. Targeting PINK1 using natural products for the treatment of human diseases. *BioMed Res. Int.* **2021**, *2021*, 4045819. [CrossRef] [PubMed]
35. Tang, C.; Han, H.; Yan, M.; Zhu, S.; Liu, J.; Liu, Z.; He, L.; Tan, J.; Liu, Y.; Liu, H.; et al. PINK1-PRKN/PARK2 pathway of mitophagy is activated to protect against renal ischemia-reperfusion injury. *Autophagy* **2018**, *14*, 880–897. [CrossRef]
36. Hu, Y.; Wang, M.; Pan, Y.; Li, Q.; Xu, L. Salvianolic acid B attenuates renal interstitial fibrosis by regulating the HPSE/SDC1 axis. *Mol. Med. Rep.* **2020**, *22*, 1325–1334. [CrossRef] [PubMed]
37. Dall'Acqua, S.; Grabnar, I.; Verardo, R.; Klaric, E.; Marchionni, L.; Luidy-Imada, E.; Sut, S.; Agostinis, C.; Bulla, R.; Perissutti, B.; et al. Combined extracts of *Echinacea angustifolia* DC. and *Zingiber officinale* Roscoe in softgel capsules: Pharmacokinetics and immunomodulatory effects assessed by gene expression profiling. *Phytomedicine Int. J. Phytother. Phytopharm.* **2019**, *65*, 153090. [CrossRef] [PubMed]
38. Dong, X.; Zhu, Y.; Wang, S.; Luo, Y.; Lu, S.; Nan, F.; Sun, G.; Sun, X. Bavachinin inhibits cholesterol synthesis enzyme FDFT1 expression via AKT/mTOR/SREBP-2 pathway. *Int. Immunopharmacol.* **2020**, *88*, 106865. [CrossRef]
39. Pandey, P.; Khan, F. Jab1 inhibition by methanolic extract of *Moringa oleifera* leaves in cervical cancer cells: A potent targeted therapeutic approach. *Nutr. Cancer* **2021**, *73*, 2411–2419. [CrossRef]
40. Pandey, P.; Khan, F.; Alzahrani, F.A.; Qari, H.A.; Oves, M. A novel approach to unraveling the apoptotic potential of rutin (bioflavonoid) via targeting Jab1 in cervical cancer cells. *Molecules* **2021**, *26*, 5529. [CrossRef]
41. Kaftan, G.; Erdoğan, M.; El-Shazly, M.; Lu, M.-C.; Shih, S.-P.; Lin, H.-Y.; Saso, L.; Armagan, G. Heteronemin promotes iron-dependent cell death in pancreatic cancer. *Res. Sq.* **2022**. [CrossRef]
42. Ba, Q.; Zhou, N.; Duan, J.; Chen, T.; Hao, M.; Yang, X.; Li, J.; Yin, J.; Chu, R.; Wang, H. Dihydroartemisinin exerts its anticancer activity through depleting cellular iron via transferrin receptor-1. *PloS ONE* **2012**, *7*, e42703. [CrossRef] [PubMed]
43. Xie, Y.; Zhou, X.; Li, J.; Yao, X.C.; Liu, W.L.; Kang, F.H.; Zou, Z.X.; Xu, K.P.; Xu, P.S.; Tan, G.S. Identification of a new natural biflavonoids against breast cancer cells induced ferroptosis via the mitochondrial pathway. *Bioorganic Chem.* **2021**, *109*, 104744. [CrossRef] [PubMed]
44. Zhou, J.; Li, G.; Zheng, Y.; Shen, H.M.; Hu, X.; Ming, Q.L.; Huang, C.; Li, P.; Gao, N. A novel autophagy/mitophagy inhibitor liensinine sensitizes breast cancer cells to chemotherapy through DNM1L-mediated mitochondrial fission. *Autophagy* **2015**, *11*, 1259–1279. [CrossRef] [PubMed]
45. Im, E.J.; Lee, C.H.; Moon, P.G.; Rangaswamy, G.G.; Lee, B.; Lee, J.M.; Lee, J.C.; Jee, J.G.; Bae, J.S.; Kwon, T.K.; et al. Sulfisoxazole inhibits the secretion of small extracellular vesicles by targeting the endothelin receptor A. *Nat. Commun.* **2019**, *10*, 1387. [CrossRef] [PubMed]
46. Si, J.; Van den Haute, C.; Lobbestael, E.; Martin, S.; van Veen, S.; Vangheluwe, P.; Baekelandt, V. ATP13A2 regulates cellular alpha-synuclein multimerization, membrane association, and externalization. *Int. J. Mol. Sci.* **2021**, *22*, 2689. [CrossRef]
47. Chimplee, S.; Roytrakul, S.; Sukrong, S.; Srisawat, T.; Graidist, P.; Kanokwiroon, K. Anticancer effects and molecular action of 7-alpha-hydroxyfrullanolide in G2/M-phase arrest and apoptosis in triple negative breast cancer cells. *Molecules* **2022**, *27*, 407. [CrossRef]
48. Liu, Y.; Chen, Y.; Zhu, R.; Xu, L.; Xie, H.Q.; Zhao, B. Rutaecarpine inhibits U87 glioblastoma cell migration by activating the aryl hydrocarbon receptor signaling pathway. *Front. Mol. Neurosci.* **2021**, *14*, 765712. [CrossRef]
49. Mao, Z.; Han, X.; Chen, D.; Xu, Y.; Xu, L.; Yin, L.; Sun, H.; Qi, Y.; Fang, L.; Liu, K.; et al. Potent effects of dioscin against hepatocellular carcinoma through regulating TP53-induced glycolysis and apoptosis regulator (TIGAR)-mediated apoptosis, autophagy, and DNA damage. *Br. J. Pharmacol.* **2019**, *176*, 919–937. [CrossRef]
50. Shang, H.S.; Shih, Y.L.; Lee, C.H.; Hsueh, S.C.; Liu, J.Y.; Liao, N.C.; Chen, Y.L.; Huang, Y.P.; Lu, H.F.; Chung, J.G. Sulforaphane-induced apoptosis in human leukemia HL-60 cells through extrinsic and intrinsic signal pathways and altering associated genes expression assayed by cDNA microarray. *Environ. Toxicol.* **2017**, *32*, 311–328. [CrossRef]
51. Shen, Y.; Takahashi, M.; Byun, H.M.; Link, A.; Sharma, N.; Balaguer, F.; Leung, H.C.; Boland, C.R.; Goel, A. Boswellic acid induces epigenetic alterations by modulating DNA methylation in colorectal cancer cells. *Cancer Biol. Ther.* **2012**, *13*, 542–552. [CrossRef]
52. Mondal, S.; Mandal, C.; Sangwan, R.; Chandra, S.; Mandal, C. Withanolide D induces apoptosis in leukemia by targeting the activation of neutral sphingomyelinase-ceramide cascade mediated by synergistic activation of c-Jun N-terminal kinase and p38 mitogen-activated protein kinase. *Mol. Cancer* **2010**, *9*, 239. [CrossRef] [PubMed]
53. Schneider, Y.; Duranton, B.; Gosse, F.; Schleiffer, R.; Seiler, N.; Raul, F. Resveratrol inhibits intestinal tumorigenesis and modulates host-defense-related gene expression in an animal model of human familial adenomatous polyposis. *Nutr. Cancer* **2001**, *39*, 102–107. [CrossRef] [PubMed]
54. Han, L.; Liu, N.; Yang, L.; Mao, Y.; Ye, S. *Astragalus membranaceus* extract promotes angiogenesis by inducing VEGF, CD34 and eNOS expression in rats subjected to myocardial infarction. *Int. J. Clin. Exp. Med.* **2016**, *9*, 5709–5718.
55. Chen, W.X.; Xu, L.Y.; Qian, Q.; He, X.; Peng, W.T.; Fan, W.Q.; Zhu, Y.L.; Tang, J.H.; Cheng, L. d Rhamnose beta-hederin reverses chemoresistance of breast cancer cells by regulating exosome-mediated resistance transmission. *Biosci. Rep.* **2018**, *38*, BSR20180110. [CrossRef] [PubMed]

56. Perni, M.; Galvagnion, C.; Maltsev, A.; Meisl, G.; Muller, M.B.; Challa, P.K.; Kirkegaard, J.B.; Flagmeier, P.; Cohen, S.I.; Cascella, R.; et al. A natural product inhibits the initiation of alpha-synuclein aggregation and suppresses its toxicity. *Proc. Natl. Acad. Sci. USA* **2017**, *114*, E1009–E1017. [CrossRef]
57. Salehi, M.; Vafadar, A.; Khatami, S.H.; Taheri-Anganeh, M.; Vakili, O.; Savardashtaki, A.; Negahdari, B.; Naeli, P.; Behrouj, H.; Ghasemi, H.; et al. Gastrointestinal cancer drug resistance: The role of exosomal miRNAs. *Mol. Biol. Rep.* **2022**, *49*, 2421–2432. [CrossRef]
58. Shi, L.; Zhu, W.; Huang, Y.; Zhuo, L.; Wang, S.; Chen, S.; Zhang, B.; Ke, B. Cancer-associated fibroblast-derived exosomal microRNA-20a suppresses the PTEN/PI3K-AKT pathway to promote the progression and chemoresistance of non-small cell lung cancer. *Clin. Transl. Med.* **2022**, *12*, e989. [CrossRef]
59. Zhang, L.; Ouyang, P.; He, G.; Wang, X.; Song, D.; Yang, Y.; He, X. Exosomes from microRNA-126 overexpressing mesenchymal stem cells promote angiogenesis by targeting the PIK3R2-mediated PI3K/Akt signalling pathway. *J. Cell. Mol. Med.* **2021**, *25*, 2148–2162. [CrossRef]
60. Sun, J.; Wei, J.; Zhang, Y.; Li, J.; Li, J.; Yan, J.; Guo, M.; Han, J.; Qiao, H. Plasma exosomes transfer miR-885-3p targeting the AKT/NFkappaB signaling pathway to improve the sensitivity of intravenous glucocorticoid therapy against Graves ophthalmopathy. *Front. Immunol.* **2022**, *13*, 819680. [CrossRef]
61. Bae, I.S.; Kim, S.H. Milk exosome-derived microRNA-2478 suppresses melanogenesis through the Akt-GSK3β pathway. *Cells* **2021**, *10*, 2848. [CrossRef] [PubMed]
62. Chen, F.; Wang, S.; Wei, Y.; Wu, J.; Huang, G.; Chen, J.; Shi, J.; Xia, J. Norcantharidin modulates the miR-30a/Metadherin/AKT signaling axis to suppress proliferation and metastasis of stromal tumor cells in giant cell tumor of bone. *Biomed. Pharmacother.* **2018**, *103*, 1092–1100. [CrossRef] [PubMed]
63. Ali, N.B.; Abdull Razis, A.F.; Ooi, J.; Chan, K.W.; Ismail, N.; Foo, J.B. Theragnostic applications of mammal and plant-derived extracellular vesicles: Latest findings, current technologies, and prospects. *Molecules* **2022**, *27*, 3941. [CrossRef] [PubMed]
64. Otsuka, K.; Yamamoto, Y.; Matsuoka, R.; Ochiya, T. Maintaining good miRNAs in the body keeps the doctor away?: Perspectives on the relationship between food-derived natural products and microRNAs in relation to exosomes/extracellular vesicles. *Mol. Nutr. Food Res.* **2017**. Available online: https://onlinelibrary.wiley.com/doi/10.1002/mnfr.201700080. [CrossRef]
65. Song, H.; Liu, B.; Dong, B.; Xu, J.; Zhou, H.; Na, S.; Liu, Y.; Pan, Y.; Chen, F.; Li, L.; et al. Exosome-based delivery of natural products in cancer therapy. *Front. Cell Dev. Biol.* **2021**, *9*, 650426. [CrossRef]
66. Xu, Y.; Feng, K.; Zhao, H.; Di, L.; Wang, L.; Wang, R. Tumor-derived extracellular vesicles as messengers of natural products in cancer treatment. *Theranostics* **2022**, *12*, 1683–1714. [CrossRef]
67. Zheng, K.; Ma, J.; Wang, Y.; He, Z.; Deng, K. Sulforaphane inhibits autophagy and induces exosome-mediated paracrine senescence via regulating mTOR/TFE3. *Mol. Nutr. Food Res.* **2020**, *64*, e1901231. [CrossRef]
68. Komatsu, M.; Waguri, S.; Koike, M.; Sou, Y.S.; Ueno, T.; Hara, T.; Mizushima, N.; Iwata, J.; Ezaki, J.; Murata, S.; et al. Homeostatic levels of p62 control cytoplasmic inclusion body formation in autophagy-deficient mice. *Cell* **2007**, *131*, 1149–1163. [CrossRef]
69. Xu, J.; Camfield, R.; Gorski, S.M. The interplay between exosomes and autophagy-partners in crime. *J. Cell Sci.* **2018**, *131*, jcs215210. [CrossRef]
70. Mitani, F.; Lin, J.; Sakamoto, T.; Uehara, R.; Hikita, T.; Yoshida, T.; Setiawan, A.; Arai, M.; Oneyama, C. Asteltoxin inhibits extracellular vesicle production through AMPK/mTOR-mediated activation of lysosome function. *Sci. Rep.* **2022**, *12*, 6674. [CrossRef]
71. Gu, S.; Song, X.; Xie, R.; Ouyang, C.; Xie, L.; Li, Q.; Su, T.; Xu, M.; Xu, T.; Huang, D.; et al. Berberine inhibits cancer cells growth by suppressing fatty acid synthesis and biogenesis of extracellular vesicles. *Life Sci.* **2020**, *257*, 118122. [CrossRef]
72. Shiau, J.Y.; Chang, Y.Q.; Nakagawa-Goto, K.; Lee, K.H.; Shyur, L.F. Phytoagent deoxyelephantopin and its derivative inhibit triple negative breast cancer cell activity through ROS-mediated exosomal activity and protein functions. *Front. Pharmacol.* **2017**, *8*, 398. [CrossRef] [PubMed]
73. Wang, B.; Guo, X.J.; Cai, H.; Zhu, Y.H.; Huang, L.Y.; Wang, W.; Luo, L.; Qi, S.H. *Momordica charantia*-derived extracellular vesicles-like nanovesicles inhibited glioma proliferation, migration, and invasion by regulating the PI3K/AKT signaling pathway. *J. Funct. Foods* **2022**, *90*, 104968. [CrossRef]
74. Lin, L.T.; Shi, Y.C.; Choong, C.Y.; Tai, C.J. The fruits of *Paris polyphylla* inhibit colorectal cancer cell migration induced by *Fusobacterium nucleatum*-derived extracellular vesicles. *Molecules* **2021**, *26*, 4081. [CrossRef] [PubMed]
75. Srivastava, A.; Rathore, S.; Munshi, A.; Ramesh, R. Organically derived exosomes as carriers of anticancer drugs and imaging agents for cancer treatment. *Semin. Cancer Biol.* **2022**, *86*, 80–100. [CrossRef]
76. Agrawal, A.K.; Aqil, F.; Jeyabalan, J.; Spencer, W.A.; Beck, J.; Gachuki, B.W.; Alhakeem, S.S.; Oben, K.; Munagala, R.; Bondada, S.; et al. Milk-derived exosomes for oral delivery of paclitaxel. *Nanomed. Nanotechnol. Biol. Med.* **2017**, *13*, 1627–1636. [CrossRef]
77. Sun, D.; Zhuang, X.; Xiang, X.; Liu, Y.; Zhang, S.; Liu, C.; Barnes, S.; Grizzle, W.; Miller, D.; Zhang, H.G. A novel nanoparticle drug delivery system: The anti-inflammatory activity of curcumin is enhanced when encapsulated in exosomes. *Mol. Ther. J. Am. Soc. Gene Ther.* **2010**, *18*, 1606–1614. [CrossRef]
78. Aqil, F.; Kausar, H.; Agrawal, A.K.; Jeyabalan, J.; Kyakulaga, A.H.; Munagala, R.; Gupta, R. Exosomal formulation enhances therapeutic response of celastrol against lung cancer. *Exp. Mol. Pathol.* **2016**, *101*, 12–21. [CrossRef]
79. Zhang, B.; Tian, L.; Xie, J.; Chen, G.; Wang, F. Targeting miRNAs by natural products: A new way for cancer therapy. *Biomed. Pharmacother.* **2020**, *130*, 110546. [CrossRef]

80. Park, Y.; Lee, K.; Kim, S.W.; Lee, M.W.; Kim, B.; Lee, S.G. Effects of induced exosomes from endometrial cancer cells on tumor activity in the presence of *Aurea helianthus* extract. *Molecules* **2021**, *26*, 2207. [CrossRef]
81. Wang, J.; Li, Y.; Wang, X.; Jiang, C. Ursolic acid inhibits proliferation and induces apoptosis in human glioblastoma cell lines U251 by suppressing TGF-β1/miR-21/PDCD 4 pathway. *Basic Clin. Pharmacol. Toxicol.* **2012**, *111*, 106–112. [PubMed]
82. Zhang, L.; Cai, Q.Y.; Liu, J.; Peng, J.; Chen, Y.Q.; Sferra, T.J.; Lin, J.M. Ursolic acid suppresses the invasive potential of colorectal cancer cells by regulating the TGF-beta1/ZEB1/miR-200c signaling pathway. *Oncol. Lett.* **2019**, *18*, 3274–3282. [CrossRef] [PubMed]
83. Zhou, C.; Ding, J.; Wu, Y. Resveratrol induces apoptosis of bladder cancer cells via miR21 regulation of the Akt/Bcl2 signaling pathway. *Mol. Med. Rep.* **2014**, *9*, 1467–1473. [CrossRef] [PubMed]
84. Alrafas, H.R.; Busbee, P.B.; Nagarkatti, M.; Nagarkatti, P.S. Resveratrol downregulates miR-31 to promote to regulatory cells during prevention of TNBS-induced colitis. *Mol. Nutr. Food Res.* **2020**, *64*, e1900633. [CrossRef]
85. Otsuka, K.; Yamamoto, Y.; Ochiya, T. Regulatory role of resveratrol, a microRNA-controlling compound, in HNRNPA1 expression, which is associated with poor prognosis in breast cancer. *Oncotarget* **2018**, *9*, 24718–24730. [CrossRef]
86. Luo, X.; Gu, J.; Zhu, R.; Feng, M.; Zhu, X.; Li, Y.; Fei, J. Integrative analysis of differential miRNA and functional study of miR-21 by seed-targeting inhibition in multiple myeloma cells in response to berberine. *BMC Syst. Biol.* **2014**, *8*, 82. [CrossRef]
87. Gao, Z.; Tan, C.; Sha, R. Berberine Promotes A549 Cell Apoptosis and Autophagy via miR-144. *Nat. Prod. Commun.* **2022**, *17*, 1934578–221124752. [CrossRef]
88. Wang, Y.; Zhang, S. Berberine suppresses growth and metastasis of endometrial cancer cells via miR-101/COX-2. *Biomed. Pharmacother. Biomed. Pharmacother.* **2018**, *103*, 1287–1293. [CrossRef]
89. Matarlo, J.S.; Krumpe, L.R.H.; Heinz, W.F.; Oh, D.; Shenoy, S.R.; Thomas, C.L.; Goncharova, E.I.; Lockett, S.J.; O'Keefe, B.R. The natural product butylcycloheptyl prodiginine binds pre-miR-21, inhibits Dicer-mediated processing of pre-miR-21, and blocks cellular proliferation. *Cell Chem. Biol.* **2019**, *26*, 1133–1142.e1134. [CrossRef]
90. Yang, J.; Zou, Y.; Jiang, D. Honokiol suppresses proliferation and induces apoptosis via regulation of the miR21/PTEN/PI3K/AKT signaling pathway in human osteosarcoma cells. *Int. J. Mol. Med.* **2018**, *41*, 1845–1854. [CrossRef]
91. Avtanski, D.B.; Nagalingam, A.; Bonner, M.Y.; Arbiser, J.L.; Saxena, N.K.; Sharma, D. Honokiol activates LKB1-miR-34a axis and antagonizes the oncogenic actions of leptin in breast cancer. *Oncotarget* **2015**, *6*, 29947–29962. [CrossRef]
92. Liu, W.; Zhang, B.; Chen, G.; Wu, W.; Zhou, L.; Shi, Y.; Zeng, Q.; Li, Y.; Sun, Y.; Deng, X.; et al. Targeting miR-21 with sophocarpine inhibits tumor progression and reverses epithelial-mesenchymal transition in head and neck cancer. *Mol. Ther. J. Am. Soc. Gene Ther.* **2017**, *25*, 2129–2139. [CrossRef]
93. Ghasemi, S.; Lorigooini, Z.; Wibowo, J.; Amini-Khoei, H. Tricin isolated from *Allium atroviolaceum* potentiated the effect of docetaxel on PC3 cell proliferation: Role of miR-21. *Nat. Prod. Res.* **2019**, *33*, 1828–1831. [CrossRef] [PubMed]
94. Chen, L.; Yang, Z.S.; Zhou, Y.Z.; Deng, Y.; Jiang, P.; Tan, S.L. Dihydromyricetin inhibits cell proliferation, migration, invasion and promotes apoptosis via regulating miR-21 in human cholangiocarcinoma cells. *J. Cancer* **2020**, *11*, 5689–5699. [CrossRef] [PubMed]
95. Zhou, C.; Hu, C.; Wang, B.; Fan, S.; Jin, W. Curcumin suppresses cell proliferation, migration, and invasion through modulating miR-21-5p/SOX6 axis in hepatocellular carcinoma. *Cancer Biother. Radiopharm.* **2020**. [CrossRef] [PubMed]
96. Wang, H.; Cai, X.; Ma, L. Curcumin modifies epithelial–mesenchymal transition in colorectal cancer through regulation of miR-200c/EPM5. *Cancer Manag. Res.* **2020**, *12*, 9405–9415. [CrossRef]
97. Liu, L.; Fu, Y.; Zheng, Y.; Ma, M.; Wang, C. Curcumin inhibits proteasome activity in triple-negative breast cancer cells through regulating p300/miR-142-3p/PSMB5 axis. *Phytomedicine Int. J. Phytother. Phytopharm.* **2020**, *78*, 153312. [CrossRef]
98. Xu, R.; Li, H.; Wu, S.; Qu, J.; Yuan, H.; Zhou, Y.; Lu, Q. MicroRNA-1246 regulates the radio-sensitizing effect of curcumin in bladder cancer cells via activating P53. *Int. Urol. Nephrol.* **2019**, *51*, 1771–1779. [CrossRef]
99. Liu, H.; Wang, J.; Tao, Y.; Li, X.; Qin, J.; Bai, Z.; Chi, B.; Yan, W.; Chen, X. Curcumol inhibits colorectal cancer proliferation by targeting miR-21 and modulated PTEN/PI3K/Akt pathways. *Life Sci.* **2019**, *221*, 354–361. [CrossRef]
100. He, J.Q.; Zheng, M.X.; Ying, H.Z.; Zhong, Y.S.; Zhang, H.H.; Xu, M.; Yu, C.H. PRP1, a heteropolysaccharide from Platycodonis Radix, induced apoptosis of HepG2 cells via regulating miR-21-mediated PI3K/AKT pathway. *Int. J. Biol. Macromol.* **2020**, *158*, 542–551. [CrossRef]
101. Shen, K.H.; Hung, J.H.; Liao, Y.C.; Tsai, S.T.; Wu, M.J.; Chen, P.S. Sinomenine inhibits migration and invasion of human lung cancer cell through downregulating expression of miR-21 and MMPs. *Int. J. Mol. Sci.* **2020**, *21*, 3080. [CrossRef] [PubMed]
102. Jin, L.; Ma, X.M.; Wang, T.T.; Yang, Y.; Zhang, N.; Zeng, N.; Bai, Z.G.; Yin, J.; Zhang, J.; Ding, G.Q.; et al. Psoralen suppresses cisplatin-mediated resistance and induces apoptosis of gastric adenocarcinoma by disruption of the miR196a-HOXB7-HER2 axis. *Cancer Manag. Res.* **2020**, *12*, 2803–2827. [CrossRef] [PubMed]
103. Takala, R.; Ramji, D.P.; Andrews, R.; Zhou, Y.; Farhat, M.; Elmajee, M.; Rundle, S.; Choy, E. Pinolenic acid exhibits anti-inflammatory and anti-atherogenic effects in peripheral blood-derived monocytes from patients with rheumatoid arthritis. *Sci. Rep.* **2022**, *12*, 8807. [CrossRef] [PubMed]
104. Younis, N.N.; Salama, A.; Shaheen, M.A.; Eissa, R.G. Pachymic acid attenuated doxorubicin-induced heart failure by suppressing miR-24 and preserving cardiac junctophilin-2 in rats. *Int. J. Mol. Sci.* **2021**, *22*, 10710. [CrossRef] [PubMed]
105. de la Parra, C.; Castillo-Pichardo, L.; Cruz-Collazo, A.; Cubano, L.; Redis, R.; Calin, G.A.; Dharmawardhane, S. Soy isoflavone genistein-mediated downregulation of miR-155 contributes to the anticancer effects of genistein. *Nutr. Cancer* **2016**, *68*, 154–164. [CrossRef] [PubMed]

106. La, X.; Zhang, L.; Li, Z.; Li, H.; Yang, Y. (-)-Epigallocatechin gallate (EGCG) enhances the sensitivity of colorectal cancer cells to 5-FU by inhibiting GRP78/NF-kappaB/miR-155-5p/MDR1 pathway. *J. Agric. Food Chem.* **2019**, *67*, 2510–2518. [CrossRef] [PubMed]
107. Kang, Q.; Zhang, X.; Cao, N.; Chen, C.; Yi, J.; Hao, L.; Ji, Y.; Liu, X.; Lu, J. EGCG enhances cancer cells sensitivity under (60)Cogamma radiation based on miR-34a/Sirt1/p53. *Food Chem. Toxicol.* **2019**, *133*, 110807. [CrossRef] [PubMed]
108. Hagiwara, K.; Gailhouste, L.; Yasukawa, K.; Kosaka, N.; Ochiya, T. A robust screening method for dietary agents that activate tumour-suppressor microRNAs. *Sci. Rep.* **2015**, *5*, 14697. [CrossRef]
109. Peng, F.; Xiong, L.; Peng, C. (-)-Sativan inhibits tumor development and regulates miR-200c/PD-L1 in triple negative breast cancer cells. *Front. Pharmacol.* **2020**, *11*, 251. [CrossRef]
110. Peng, F.; Tang, H.; Du, J.; Chen, J.; Peng, C. Isoliquiritigenin suppresses EMT-induced metastasis in triple-negative breast cancer through miR-200c/c-Jun/β-Catenin. *Am. J. Chin. Med.* **2021**, *49*, 505–523. [CrossRef]
111. Geng, W.; Li, C.; Zhan, Y.; Zhang, R.; Zheng, J. Thymoquinone alleviates liver fibrosis via miR-30a-mediated epithelial-mesenchymal transition. *J. Cell. Physiol.* **2020**, *236*, 3629–3640. [CrossRef] [PubMed]
112. Wu, L.; Yang, K.; Gui, Y.; Wang, X. Nicotine-upregulated miR-30a arrests cell cycle in G1 phase by directly targeting CCNE2 in human periodontal ligament cells. *Biochem. Cell Biol.* **2020**, *98*, 354–361. [CrossRef] [PubMed]
113. Phuah, N.H.; Azmi, M.N.; Awang, K.; Nagoor, N.H. Down-regulation of microRNA-210 confers sensitivity towards 1′s-1′-acetoxychavicol acetate (ACA) in cervical cancer cells by targeting SMAD4. *Mol. Cells* **2017**, *40*, 291–298. [CrossRef] [PubMed]
114. Mollaei, H.; Safaralizadeh, R.; Babaei, E.; Abedini, M.R.; Hoshyar, R. The anti-proliferative and apoptotic effects of crocin on chemosensitive and chemoresistant cervical cancer cells. *Biomed. Pharmacother. Biomed. Pharmacother.* **2017**, *94*, 307–316. [CrossRef] [PubMed]
115. Tang, Y.; Yang, H.; Yu, J.; Li, Z.; Xu, Q.; Ding, B.; Jia, G. Crocin induces ROS-mediated papillary thyroid cancer cell apoptosis by modulating the miR-34a-5p/PTPN4 axis in vitro. *Toxicol. Appl. Pharmacol.* **2022**, *437*, 115892. [CrossRef] [PubMed]
116. Hsia, S.M.; Yu, C.C.; Shih, Y.H.; Yuanchien Chen, M.; Wang, T.H.; Huang, Y.T.; Shieh, T.M. Isoliquiritigenin as a cause of DNA damage and inhibitor of ataxia-telangiectasia mutated expression leading to G2/M phase arrest and apoptosis in oral squamous cell carcinoma. *Head Neck* **2016**, *38* (Suppl. 1), E360–E371. [CrossRef] [PubMed]
117. Ye, W.; Ni, Z.; Yicheng, S.; Pan, H.; Huang, Y.; Xiong, Y.; Liu, T. Anisomycin inhibits angiogenesis in ovarian cancer by attenuating the molecular sponge effect of the lncRNAMeg3/miR421/PDGFRA axis. *Int. J. Oncol.* **2019**, *55*, 1296–1312. [CrossRef]
118. Zhang, F.; Ni, Z.J.; Ye, L.; Zhang, Y.Y.; Thakur, K.; Cespedes-Acuna, C.L.; Han, J.; Zhang, J.G.; Wei, Z.J. Asparanin A inhibits cell migration and invasion in human endometrial cancer via Ras/ERK/MAPK pathway. *Food Chem. Toxicol.* **2021**, *150*, 112036. [CrossRef]
119. Kang, J.; Kim, E.; Kim, W.; Seong, K.M.; Youn, H.; Kim, J.W.; Kim, J.; Youn, B. Rhamnetin and cirsiliol induce radiosensitization and inhibition of epithelial-mesenchymal transition (EMT) by miR-34a-mediated suppression of Notch-1 expression in non-small cell lung cancer cell lines. *J. Biol. Chem.* **2013**, *288*, 27343–27357. [CrossRef]
120. Paccez, J.D.; Duncan, K.; Sekar, D.; Correa, R.G.; Wang, Y.; Gu, X.; Bashin, M.; Chibale, K.; Libermann, T.A.; Zerbini, L.F. Dihydroartemisinin inhibits prostate cancer via JARID2/miR-7/miR-34a-dependent downregulation of Axl. *Oncogenesis* **2019**, *8*, 14. [CrossRef]
121. Liang, X.; Xu, C.; Cao, X.; Wang, W. Isovitexin suppresses cancer stemness property and induces apoptosis of osteosarcoma cells by disruption of the DNMT1/miR-34a/Bcl-2 axis. *Cancer Manag. Res.* **2019**, *11*, 8923–8936. [CrossRef]
122. Bai, J.; Wu, J.; Tang, R.; Sun, C.; Ji, J.; Yin, Z.; Ma, G.; Yang, W. Emodin, a natural anthraquinone, suppresses liver cancer in vitro and in vivo by regulating VEGFR2 and miR-34a. *Investig. New Drugs* **2020**, *38*, 229–245. [CrossRef]
123. Xiao, Y.; Liu, L.; Zheng, Y.; Liu, W.; Xu, Y. Kaempferol attenuates the effects of XIST/miR-130a/STAT3 on inflammation and extracellular matrix degradation in osteoarthritis. *Future Med. Chem.* **2021**, *13*, 1451–1464. [CrossRef]
124. Yan, Z.; Huang, Q.-L.; Chen, J.; Liu, F.; Wei, Y.; Chen, S.-L.; Wu, C.-Y.; Li, Z.; Lin, X.-P. Chicoric acid alleviates LPS-induced inflammatory response through miR-130a-3p/IGF-1pathway in human lung A549 epithelial cells. *Eur. J. Inflamm.* **2021**, *19*, 20587392211038244. [CrossRef]
125. Xu, T.; Qin, L.; Zhu, Z.; Wang, X.; Liu, Y.; Fan, Y.; Zhong, S.; Wang, X.; Zhang, X.; Xia, L.; et al. MicroRNA-31 functions as a tumor suppressor and increases sensitivity to mitomycin-C in urothelial bladder cancer by targeting integrin alpha5. *Oncotarget* **2016**, *7*, 27445–27457. [CrossRef]
126. Chen, G.; Ma, Y.; Jiang, Z.; Feng, Y.; Han, Y.; Tang, Y.; Zhang, J.; Ni, H.; Li, X.; Li, N. Lico A causes ER stress and apoptosis via up-regulating miR-144-3p in human lung cancer cell line H292. *Front. Pharmacol.* **2018**, *9*, 837. [CrossRef]
127. Zeng, L.; Sun, Y.; Li, X.; Wang, J.; Yan, L. 10Hydroxycamptothecin induces apoptosis in human fibroblasts by regulating miRNA23b3p expression. *Mol. Med. Rep.* **2019**, *19*, 2680–2686. [CrossRef]
128. Bae, M.; Kim, M.B.; Lee, J.Y. Astaxanthin attenuates the changes in the expression of microRNAs involved in the activation of hepatic stellate cells. *Nutrients* **2022**, *14*, 962. [CrossRef]
129. Jin, Y.; Zhan, X.B.; Zhang, B.; Chen, Y.; Liu, C.F.; Yu, L.L. Polydatin exerts an antitumor effect through regulating the miR-382/PD-L1 axis in colorectal cancer. *Cancer Biother. Radiopharm.* **2020**, *35*, 83–91. [CrossRef]
130. Hu, Y.; Luo, X.; Zhou, J.; Chen, S.; Gong, M.; Deng, Y.; Zhang, H. Piperlongumine inhibits the progression of osteosarcoma by downregulating the SOCS3/JAK2/STAT3 pathway via miR-30d-5p. *Life Sci.* **2021**, *277*, 119501. [CrossRef]

131. Xie, C.; Du, L.Y.; Guo, F.; Li, X.; Cheng, B. Exosomes derived from microRNA-101-3p-overexpressing human bone marrow mesenchymal stem cells suppress oral cancer cell proliferation, invasion, and migration. *Mol. Cell. Biochem.* **2019**, *458*, 11–26. [CrossRef]
132. Xue, P.; Huang, S.; Han, X.; Zhang, C.; Yang, L.; Xiao, W.; Fu, J.; Li, H.; Zhou, Y. Exosomal miR-101-3p and miR-423-5p inhibit medulloblastoma tumorigenesis through targeting FOXP4 and EZH2. *Cell Death Differ.* **2022**, *29*, 82–95. [CrossRef]
133. Tao, L.; Xu, C.; Shen, W.; Tan, J.; Li, L.; Fan, M.; Sun, D.; Lai, Y.; Cheng, H. HIPK3 inhibition by exosomal hsa-miR-101-3p is related to metabolic reprogramming in colorectal cancer. *Front. Oncol.* **2021**, *11*, 758336. [CrossRef]
134. Sakha, S.; Muramatsu, T.; Ueda, K.; Inazawa, J. Exosomal microRNA miR-1246 induces cell motility and invasion through the regulation of DENND2D in oral squamous cell carcinoma. *Sci. Rep.* **2016**, *6*, 38750. [CrossRef]
135. Zheng, M.; Hou, L.; Ma, Y.; Zhou, L.; Wang, F.; Cheng, B.; Wang, W.; Lu, B.; Liu, P.; Lu, W.; et al. Exosomal let-7d-3p and miR-30d-5p as diagnostic biomarkers for non-invasive screening of cervical cancer and its precursors. *Mol Cancer* **2019**, *18*, 76. [CrossRef]
136. Lin, X.J.; Fang, J.H.; Yang, X.J.; Zhang, C.; Yuan, Y.; Zheng, L.; Zhuang, S.M. Hepatocellular carcinoma cell-secreted exosomal microRNA-210 promotes angiogenesis in vitro and in vivo. *Mol. Therapy. Nucleic Acids* **2018**, *11*, 243–252. [CrossRef]
137. Wang, L.; He, J.; Hu, H.; Tu, L.; Sun, Z.; Liu, Y.; Luo, F. Lung CSC-derived exosomal miR-210-3p contributes to a pro-metastatic phenotype in lung cancer by targeting FGFRL1. *J. Cell. Mol. Med.* **2020**, *24*, 6324–6339. [CrossRef]
138. Ge, L.; Zhou, F.; Nie, J.; Wang, X.; Zhao, Q. Hypoxic colorectal cancer-secreted exosomes deliver miR-210-3p to normoxic tumor cells to elicit a protumoral effect. *Exp. Biol. Med.* **2021**, *246*, 1895–1906. [CrossRef]
139. Min, Q.H.; Wang, X.Z.; Zhang, J.; Chen, Q.G.; Li, S.Q.; Liu, X.Q.; Li, J.; Liu, J.; Yang, W.M.; Jiang, Y.H.; et al. Exosomes derived from imatinib-resistant chronic myeloid leukemia cells mediate a horizontal transfer of drug-resistant trait by delivering miR-365. *Exp. Cell Res.* **2018**, *362*, 386–393. [CrossRef]
140. Mollaei, H.; Hoshyar, R.; Abedini, M.R.; Safaralizadeh, R. Crocin enhances cisplatin-induced chemosensitivity in human cervical cancer cell line. *Int. J. Cancer Manag.* **2019**, *12*, e94909.
141. Wang, X.; Hao, R.; Wang, F.; Wang, F. ZFAS1 promotes cisplatin resistance via suppressing miR-421 expression in oral squamous cell carcinoma. *Cancer Manag. Res.* **2020**, *12*, 7251–7262. [CrossRef] [PubMed]
142. Jingyue, S.; Xiao, W.; Juanmin, Z.; Wei, L.; Daoming, L.; Hong, X. TFAP2E methylation promotes 5fluorouracil resistance via exosomal miR106a5p and miR421 in gastric cancer MGC803 cells. *Mol. Med. Rep.* **2019**, *20*, 323–331. [CrossRef] [PubMed]
143. Li, Y.Y.; Tao, Y.W.; Gao, S.; Li, P.; Zheng, J.M.; Zhang, S.E.; Liang, J.; Zhang, Y. Cancer-associated fibroblasts contribute to oral cancer cells proliferation and metastasis via exosome-mediated paracrine miR-34a-5p. *EBioMedicine* **2018**, *36*, 209–220. [CrossRef] [PubMed]
144. Zuo, L.; Tao, H.; Xu, H.; Li, C.; Qiao, G.; Guo, M.; Cao, S.; Liu, M.; Lin, X. Exosomes-coated miR-34a displays potent antitumor activity in pancreatic cancer both in vitro and in vivo. *Drug Des. Dev. Ther.* **2020**, *14*, 3495–3507. [CrossRef]
145. Liang, Y.; Zhang, D.; Li, L.; Xin, T.; Zhao, Y.; Ma, R.; Du, J. Exosomal microRNA-144 from bone marrow-derived mesenchymal stem cells inhibits the progression of non-small cell lung cancer by targeting CCNE1 and CCNE2. *Stem Cell Res. Ther.* **2020**, *11*, 87. [CrossRef]
146. Tian, X.; Liu, Y.; Wang, Z.; Wu, S. miR-144 delivered by nasopharyngeal carcinoma-derived EVs stimulates angiogenesis through the FBXW7/HIF-1alpha/VEGF-A axis. *Mol. Ther. Nucleic Acids* **2021**, *24*, 1000–1011. [CrossRef]
147. Zhou, C.; Chen, Y.; He, X.; Zheng, Z.; Xue, D. Functional implication of exosomal miR-217 and miR-23b-3p in the progression of prostate cancer. *OncoTargets Ther.* **2020**, *13*, 11595–11606. [CrossRef]
148. Chen, D.; Wu, X.; Xia, M.; Wu, F.; Ding, J.; Jiao, Y.; Zhan, Q.; An, F. Upregulated exosomic miR23b3p plays regulatory roles in the progression of pancreatic cancer. *Oncol. Rep.* **2017**, *38*, 2182–2188. [CrossRef]
149. Hou, C.X.; Sun, N.N.; Han, W.; Meng, Y.; Wang, C.X.; Zhu, Q.H.; Tang, Y.T.; Ye, J.H. Exosomal microRNA-23b-3p promotes tumor angiogenesis and metastasis by targeting PTEN in salivary adenoid cystic carcinoma. *Carcinogenesis* **2022**, *43*, 682–692. [CrossRef]
150. Sun, L.P.; Xu, K.; Cui, J.; Yuan, D.Y.; Zou, B.; Li, J.; Liu, J.L.; Li, K.Y.; Meng, Z.; Zhang, B. Cancer associated fibroblast derived exosomal miR3825p promotes the migration and invasion of oral squamous cell carcinoma. *Oncol. Rep.* **2019**, *42*, 1319–1328. [CrossRef]
151. Jiang, Y.; Ji, X.; Liu, K.; Shi, Y.; Wang, C.; Li, Y.; Zhang, T.; He, Y.; Xiang, M.; Zhao, R. Exosomal miR-200c-3p negatively regulates the migraion and invasion of lipopolysaccharide (LPS)-stimulated colorectal cancer (CRC). *BMC Mol. Cell. Biol.* **2020**, *21*, 48. [CrossRef] [PubMed]
152. Li, L.; Li, C.; Wang, S.; Wang, Z.; Jiang, J.; Wang, W.; Li, X.; Chen, J.; Liu, K.; Li, C.; et al. Exosomes derived from hypoxic oral squamous cell carcinoma cells deliver miR-21 to normoxic cells to elicit a prometastatic phenotype. *Cancer Res.* **2016**, *76*, 1770–1780. [CrossRef] [PubMed]
153. Liu, T.; Chen, G.; Sun, D.; Lei, M.; Li, Y.; Zhou, C.; Li, X.; Xue, W.; Wang, H.; Liu, C.; et al. Exosomes containing miR-21 transfer the characteristic of cisplatin resistance by targeting PTEN and PDCD4 in oral squamous cell carcinoma. *Acta Biochim. Biophys. Sin.* **2017**, *49*, 808–816. [CrossRef] [PubMed]
154. Shi, S.S.; Zhang, H.P.; Yang, C.Q.; Li, L.N.; Shen, Y.; Zhang, Y.Q. Exosomal miR-155-5p promotes proliferation and migration of gastric cancer cells by inhibiting TP53INP1 expression. *Pathol. Res. Pract.* **2020**, *216*, 152986. [CrossRef] [PubMed]
155. Li, X.; Chen, Z.; Ni, Y.; Bian, C.; Huang, J.; Chen, L.; Xie, X.; Wang, J. Tumor-associated macrophages secret exosomal miR-155 and miR-196a-5p to promote metastasis of non-small-cell lung cancer. *Transl. Lung Cancer Res.* **2021**, *10*, 1338–1354. [CrossRef]

156. Gu, W.; Gong, L.; Wu, X.; Yao, X. Hypoxic TAM-derived exosomal miR-155-5p promotes RCC progression through HuR-dependent IGF1R/AKT/PI3K pathway. *Cell Death Discov.* **2021**, *7*, 147. [CrossRef]
157. Wang, D.; Wang, X.; Song, Y.; Si, M.; Sun, Y.; Liu, X.; Cui, S.; Qu, X.; Yu, X. Exosomal miR-146a-5p and miR-155-5p promote CXCL12/CXCR7-induced metastasis of colorectal cancer by crosstalk with cancer-associated fibroblasts. *Cell Death Dis.* **2022**, *13*, 380. [CrossRef]
158. Kirave, P.; Gondaliya, P.; Kulkarni, B.; Rawal, R.; Garg, R.; Jain, A.; Kalia, K. Exosome mediated miR-155 delivery confers cisplatin chemoresistance in oral cancer cells via epithelial-mesenchymal transition. *Oncotarget* **2020**, *11*, 1157–1171. [CrossRef]
159. Xing, Y.; Ruan, G.; Ni, H.; Qin, H.; Chen, S.; Gu, X.; Shang, J.; Zhou, Y.; Tao, X.; Zheng, L. Tumor immune microenvironment and its related miRNAs in tumor progression. *Front. Immunol.* **2021**, *12*, 624725. [CrossRef]
160. Yuan, Y.; Wang, Z.; Chen, M.; Jing, Y.; Shu, W.; Xie, Z.; Li, Z.; Xu, J.; He, F.; Jiao, P.; et al. Macrophage-derived exosomal miR-31-5p promotes oral squamous cell carcinoma tumourigenesis through the large tumor suppressor 2-mediated Hippo signalling pathway. *J. Biomed. Nanotechnol.* **2021**, *17*, 822–837. [CrossRef]
161. Yu, F.; Liang, M.; Huang, Y.; Wu, W.; Zheng, B.; Chen, C. Hypoxic tumor-derived exosomal miR-31-5p promotes lung adenocarcinoma metastasis by negatively regulating SATB2-reversed EMT and activating MEK/ERK signaling. *J. Exp. Clin. Cancer Res. CR* **2021**, *40*, 179. [CrossRef] [PubMed]
162. He, J.; He, J.; Min, L.; He, Y.; Guan, H.; Wang, J.; Peng, X. Extracellular vesicles transmitted miR-31-5p promotes sorafenib resistance by targeting MLH1 in renal cell carcinoma. *Int. J. Cancer. J. Int. Cancer* **2020**, *146*, 1052–1063. [CrossRef] [PubMed]
163. Hsu, H.H.; Kuo, W.W.; Shih, H.N.; Cheng, S.F.; Yang, C.K.; Chen, M.C.; Tu, C.C.; Viswanadha, V.P.; Liao, P.H.; Huang, C.Y. FOXC1 regulation of miR-31-5p confers oxaliplatin resistance by targeting LATS2 in colorectal cancer. *Cancers* **2019**, *11*, 1576. [CrossRef] [PubMed]
164. Wang, X.; Qin, X.; Yan, M.; Shi, J.; Xu, Q.; Li, Z.; Yang, W.; Zhang, J.; Chen, W. Loss of exosomal miR-3188 in cancer-associated fibroblasts contributes to HNC progression. *J. Exp. Clin. Cancer Res. CR* **2019**, *38*, 151. [CrossRef] [PubMed]
165. Zhao, M.; Luo, R.; Liu, Y.; Gao, L.; Fu, Z.; Fu, Q.; Luo, X.; Chen, Y.; Deng, X.; Liang, Z.; et al. miR-3188 regulates nasopharyngeal carcinoma proliferation and chemosensitivity through a FOXO1-modulated positive feedback loop with mTOR-p-PI3K/AKT-c-JUN. *Nat. Commun.* **2016**, *7*, 11309. [CrossRef]
166. Wang, C.; Liu, E.; Li, W.; Cui, J.; Li, T. MiR-3188 inhibits non-small cell lung cancer cell proliferation through FOXO1-mediated mTOR-p-PI3K/AKT-c-JUN signaling pathway. *Front. Pharmacol.* **2018**, *9*, 1362. [CrossRef]
167. He, L.; Ping, F.; Fan, Z.; Zhang, C.; Deng, M.; Cheng, B.; Xia, J. Salivary exosomal miR-24-3p serves as a potential detective biomarker for oral squamous cell carcinoma screening. *Biomed. Pharmacother.* **2020**, *121*, 109553. [CrossRef]
168. Zhang, H.W.; Shi, Y.; Liu, J.B.; Wang, H.M.; Wang, P.Y.; Wu, Z.J.; Li, L.; Gu, L.P.; Cao, P.S.; Wang, G.R.; et al. Cancer-associated fibroblast-derived exosomal microRNA-24-3p enhances colon cancer cell resistance to MTX by down-regulating CDX2/HEPH axis. *J. Cell. Mol. Med.* **2021**, *25*, 3699–3713. [CrossRef]
169. Kulkarni, B.; Gondaliya, P.; Kirave, P.; Rawal, R.; Jain, A.; Garg, R.; Kalia, K. Exosome-mediated delivery of miR-30a sensitize cisplatin-resistant variant of oral squamous carcinoma cells via modulating Beclin1 and Bcl2. *Oncotarget* **2020**, *11*, 1832–1845. [CrossRef]
170. Tao, K.; Liu, J.; Liang, J.; Xu, X.; Xu, L.; Mao, W. Vascular endothelial cell-derived exosomal miR-30a-5p inhibits lung adenocarcinoma malignant progression by targeting CCNE2. *Carcinogenesis* **2021**, *42*, 1056–1067. [CrossRef]
171. Du, Q.; Ye, X.; Lu, S.R.; Li, H.; Liu, H.Y.; Zhai, Q.; Yu, B. Exosomal miR-30a and miR-222 derived from colon cancer mesenchymal stem cells promote the tumorigenicity of colon cancer through targeting MIA3. *J. Gastrointest. Oncol.* **2021**, *12*, 52–68. [CrossRef] [PubMed]
172. Kong, X.; Zhang, J.; Li, J.; Shao, J.; Fang, L. MiR-130a-3p inhibits migration and invasion by regulating RAB5B in human breast cancer stem cell-like cells. *Biochem. Biophys. Res. Commun.* **2018**, *501*, 486–493. [CrossRef] [PubMed]
173. Yin, G.; Kong, W.; Zheng, S.; Shan, Y.; Zhang, J.; Ying, R.; Wu, H. Exosomal miR-130a-3p promotes the progression of differentiated thyroid cancer by targeting insulin-like growth factor 1. *Oncol. Lett.* **2021**, *21*, 283. [CrossRef]
174. Dickman, C.T.; Lawson, J.; Jabalee, J.; MacLellan, S.A.; LePard, N.E.; Bennewith, K.L.; Garnis, C. Selective extracellular vesicle exclusion of miR-142-3p by oral cancer cells promotes both internal and extracellular malignant phenotypes. *Oncotarget* **2017**, *8*, 15252–15266. [CrossRef] [PubMed]
175. Plousiou, M.; De Vita, A.; Miserocchi, G.; Bandini, E.; Vannini, I.; Melloni, M.; Masalu, N.; Fabbri, F.; Serra, P. Growth inhibition of retinoblastoma cell line by exosome-mediated transfer of miR-142-3p. *Cancer Manag. Res.* **2022**, *14*, 2119–2131. [CrossRef] [PubMed]
176. Hu, Z.; Zhang, H.; Liu, W.; Yin, Y.; Jiang, J.; Yan, C.; Wang, Y.; Li, L. Mechanism of HBV-positive liver cancer cell exosomal miR-142-3p by inducing ferroptosis of M1 macrophages to promote liver cancer progression. *Transl. Cancer Res.* **2022**, *11*, 1173–1187. [CrossRef]
177. Lou, C.; Shi, J.; Xu, Q. Exosomal miR-626 promotes the malignant behavior of oral cancer cells by targeting NFIB. *Mol. Biol. Rep.* **2022**, *49*, 4829–4840. [CrossRef]
178. Singh, R.; Pochampally, R.; Watabe, K.; Lu, Z.; Mo, Y.Y. Exosome-mediated transfer of miR-10b promotes cell invasion in breast cancer. *Mol. Cancer* **2014**, *13*, 256. [CrossRef]
179. Yan, T.; Wang, X.; Wei, G.; Li, H.; Hao, L.; Liu, Y.; Yu, X.; Zhu, W.; Liu, P.; Zhu, Y.; et al. Exosomal miR-10b-5p mediates cell communication of gastric cancer cells and fibroblasts and facilitates cell proliferation. *J. Cancer* **2021**, *12*, 2140–2150. [CrossRef]

180. Higaki, M.; Shintani, T.; Hamada, A.; Rosli, S.N.Z.; Okamoto, T. Eldecalcitol (ED-71)-induced exosomal miR-6887-5p suppresses squamous cell carcinoma cell growth by targeting heparin-binding protein 17/fibroblast growth factor-binding protein-1 (HBp17/FGFBP-1). *Vitr. Cell. Dev. Biol. Anim.* **2020**, *56*, 222–233. [CrossRef]
181. Chen, T.; Liu, Y.; Chen, J.; Zheng, H.; Chen, Q.; Zhao, J. Exosomal miR-3180-3p inhibits proliferation and metastasis of non-small cell lung cancer by downregulating FOXP4. *Thorac. Cancer* **2021**, *12*, 372–381. [CrossRef] [PubMed]

Disclaimer/Publisher's Note: The statements, opinions and data contained in all publications are solely those of the individual author(s) and contributor(s) and not of MDPI and/or the editor(s). MDPI and/or the editor(s) disclaim responsibility for any injury to people or property resulting from any ideas, methods, instructions or products referred to in the content.

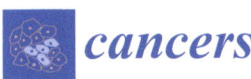

Review

Non-Coding RNAs in Airway Diseases: A Brief Overview of Recent Data

Giusy Daniela Albano, Rosalia Gagliardo, Angela Marina Montalbano and Mirella Profita *

Istituto di Farmacologia Traslazionale, Consiglio Nazionale delle Ricerche, Italy (IFT-CNR), 90146 Palermo, Italy
* Correspondence: mirella.profita@ift.cnr.it

Simple Summary: Nc-RNA are microRNA, long-coding RNA, and circulating-RNA. In this review we report most recent data regarding the role of nc-RNA in airway diseases, with a particular attention to microRNA. They are short, endogenously initiated non-coding RNAs involved in post-transcriptionally control gene expression via either translational repression or mRNA degradation. MiRNAs play significant roles in control of cell mechanisms involved in developmental timing and host-pathogen interactions as well as cell differentiation, proliferation, apoptosis, and tumorigenesis. Today the knowledge of the functions of the micro-RNA are of fundamental importance to define the subtypes of inflammatory diseases of the lung and to understand the effectiveness of the treatment.

Abstract: Inflammation of the human lung is mediated in response to different stimuli (e.g., physical, radioactive, infective, pro-allergenic, or toxic) such as cigarette smoke and environmental pollutants. These stimuli often promote an increase in different inflammatory activities in the airways, manifesting themselves as chronic diseases (e.g., allergic airway diseases, asthma chronic bronchitis/chronic obstructive pulmonary disease, or even lung cancer). Non-coding RNA (ncRNAs) are single-stranded RNA molecules of few nucleotides that regulate the gene expression involved in many cellular processes. ncRNA are molecules typically involved in the reduction of translation and stability of the genes of mRNAs s. They regulate many biological aspects such as cellular growth, proliferation, differentiation, regulation of cell cycle, aging, apoptosis, metabolism, and neuronal patterning, and influence a wide range of biologic processes essential for the maintenance of cellular homeostasis. The relevance of ncRNAs in the pathogenetic mechanisms of respiratory diseases has been widely established and in the last decade many papers were published. However, once their importance is established in pathogenetic mechanisms, it becomes important to further deepen the research in this direction. In this review we describe several of most recent knowledge concerning ncRNA (overall miRNAs) expression and activities in the lung.

Keywords: microRNAs; asthma; COPD; lung cancer; pollutions; extracellular vesicles

1. Lung Diseases

Lung diseases are types of disorders affecting the normal pulmonary functions preventing the ability to breathe. Many respiratory diseases begin with the onset of inflammatory reactions with a key role in the pathological conditions of the lung, as the reduced airflow of asthmatic and Chronic Obstructive Pulmonary Disease (COPD) patients [1].

The causes of the asthma pathogenesis are genetic, immune, or associated with environmental factors (pollutants, allergens, and pathogens). Asthma is characterized by airway hyper-responsiveness (AHR) and leads to intermittent and usually reversible airway obstruction. The symptoms of asthma are generated by drugs, exercise, or intrinsic problems; they can be repeated wheezing, chest tightness, cough, and other symptoms all related with reversible airflow restriction. Asthma pathogenesis is regulated by the co-participation of various immune cells and cytokines that are highly heterogeneous and affect numerous aspects of asthma regarding pathologic processes and clinical manifestations. Airway inflammation is characterized by T-helper 2 cells (Th2 cells) immune response and type 2 cytokines (e.g., IL-4, IL-5 and IL-13) release, eliciting airway eosinophilia, bronchial hyperresponsiveness, mucus overproduction, airway remodeling, and immunoglobulins E (IgE) synthesis in asthma. In addition, subject with asthma show in the airway epithelial cell exfoliation, fibrosis, vasodilation of the walls, and exudation of plasma [2]. The World Health Organization described that people suffering from asthma are currently 235 million, worldwide, and children are a bigger and most vulnerable group of asthmatic population [3]. Pharmacological treatment of asthma includes its action against allergens and irritants, as well as the use of β-adrenergic receptor agonists such as bronchodilators, glucocorticoids, and antileukotrienes to suppress inflammation or immunotherapy. These conventional therapies of asthma patients keep under control the symptoms but are not able to cure completely the disease [4].

Cigarette smokers are approximately 90% of the COPD patients. Smoke habits are the first cause of risk factor for the development of COPD [5,6]. The inflammation in COPD involves the innate and adaptive immune responses. It is one of the major public health problems worldwide since it is the major cause of chronic morbidity and mortality. The subjects with COPD are older than forty years of age and had a progressive and irreversible airway obstruction, characterized by deterioration of pulmonary function time related [7], causing the destruction of the lung parenchyma. This characterizes inflammation of central and distal airways, pulmonary emphysema, respiratory bronchiolitis representing the hallmarks of COPD [5,6]. The inflammation in COPD subjects includes the recruitment of different cell types as neutrophils, macrophages, lymphocytes, and the activation of epithelial cells in the airways [5,6]. To what extent central airways may mirror events, occurring in distal lung is uncertain. $β_2$-AR-agonist and anticholinergic drugs are as concurrent therapy used in the treatment of COPD to maximize bronchodilation and have a potential anti-inflammatory role [8]. The older compounds are modified to make novel therapeutic agents more potent, long lasting, enclosed in new inhalation devices [9].

Asthma and COPD are diseases with similarities [10]. However, they are different regarding etiology, type of inflammatory cells, mediators, consequences of inflammation, response to therapy [8] (Figure 1). COPD can originate in smoker subjects aged over 40 and its incidence increases in over 60-year-olds. Aging accelerates the decline of normal lung function in COPD patients showing a premature lung function loss.

The mechanisms of aging can be non-programmed or programmed. The first is related to the failure of the repair of DNA in the organs due to the increase in oxidative stress. The second is related to telomere shortening for a repeated cell division. Both aging defects are present in COPD patients per se, as physiological conditions disease. They may be involved in the progression of diseases toward lung cancer (LC). The premature aging of the lung, genetic predispositions, common pathogenic factors as growth factors, activation of intracellular pathways, or epigenetic modifications are common mechanisms that can be a cause of high prevalence of LC in patients with COPD [11].

The major risk factor for lung cancer is cigarette smoking. The smoking habit, common to COPD and LC alters the defense mechanisms regarding the antioxidant production such as superoxide dismutase, anti-proteases, and DNA repair mechanisms. If the damage to these mechanisms becomes too high in COPD patients, mutations leading to LC can occur [12]. In LC, increasing oxidative stress, reduction of DNA repair mechanisms and the resulting DNA damage, chronic exposure to pro-inflammatory cytokines, and increased cellular proliferation are common to COPD. LC is also a leading cause of morbidity and mortality in patients with COPD [13]. Mutations in oncogenes lead to an abnormal cell proliferation causing LC. The benign tumor was transformed to an invasive cancer by additional mutations that initiate spread invasiveness and anaplasia of the cells. It usually originates from the basal epithelial cells and are classified into two types, non-small-cell lung cancer (NSCLC) and small-cell lung cancer (SCLC) [14].

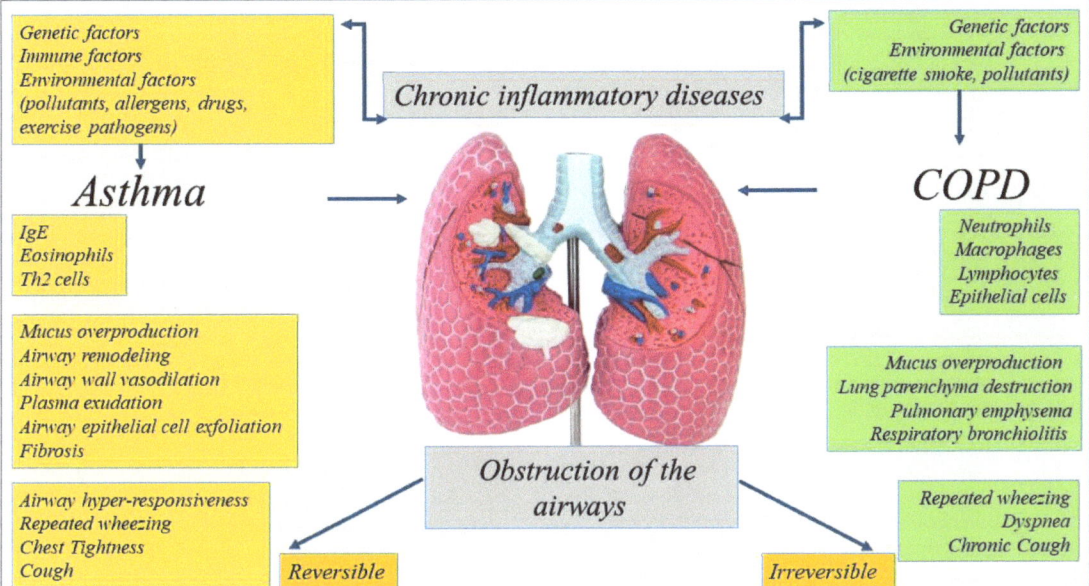

Figure 1. Representation of the etiology, inflammation, and symptoms of chronic inflammatory diseases of the lung. Asthma and COPD are diseases with similarities. However, they are different regarding etiology, type of inflammatory cells, mediators, consequences of inflammation.

Understanding the cellular and molecular processes driving the modifications in primary cells from patients, together with original and new models of disease is essential for the development of new treatments in lung diseases. Today, knowledge on immunobiology of inflammatory and structural cells of the lung is insufficient to explain the progression of lung disease to cancer [15].

2. Nc-RNA Biogenesis

The nc-RNA are classified in two categories housekeeping and regulatory. The regulatory included two noteworthy ncRNA: miRNAs or miRs (transcripts of 19–25 nucleotides) and long-ncRNAs (transcripts of 200 nucleotides) (lnc-RNAs) and circular RNAs (circ-RNAs). MiRNAs generally regulate post-transcriptional gene expression in physiological and pathological processes targeting the messenger RNA (mRNA) cleavage and degradation, and/or by inducing mechanism of translational repression or mRNA degradation [16]. lncRNAs, interacting with DNA, RNA, or protein through various mechanisms, positively or negatively control the stage of gene expression [17–19]. Finally, circ-RNAs have multiple biological functions as miRNA sponge, transcription regulator, protein translation, interaction with protein, RNA maturation, and so on [20]. The biogenesis, characteristics, types, and mechanism of action ncRNAs have a relevant role in developmental and homeostasis of human tissues [17–19,21]. In this section we described the biogenesis of miRNA mainly reported as nc-RNA in airway diseases in this review.

A conserved family of small endogenous noncoding RNA (nc-RNA) molecules (18–22 nucleotides in length) named microRNAs (miRNAs) was found in eukaryotes and have been extensively studied in human diseases and in cancer [22–24]. Many human diseases show aberrant expression of miRNAs [25,26]. MiRNAs are critical for normal animal development and are involved in a variety of biological processes such as proliferation, apoptosis, differentiation, and survival, playing an important role in gene expression regulation [27,28], also in the biological processes of the lung diseases [29].

MiRNA family are long transcripts called clusters, with repeated similar regions [30]. The discovery of new miRNAs and the description of their role in the pathogenesis of diseases are constantly evolving [31,32]. MiRNA action often suppresses expression of target gene interacting with the 3′ UTR of target mRNAs [33], or it has also been reported that miRNAs interact with 5′ UTR, coding sequence, and gene promoters. They shuttled between different subcellular compartments to control the rate of translation transcription [34].

MiRNA biogenesis is classified as canonical and non-canonical. However, the dominant pathway is the canonical miRNAs processing. The biogenesis of miRNAs starts in the nucleus with the processing of RNA polymerase II/III transcripts post- or co-transcriptionally. Pol II initiates the transcription of miRNA genes to produce pri-miRNA. Then, DiGeorge Syndrome Critical Region 8 (DGCR8), a microprocessor complex with a RNA binding protein ribonuclease III, transforms the pri-miRNA in pre-miRNA. Subsequently, DGCR8 targets N6-methyladenylated GGAC and other motifs into pri-miRNA, Drosha cleaves the pri-miRNA duplex in the hairpin structure of pri-miRNA [35]. Subsequently, by the exportin 5 (XPO5)/RanGTP complex action, pre-miRNA translocated from the nucleus to the cytoplasm and was transformed in mature miRNA/miRNA duplex by RNase III endonuclease Dicer and the RNA-binding protein TRBP the action. Then helicases separate the duplex by Argonaute (AGO2), and the strand guide of miRNA incorporates RISC to form a complex that recognizes specific mRNA by sequence complementarity leading to either mRNA degradation or translational inhibition [36,37] (Figure 2).

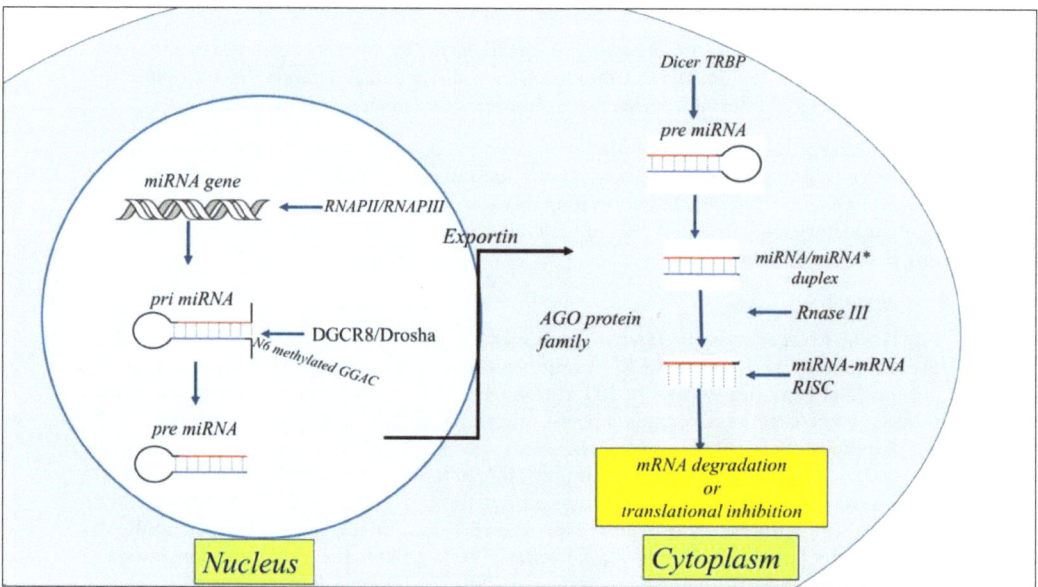

Figure 2. Schematic representation of the general steps of miRNA biogenesis. The biogenesis of miRNAs starts in the nucleus with the processing of RNA polymerase II/III transcripts post- or co-transcriptionally into pri-miRNAs. Then, a ribonuclease III enzyme transforms the pri-miRNAs in pre-miRNAs, which are transported into the cytoplasm by Exportin 5 (XPO5)/RanGTP complex action. Reaching the cytoplasm pre-miRNA is transformed in mature miRNA/miRNA* duplex by RNase III endonuclease Dicer and the RNA-binding protein TRBP the action. miRNA then forms a miRNA-mRNA RISC complex to induce mRNA degradation or translational repression.

The multiple non-canonical pathways of miRNA biogenesis involved different combinations of proteins used in the canonical pathway as Drosha, Dicer, exportin 5, and AGO2. miRNA biogenesis is grouped into two principal pathways defined Drosha/DGCR8-independent and Dicer-independent. Drosha/DGCR8-independent pathway produces pre-miRNAs like Dicer substrates. These pre-miRNA such as mirtrons nascent through exportin 1 are exported to the cytoplasm without the need for Drosha cleavage [35].

3. Nc-RNAs in Asthma

The throughput epigenetic analysis technologies, together with traditional biological function and clinical studies improved the genetic knowledge and finding epigenetic biomarkers of asthma provided new frontiers in the precision medicine of the lung [38]. The knowledge of nc-RNA regulatory networks opens new perspectives for the understanding the pathogenesis of asthma [39]. Asthma is a heterogeneous chronic inflammatory disorder in which different endotypes contribute to defining clinical inflammatory phenotypes. It is classified as mild, moderate, and severe. Nc-RNAs, in particular microRNA profiling in asthma is involved in the definition of subtyping asthma as potential biomarkers and therapeutic targets [40]. Altered expression of nc-RNAs in blood, in exhaled breath condensate, or in induced sputum condensate of sputum indicate the progression of asthma and the immune response in the lung.

Nc-RNAs regulate the gene expression at the post-transcriptional level and by targeting mRNAs affect the synthesis of cytokines and signaling pathways in airway inflammation [41,42]. mRNAs induce the activation of structural cells (bronchial epithelial cells, fibroblasts, endothelial cells, and smooth muscle cells) and immune cells playing an essential role in cell proliferation, differentiation, signal transduction, stress response, cell apoptosis, and other cellular and molecular aspects of asthma diseases.

MiRNAs might be considered as novel biomarkers of disease [42]. For examples miR-21 and miR-155 are important regulators of gene expression of many immunological molecules. Higher levels of miR-21 and miR-155 are detected in the serum of asthmatic patients compared to control subjects. Both miRNAs might be considered as potential non-invasive biomarkers useful for the diagnosis and response to the therapy in eosinophilic asthma [43].

The inflammatory processes of asthma are regulated by the activation and differentiation of Th2 cells, secretion of cytokines, and functions of eosinophils. let-7 family, miR-193b, miR-375 (downregulated), and miR-21, miR-223, miR-146a, miR-142-5p, miR-142-3p, miR-146b and miR-155 (upregulated) represent a core set of nc-RNA involved in asthma. Many of them are involved in T-cell differentiation increasing Th2 cell phenotype and Th2 cytokines secretions active in the origin of hyperplasia and hypertrophy of bronchial smooth muscle cells [44–46]. miR-21 is involved in the switch of Th1 versus Th2 responses, and defines the mechanisms of immunoinflammatory responses, limiting in vivo immune response-mediated activation of the IL-12/IFN-gamma pathway [47]. miR-146a is a candidate molecule with an association with impact of genetic variation in asthma [48]. It together with miR-26a and miR-31 is increased in the lung tissues of asthma mice, and in bronco alveolar lining fluid (BALF) of asthma children [49]. Furthermore, miR-146a define endotypes of asthma in moderate asthma (MA) and severe asthma (SA). MiR-146a and lower production of resolvin D1 create a dysregulation of inflammation in children, promoting remodeling processes and leading to lung function impairment [50]. MiR-155 and miR-221 are associated with Th2 responses [51] and with cells involved in allergic response (eosinophils, macrophages mast cells) in asthma and rhinitis [39,52–54].

Follicular helper (Th) and regulatory T (Treg) cells are involved in allergic asthma [55]. MiR-17 affects T-cell-like characteristics and via the de-repression of genes encoding effector cytokines transform them in Treg cells. It modulates regulatory T-cell function through targeting eosinophils and by targeting co-regulators of the Foxp3 transcription factor Foxp3 co-regulators [56]. PU.1 transcription factor is a negative regulator of Th2 cytokine release.

It is upregulated in the airways of allergen-challenged miR-155 knockout mice. These data underline that miR-155 regulates Th2 responses in allergic airway inflammation by transcription factor PU.1 [53]. Furthermore, miR-155 regulates type 2 innate lymphoid cells ILC2s and IL-33 signaling in allergic airway inflammation [57].

Remodeling and oxidative stress in asthma are regulated by many miRNAs. MiR-26, −133a, −140, −206, and −221, are associated with an effect on smooth muscle cell function and proliferation [39]. MiR-143-3p inhibits airway remodeling in asthma, suppressing transforming growth factor (TGF)-β1-induced cell proliferation and protein deposition of extracellular matrix (ECM) production proliferation via negative regulation of nuclear factor of activated T cells 1 (NFATc1) signaling [58]. MiR-192-5p is down-regulated in asthmatics and attenuates airway remodeling and autophagy in asthma by targeting MMP-16 and ATG7 [59].

The action of miRNAs can favor the progression of asthma phenotype from mild to severe stage [60]. However, despite the relevant role of miRNAs in asthma, few studies define their immunological activity in severe asthma. It is observed that miR-221 downregulates the action of TGF-β, on the aberrant airway smooth muscle proliferation and size, and consequently proinflammatory effects [61]; miR-28–5p and miR-146a/b downregulation led to circulating CD8+ T-cell activation in severe asthma [62]; and miR-223–3p, miR-142–3p, and miR-629–3p are well correlated with neutrophils in severe asthma [63]. All these findings facilitate the conclusions in this field [64] underlining that miRNA expression profiles might represent a risk factor for the development of a severe stage of asthma disease [28].

MiR-1278 inhibited inflammation in asthmatic mice and counteracted the effect of TGF-β1 in the cell proliferation and reduced apoptosis in airway smooth muscle cells (ASMCs). In particular this study showed that miR1278/SHP-1/STAT3 pathway is involved in airway smooth muscle cell proliferation in a model of severe asthma [28]. Recent overviews underline the emerging role of ncRNAs in childhood asthma. For instance, lncRNA CASC2 and BAZ2B are increased in the serum of childhood asthma [65,66]. CASC2 is involved in childhood asthma through inhibiting ASMCs proliferation, migration, and inflammation via miR-31-5p activity [65]. *BAZ2B* correlates with M2 macrophage activation and inflammation in children with asthma, and positively correlates with the exacerbating progression of diseases [66].

Circulating miRNAs such as miR-155-5p and miR-532-5p are predictive of asthma ICS treatment response over time and are significantly associated with changes in dexamethasone-induced trans-repression of NF-κB. Accordingly miR-155-5p and miR-532-5p might be considered as predictive of ICS response in clinical trial [67]. MiRNA-155 and Let-7a are differentially expressed in the plasma asthmatics than in control children, and levels well correlate with the degree of asthma severity. MiRNA-155 and let-7a could be used as serological non-invasive biomarkers for diagnosis of asthma and degree of severity [68]. Furthermore, it is underlined that circulating miR-146b, miR-206, and miR-720 are predictive of clinical exacerbation in asthmatic children, representing diagnostic biomarkers and therapeutic targets in childhood asthma [69] (Figure 3).

All these findings suggest that the regulatory networks of ncRNA provide new tools for the diagnosis and treatment of asthmatic patients to control inflammation, remodeling, and bronchial hyperresponsiveness in asthma controlling the activity of immune cells, ASMCs, and bronchial epithelial cells.

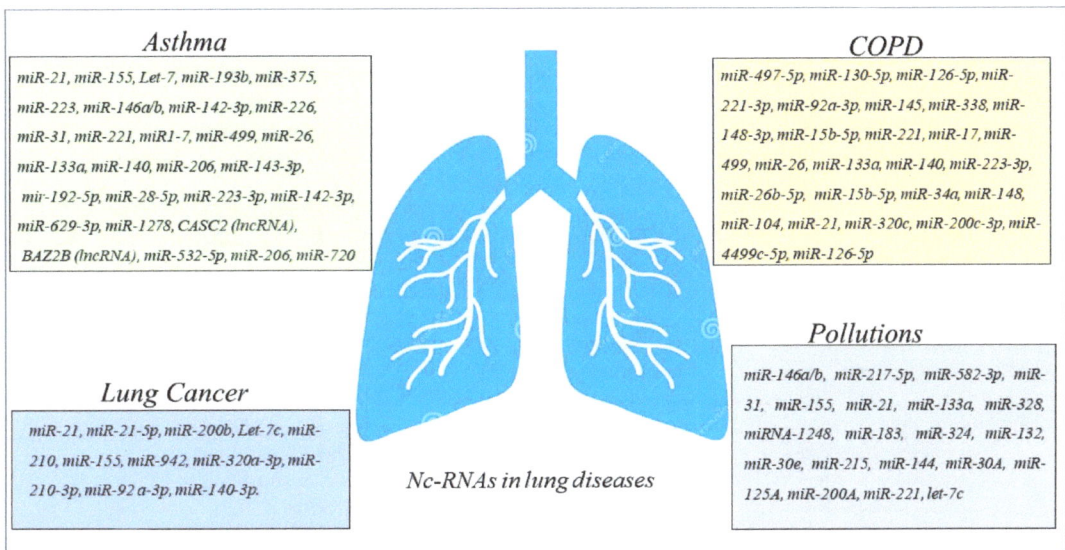

Figure 3. Schematic panel describing nc-RNAs involved in airway diseases and indicated in the review. The miRNAs and lnc-RNAs are expressed in lung diseases such as asthma, COPD, LC, or in lung diseases associated with environmental pollution.

4. ncRNAs in COPD

Many studies show that miRNAs production is increased in the pathogenesis of COPD [70]. MiRNAs involved in the myogenesis (proliferation and differentiation of satellite cells) alleviate the negative impact of skeletal muscle dysfunction and mass loss in COPD regardless of the degree of the airway obstruction [71].

miRNA-mRNA regulatory network is identified by GEO2R tool in the circulating plasma of COPD patients. Hub genes are potentially modulated by miR-497-5p, miR-130b-5p, and miR-126-5p and among the top 12 hub genes, MYC and FOXO1 expressions are consistent with that in the GSE56768 dataset [72]. Recent studies describe increased levels of miR-221-3p and miR-92a-3p in the serum of COPD patients than in healthy subjects, suggesting that both miR-221-3p and miR-92a-3p might be considered molecular markers to discriminate stable COPD and COPD with acute exacerbations. In addition, the same authors underline that miR-221-3p and miR-92a-3p are involved in the description of CSE-induced hyperinflammation of COPD [27].

Asthma-COPD overlap syndrome is an inflammatory disease of the airways that describe a new phenotype including both asthma and COPD characteristics. miRNA molecular pathways can help the scientists to better understand the pathophysiological features in many diseases. MiRNA expression profile of serum and sputum supernatants shows the increased expression of miRNA-338 in the sputum supernatants of patients with different obstructive diseases than in peripheral blood, while miRNA-145 increases only in the sputum supernatants of asthmatic subjects. However, both miRNAs are higher in the sputum supernatants of patients with asthma and COPD compared with control subjects. These data describe miRNAs as potential biomarkers in the discrimination of asthma-COPD overlap syndrome, asthma, and COPD [73]. The expression of five miRNAs (miR-148a-3p, miR-15b-5p, miR-223-3p, miR-23a-3p, and miR-26b-5p) is lower in patients with asthma-COPD overlap syndrome. Moreover, these miRNAs might be able to discriminate patients with asthma-COPD overlap and patients with either asthma or COPD. Between these miRNAs, miR-15b-5p is the most accurate and associated with the levels of Periostin and chitinase-3-like protein 1 (YKL-40) in the serum of patients representing a potential marker to identify asthma-COPD overlap patients [74].

The mechanism of cellular senescence is important to drive pathogenesis of COPD. MiRNA-34a is involved in this cell mechanism and reduces sirtuin-1/6 as markers of senescence through PI3K–mTOR signaling. In this manner its activity reduces secretory phenotype associated with senescence, and reverses cell cycle arrest in epithelial cells from peripheral airways of COPD patients [75].

MiRNA data analysis was performed using the TAC software, and reveals 148 miRNAs that are differentially expressed in PBMCs from patients with COPD compared with normal controls. Among the 148 miRNAs, 104 miRNAs are upregulated, and 44 miRNAs are downregulated [76]. The data show that miRNAs differentially expressed might be involved in the regulation of cell processes playing a fundamental role in the pathogenesis of COPD. Accordingly, it is possible to think that future investigation in this direction might provide further insight into the mechanism of COPD.

The miRNAs analyses show increased levels of miRNA-21 in airway epithelium and lung macrophages of the lungs of mice with CS-induced experimental COPD. miRNA-21 inhibitor (Antago-miR21) reduces the miRNA-21 expression in CS-induced lung of mice, suppressing the infiltration of inflammatory cells (macrophages, neutrophils, and lymphocytes). Furthermore, the treatment of with Antago-miR21 CS-induced mice decreases hysteresis, transpulmonary resistance, and tissue damping improving lung function in the mouse models of COPD [77]. Accordingly, it is observed that COPD patients with periodically experience acute exacerbation have increased levels of miR-21 inversely correlated with FEV1. These data support the concept that systemic levels of miR-21 can be involved in the pathogenesis of airway diseases and represent a therapeutic target to control the physiology of the lung [78].

In a little cohort of subjects, classified as COPD, smokers, and non-smokers, joint upregulation in miR-320c, miR-200c-3p, and miR-449c-5p levels in the miRNA profiling of BAL samples is detected. These findings might suggest that 3-miRNA signature might be potentially used as biomarkers useful to distinguish COPD patients from smokers and non-smoker subjects [79].

The high-throughput RNA sequencing describes a differential expression of 282 mRNAs, 146 lncRNAs, 85 miRNAs, and 81 circRNAs in peripheral blood of COPD patients compared with control. GSEA analysis shows that these differentially expressed RNAs correlate with several critical biological processes such as "ncRNA metabolic process", "ncRNA processing", "ribosome biogenesis", "rRNAs metabolic process", "tRNA metabolic process", and "tRNA processing". All of them might participate in the progression of COPD. These data determine the construction of the lncRNA-mRNA co-expression network, and the constructed circRNA-miRNA-mRNA in COPD opens new perspective in the nc-RNA involvement as potential regulatory roles in COPD [80]. lncRNA-proliferation, apoptosis, inflammation, migration, and epithelial-mesenchymal transition (EMT) are cell processes controlled by miRNA-mRNA network. Many lncRNA-miRNA-mRNA are biomarker indicators of comorbidities and may be considered as therapeutic targets for chronic inflammatory diseases of the airways of both COPD and asthma [81]. Numerous biological processes are due to the irreversible molecular changes caused by cigarette smoking in COPD patients. Several studies show its direct correlation with the dysregulation of different miRNAs suggesting the diagnostic/prognostic potential of miRNA-based biomarkers and their efficacy as therapeutic targets [82] (Figure 3).

In conclusion a relevant number of recent studies support the concept about the potential role of miRNAs network in the regulation of different cellular processes, such as proliferation, apoptosis, inflammation, migration, and EMT in COPD patients. These data support the concept of their biological activities in the relevant pathophysiological processes of chronic inflammatory airway diseases. In this scenario, we comprehensively underline the miRNA network activities in different cell types and their potential roles as biomarkers, indicators of comorbidities, or therapeutic targets for COPD (Figure 3).

5. ncRNAs in Lung Cancer

COPD and epigenetic events are involved in the development of LC [83]. miRNAs (miR-21, miR-200b, miR-210, and miR-let7c) and DNA methylation have higher levels in patients with LC showing a history of COPD than in patients with LC alone. Often, patients with LC show a declared history of an underlying respiratory disease. The identification of airway diseases in all patients with LC can represent a differential biological profile, involved in the determination of tumor progression and therapeutic response. In these patients, biomarkers of mechanisms involved in tumor growth, angiogenesis, migration, and apoptosis are differentially expressed in tumors of patients with underlying respiratory disease. Additionally, epigenetic events offer a niche for pharmacological therapeutic targets [83].

Several miRNAs are linked to both inflammatory and proliferative processes both observed in inflammatory and cancer diseases of the lung. For instance, miR-21 had a role in both inflammation and cancer and is linked to cigarette smoking-related conditions of both, patients with COPD and LC. MiR-21 is downregulated in skeletal muscle of patients with COPD patients than in non-smoking controls and its levels of expression well correlated with clinical features [83]. MiR-21 are highlighted for its critical role in LC, such as adenocarcinoma, non-small cell lung cancer. Accordingly, miR-21 is involved in various cell processes including cell death to cancer stemness. The expression of miR-21 is higher in biofluids and tissues of cancer, representing valuable potential markers of diagnosis and prognosis of LC [84]. Likewise, epidermal growth factor receptor (EGFR)-mutated lung had considerably increased miR-21 expression compared to those without mutations. EGFR can affect miRNA maturation by posttranslational modification of AGO2 highlighting the relevant relationship between a LC mutation and miR-21 status [85]. MiR-21 is commonly overexpressed in LC, where mutations are strongly related with miR-21 and its target proteins. Non-small-cell lung cancer (NSCLC) is consistent of R175H- and R248Q-mutant p53, and miR-21 is upregulated. Patients with elevated expression of p53 mutations and higher levels of miR-21 had a lower overall survival rate [86].

miRNA-155 is a marker of early diagnosis and monitoring of cancer diseases. It is highly expressed in tumor cells of LC. An electrochemical sensor propelled by exonuclease III, which is coupled with multiple signal amplification strategies for highly efficient microRNA-155 detection with a limit of detection of 0.035 fM. Overall, the strategy for miRNA detection offers good prospects for early cancer screening [87]. miR-942 is indicated as a prognostic marker for early discovery of tumor progression, metastasis, and development. Dysregulation of miR-942 amounts is identified in patients with non-small-cell LC, and they indicate as biomarkers in cancer discovery and assist in therapy control due to their epigenetic involvement in gene expression and other biological cell processes. In this manner, due to its involvement in cell proliferation, migration, and invasion through cell cycle pathways, miRNA-942 is considered as a potential candidate for prediction of LC [88].

miR-320a-3p, miR-210-3p, miR-92a-3p, miR-21-5p, and miR-140-3p are indicated in the literature with a predictive performance in the identification and in the pre-diagnostic setting of LC cases. They are increased in the serum of patients with LC in comparison with control subjects. miR-320a-3p, miR-210-3p, miR-92a-3p, miR-21-5p, and miR-140-3p compared to of surfactant protein B (Pro-SFTPB), cancer antigen 125 (CA125), carcinoembryonic antigen (CEA), and cytokeratin-19 fragment (CYFRA21-1) precursor forms improved sensitivity at statistical analysis to detect the condition of LC diseases. These data demonstrate that miRNAs in combination with a panel of proteins might be considered as useful tools for an early detection of LC [89] (Figure 3).

6. Environmental Pollution and ncRNAs in the Airways

Among the emerging biomarkers associated with the effects of environmental contaminants in the respiratory system, there are markers of oxidative stress (ROS, MDA, GSH, etc.,), inflammation (interleukins, PHENO, CC16, etc.), DNA damage (8-OHdG, γH2AX,

OGG1). In addition to these biomarkers, the action of pollutants on respiratory system is indicated to indicators of epigenetic modulation (DNA methylation, histone modification, miRNA) playing a fundamental role. However, studies that investigate miRNA expressions and functions in lung diseases association with air pollution are scarce. Interventions in public health requires the detection of specific biomarkers to define $PM_{2.5}$-elicited inflammation, fibrogenesis, and carcinogenesis. Some inconsistent findings may possibly relate to the inter-study differentials in the airborne $PM_{2.5}$ sample, exposure mode, and targeted subjects, as well as methodological issues. The identification of novel, specific biomarkers by a scientific approach obtained with omic-techniques might be useful to define the causal relationship between $PM_{2.5}$ pollution and deleterious lung outcomes by [90].

Exposure to airborne fine particulate matter as PM2.5 has short- and long-term adverse effects on lung functions. However, early impairment of lung function is not easily detectable in time. In particular, miRNAs are classified as novel biomarkers for PM-related injury in lung diseases, and currently are widely used in epidemiological and toxicological studies to understand the biological mechanisms underlying the adverse health outcomes of PM2.5 [91]. MiR-146a and miR-146b are elevated remarkably in bronchoalveolar lavage fluid (BALF) and lung tissue homogenate of BALB/c mice exposed to PM2.5. These data suggest the relationship between MiR-146a and miR-146b and pulmonary dysfunction after the exposure to the toxicants [92]. MiR-217-5p suppresses inflammation, oxidative stress, and lung injury in macrophages and lung tissue in a mouse model, showing activated STAT1-signal after the exposure to PM2.5 [93]. The trigger with $PM_{2.5}$ significantly enhances the biological behaviors of A549 cells promoting EMT transformation. The knockdown of miR-582-3p changes the effects of $PM_{2.5}$ on malignant biological behavior in A549 cells reducing Wnt/β-catenin signaling pathway and EMT. These data suggest that the over expression of miR-582-3p after the exposure to $PM_{2.5}$ in the environment might be involved in the mechanisms of LC [94]. $PM_{2.5}$ and related epigenetic modifications are involved in asthma pathogenesis; however, the mechanism remains unclear. The exposure to traffic-related $PM_{2.5}$ aggravated pulmonary inflammation in rats and increased the level of miR146a while decreased the level of miR-31. These epigenetic modifications provide a new target for asthma treatment and control, associated with their negative action on the regulatory T (Treg) cells function and T-helper type 1 (Th1)/Th2 cells imbalance causing exacerbation of inflammation [95]. Increased levels of miR-155 in the serum of asthmatic children correlate with particulate matter level exposure. Recently, it is reported that miRNA post-transcriptional regulation that involves RNA-based epigenetic mechanisms represents a key epigenetic factor of asthma pathogenesis associated with air pollution [96].

The use of miRNAs as biomarkers and as preventive targets for childhood asthma represent an attractive RNA hypothesis. In fact, children with severe bronchiolitis exposed to higher levels of air pollution show higher risk of developing asthma than children exposed to lower levels [97]. Air pollution aggravate type 2 responses, and lead to an increase in neutrophils as a source of miRNAs in the airway [96]. However, studies on adult asthma identify that numerous miRNAs may be involved in a better identification and understanding of the effect of environmental pollution in airway disease. In bronchial brushing, the exposure of atopic individuals to diesel exhaust and allergen shows miR-183, -324, and -132 expression modulated by allergen but not by diesel exhaust [98]. Moreover, diesel exhaust exposure increases expression of miR-21, miR-30e, miR-215, and miR-144 in the plasma of mild asthmatics enrolled in a randomized crossover study. Importantly, miR-21 and miR-144 expression is associated with increased oxidative stress markers and with a reduced antioxidant gene expression [99].

An increasing body of studies has focused on the effect of $PM_{2.5}$ on lung adenocarcinoma; however, also in this case the mechanism remains unclear. It is described that the exposure in patient-derived xenograft (PDX) models to PM2.5 can generate tumorigenesis and metastasis in lung adenocarcinoma of patient-derived xenograft (PDX) models, and migration and invasion in lung adenocarcinoma cell lines. PM2.5 are involved in the regulation of miRNAs including miR-30A, miR-125A, miR-200A, miR-200C, miR-221, and Let-7c of cancer stem cells (CSCs) pathway in lung adenocarcinoma cells [100] (Figure 3).

7. ncRNAs as Therapeutic Approach in Lung Diseases

Inflammatory diseases of the airways represent a relevant problem for lung health often related to the activation of molecular mechanisms. For this reason, it is necessary to define new pharmacological approaches to overcome the effectiveness of existing conventional therapeutic therapies and to address fundamental issues concerning specific molecular pathways [101]. The efficacy of therapy targeting pro-inflammatory miRNAs in mouse models of mild/moderate and severe asthma is recently established [102]. The suggested approaches are principally directed toward miRNAs and antagonists that mimics or blocks the specific activities to be used in vivo. However, their use in the local tissue of the lung might represent a limit for their use as therapeutic treatment limiting the adequate clinical applications. The knowledge of chemically nature of miRNAs is useful to understand the stability of themselves miRNA or antagomir in the blood, cell permeability, and optimized its target specificity. The knowledge of the miRNA's nature might guide an adequate lung cell uptake, high target specificity, and efficacy with tolerable off-target effects. Innovative approaches to enhance RNA stability, tissue targeting, cell penetration, and intracellular endosomal escape are critical to realize the full potentials of RNA drugs.

It is observed that circulating miRNA would reveal candidate biomarkers related to airway hyperresponsiveness (AHR) and provide biologic insights into asthma epigenetic influences. Eight serum miRNAs, including miR-296–5p, are associated with PC20 in the Childhood Asthma Management Program (CAMP) cohort [103]. In ovalbumin (OVA)-induced asthma model established in female BALB/c mice, it is observed that targeting miRNA-182-5p is a possible new strategy to treat asthma. In fact, the treatment of female BALB/c mice with miRNA-182-5p agomir significantly reduces the levels of IL-4, IL-5, OVA-induced IL-13, and eosinophil percentage in bronchoalveolar lavage fluid, including Th2 inflammatory factors downregulation. Furthermore, miRNA-182-5p agomir reduces the peribronchial inflammatory cell infiltration, goblet cell proliferation, and collagen deposition [104]. To help with the concept of personalized medicine, it is necessary to identify novel biomarkers involved in the disease. The objective is to improve the knowledge of disease phenotype and its classification, to better identify the pharmacological treatment. MiR-144-3p is increased in both lungs and serum of asthma patients. It was observed that the levels of miR-144-3p in the lung correlated with blood eosinophilia and with the expression of genes, strongly related to the pathophysiology of asthma, while the levels of miR144-3p in serum is associated with higher doses of corticosteroids in severe asthmatic patients. These data suggest that miR-144-3p reaches higher levels in severe diseases in association to corticosteroid treatment [105].

MiRNAs operate as posttranscriptional regulators, providing another level of control of GC receptor levels. Many actual experimental data describe miRNAs as useful biomarkers providing a promising approach to better characterize and treat patients with airway diseases [106]. miR-21 play a significant role in the pathogenesis of asthma and in steroid-insensitive experimental asthma steroid resistance via PI3K activation. These findings propose that the development of miRNA-based drugs could constitute a promising therapy to improve treatment of GC-resistant asthma by amplifying phosphoinositide 3-kinase-mediated suppression of histone deacetylase 2 [107].

The emerging attention on ncRNAs in airway disease is focused on the use of siRNAs as regulatory ncRNAs [108]. The therapeutic effects of synthetic siRNA are demonstrated in allergen-induced asthma models [29]. These data suggest improving and to deepen the knowledge of the role of the ncRNAs, to describe a new direction in the field of targeted asthma in adult and children therapy and in COPD [29]. In asthma and COPD GC resistance is controlled by many molecular and cellular pathobiological mechanisms. Actually, patients with GC resistance are treated with broad-spectrum anti-inflammatory drugs that often have major side effects [106]. Recently, the effect of ncRNAs on asthma and COPD attracted the attention of researchers as a new molecular mechanism to target, with the aim to contribute a better treatment of inflammatory airway diseases. Studies on this field are lacking though. MiRNAs are non-coding molecules that act both as regulators of the epigenetic landscape and as biomarkers for diseases, including asthma and COPD. Numerous ncRNAs such as miRNAs, lncRNAs, and circRNAs, are linked to COPD, but today only few nc-RNAs are functionally characterized. The use of nc-RNA including miR-195, miR-181c, and TUG1 as therapeutic targets might be considered as promising in the control of COPD in vivo. The development of innovative drugs includes siRNA therapeutics targeting mRNAs critical for the pathogenesis of COPD. For instance, siRNAs targeting RIP2, RPS3, MAP3K19, and CHST3 mRNAs are successfully validated in an in vivo COPD model. Furthermore, it is described that the best route for the administration of RNA therapeutics in the lungs of COPD patients is inhalation [109]. TLR2/4 signaling are controlled by miR-27-3p expression, a nc-RNA involved in the production of pro-inflammatory cytokines through targeting the $3'$-UTR sequences of ppARγ, suppressing ppARγ activation and miR-27-3p in alveolar macrophages (AMs). These data provide the information that miR-27-3p might be considered as a therapeutic method able to control the airway inflammation in COPD patients [110].

Fibroblasts from the lung of COPD patients show changes associated with an altered production of growth factors, fibronectin, and inflammatory cytokines [111]. For instance, vascular endothelial growth factors (VEGF) contribute to disturb vasculature in the lung. It is observed that the levels of miR-503 expression are lower in fibroblasts compared to the lung of a COPD [112] patient and show a positive correlation with increased levels of VEGF release. These data suggest that miR-503 production is involved in the control vascular homeostasis in COPD and helps to consider this miRNA as a therapeutic target in COPD [113,114]. DNA-based gene therapy has a reversible alternative with RNA therapeutics that is highly specific and safer. Fomivirsen, mipomersen, defibrotide, eteplirsen, nusinersen, inotersen, and patisiran are seven oligonucleotide-based drugs approved for a variety of disease conditions. These RNA drugs along with many others are candidate to be tested in clinical trials [115] and might also work in COPD [109].

Treatment of NSCL lung cancer is conditioned by NSCLC cell resistance to cisplatin. This topic represents a very important therapeutic challenge. The lnc-miRNA LINC02389 regulates cell proliferation and promoted cell apoptosis in NSCLC. Cisplatin-resistant cells is guided by an overexpression of oxidative stress biomarkers and regulated by LINC02389. The lnc-miRNA is highly expressed in NSCLC tissues and is associated with poor prognosis of NSCLC patients. Cisplatin-resistant NSCLC cells shows LINC02389 overexpressed, while miR-7-5p is downregulated. In these cells, LINC02389 negatively correlates with the expression of miR-7-5p. This last exerts an opposite effect and is as spongin for LINC02389 in NSCLC. These data might suggest therapeutic solution by regulating the expression of miR-7-5p in cisplatin resistance in NSCLC [116].

MiRNAs can be explored in early diagnosis and treatment strategies to prevent LC. Many of them have a relevant role in the specific cell cycle core regulation. These observations indicate the need to provide information with the aim to create new perspectives on cell-cycle-associated miRNA studies as target and therapeutics in LC treatment. This last consideration is well supported in the review of Fariha et al. [117]. The need to create more and more new perspectives are dictated by the importance of miRNAs in the pathogenesis of LC. For instance, miR-10b, miR-21, miR-150, miR-222, miR-96, miR-1290, miR-499 are miRNAs overexpressed in LC. Many authors suggest the use of antagomir, better known as anti-miRNAs, to block their negative action in LC. In fact, specific antagomirs are studied to contrast the activities of miR-10b, miR-21, miR-150, miR-222, miR-96, miR-1290, miR-499 blocking the interaction between the RISC complex and the target mRNA, thereby preventing mRNA translation [118].

8. Extracellular Vesicles and nc-RNA in Airway Diseases

Highest vascular density is a characteristic of the lung. In the lung cells as macrophages, fibroblasts, epithelial cells, and endothelium are involved in the circulation of extracellular vesicles (EVs), including exosomes, microvesicles, and apoptotic bodies [119]. Exosomes are small vesicles with a lipidic nature, deputies to the transport of proteins, lipids, and RNA molecules. Their immunological function is facilitated cell-to-cell communication under normal and diseased conditions. miRNAs and proteins present in EVs are ideal non-invasive predictive useful tools to contribute to an early diagnosis, prognosis, and therapeutic targets in lung disease, since they are factors associated with important information on biological responses. EVs released from various cells serve as mediators of information exchange between different cells to regulate a more accurate molecular mechanism involved in the process of cell-to-cell communication. MiRNAs are shuttled by EVs playing a pivotal role in the pathogenesis of respiratory diseases. EV miRNAs show promise as diagnostic biomarkers and therapeutic targets in several lung diseases [120] (Figure 4).

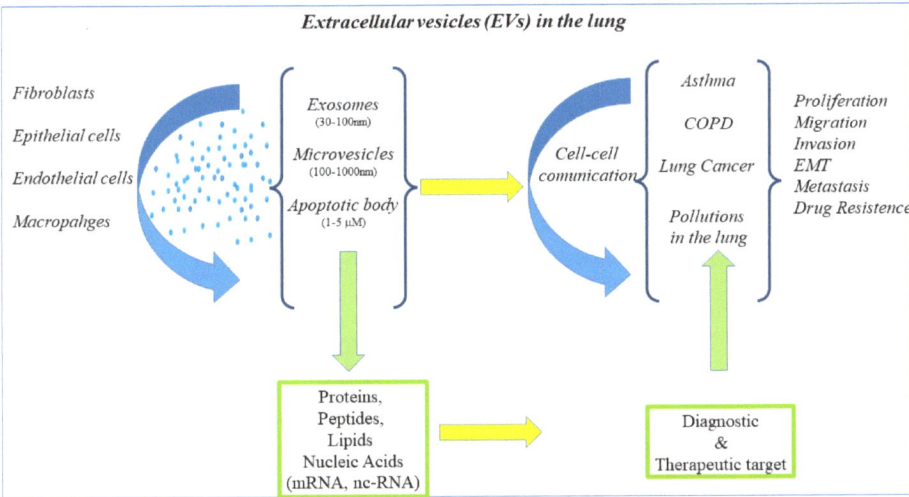

Figure 4. Cells of the lung release EVs of different size containing proteins, lipids, and nucleic acid involved in the mechanisms of cell–cell communication underlies the immunological response of respiratory disease such as asthma, COPD, LC, and airway diseases related to pollutions. EVs content show promise as diagnostic biomarkers and therapeutic targets in several lung diseases. BALF- and lung-tissue-derived EVs of healthy non-smokers, smokers have a miRNA profile with three differently expressed miRNAs in BALF, and one in the lung-derived EVs from COPD patients as compared to healthy non-smokers. MiR-122-5p is three- or five-fold downregulated among the lung-tissue-derived EVs of COPD patients as compared to healthy non-smokers and smokers, respectively. These data strongly suggest that miRNAs in the lungs of subjects with chronic lung diseases might be considered as potential biomarkers useful for therapeutic targets [121].

Nc-RNAs play critical roles in physiological and pathological processes of LC. EVs contain nc-RNAs packaged and are transported between LC cells and stromal cells. In this manner, EVs can regulate multiple activities of malignant cells of LC such as proliferation, migration, invasion, epithelial-mesenchymal transition, metastasis, and treatment resistance. In fact, it is possible to detect EVs in various body fluids associated with the stage, grade, and metastasis of LC, and potentially serve as diagnostic and prognostic biomarkers of disease playing a pivotal role in the clinical treatment of LC [122]. miR-153-3p-EVs are involved in damaging respiratory functions and produce a mass of inflammatory cells around the lung tissue of mice. It is observed that antagomir-153-3p treatment controls the deterioration of respiratory functions and inhibits the growth of lung tumors in mice. This study suggests the potential molecular mechanism of miR-153-3p-EVs in the development of metastasis of adenocarcinoma and provides a potential strategy for the treatment of metastasis in the lung [123].

MiRNA EVs cargo is different between patients with small-cell lung cancer (SCLC) and NSCLC. Particularly, miR-331-5p, miR-451a, miR-363-3p can distinguish SCLC and NSCLC tumor with highest rates of specificity and sensitivity [124]. Furthermore, EVs cargo with 7 miRNAs (miR-451a, miR-486-5p, miR-363-3p, miR-660-5p, miR-15b-5p, miR-25-3p, and miR-16-2-3p) differentiate NSCLC patients and healthy subjects [125].

Let-7i-5p is significantly overexpressed in $PM_{2.5}$-EVs and asthmatic plasma; and its levels of expression well correlated with $PM_{2.5}$ exposure in children with asthma. Mechanistically, let-7i-5p is packaged into $PM_{2.5}$-EVs by interacting with ELAVL1 and internalized by both "horizontal" recipient HBE cells and "longitudinal" recipient-sensitive HBSMCs. The result is the activation of MAPK signaling pathway via suppression of DUSP1 as its target. Furthermore, an injection of EV-packaged let-7i-5p into $PM_{2.5}$-treated juvenile mice aggravated asthma symptoms. The conclusion is that PM generates childhood asthma attacks via extracellular vesicle-packaged let-7i-5p-mediated modulation of MAPK pathway [126].

9. Conclusions

Lung diseases are a cause of morbidity and mortality in the world for all age groups. However, the underlying molecular mechanisms involved in airway diseases are not fully explored; overall, those associated with the epigenetic modification of ncRNAs differentially expressed in diverse samples of tissue and blood. We reported here some data on the role of ncRNAs in lung disease, to underline the most recent knowledge regarding their biological and molecular functions. They might be known for their capability of being biomarkers or for having a specific role in the pathogenesis of lung diseases.

ncRNA have recently attracted much attention for their roles in the regulation of a variety of biological processes. Today few biomarkers and drugs targeting ncRNAs have been identified as potential tools for clinical diagnosis and treatment, so that it becomes more and more important to verify the applicability of ncRNAs in clinical management of lung diseases. Researchers should combine innovative data-driven model elaboration and model-driven experimental design to elucidate how all ncRNAs cooperate in the pathogenesis and diagnosis of lung diseases. Finally, it goes without saying the need to develop a new approach aimed at the combination of bioinformatics, basic immunology, RNA biology, genomics, and proteomics, to better understand the role of ncRNAs regulatory networks in the pathogenesis of lung diseases. The final goal must be making a new direction in the diagnostics and pharmacological therapeutics for the lung.

Author Contributions: Conceptualization, R.G. and M.P.; methodology and validation, G.D.A. and M.P.; writing—original draft preparation M.P., R.G., A.M.M. and G.D.A.; writing—review and editing, M.P. All authors have read and agreed to the published version of the manuscript.

Funding: This research received no external funding.

Acknowledgments: The authors of the manuscript thank the National Research Council for their support.

Conflicts of Interest: The authors declare no conflict of interest.

References

1. Dey, S.; Eapen, M.S.; Chia, C.; Gaikwad, A.V.; Wark, P.A.B.; Sohal, S.S. Pathogenesis, Clinical Features of Asthma COPD Overlap, and Therapeutic Modalities. *Am. J. Physiol. Lung Cell. Mol. Physiol.* **2022**, *322*, L64–L83. [CrossRef] [PubMed]
2. Russell, R.J.; Brightling, C. Pathogenesis of Asthma: Implications for Precision Medicine. *Clin. Sci.* **2017**, *131*, 1723–1735. [CrossRef] [PubMed]
3. Zahran, H.S.; Bailey, C.M.; Damon, S.A.; Garbe, P.L.; Breysse, P.N. Vital Signs: Asthma in Children—United States, 2001–2016. *MMWR. Morb. Mortal. Wkly. Rep.* **2018**, *67*, 149–155. [CrossRef] [PubMed]
4. Kwah, J.H.; Peters, A.T. Asthma in Adults: Principles of Treatment. *Allergy Asthma Proc.* **2019**, *40*, 396–402. [CrossRef]

5. Barnes, P.J. Inflammatory Mechanisms in Patients with Chronic Obstructive Pulmonary Disease. *J. Allergy Clin. Immunol.* **2016**, *138*, 16–27. [CrossRef]
6. Barnes, P.J.; Burney, P.G.J.; Silverman, E.K.; Celli, B.R.; Vestbo, J.; Wedzicha, J.A.; Wouters, E.F.M. Chronic Obstructive Pulmonary Disease. *Nat. Rev. Dis. Prim.* **2015**, *1*, 15076. [CrossRef]
7. Negewo, N.A.; Gibson, P.G.; McDonald, V.M. COPD and Its Comorbidities: Impact, Measurement and Mechanisms. *Respirology* **2015**, *20*, 1160–1171. [CrossRef]
8. Mathioudakis, A.G.; Vanfleteren, L.E.G.W.; Lahousse, L.; Higham, A.; Allinson, J.P.; Gotera, C.; Visca, D.; Singh, D.; Spanevello, A. Current Developments and Future Directions in COPD. *Eur. Respir. Rev. Off. J. Eur. Respir. Soc.* **2020**, *29*, 200289. [CrossRef]
9. Hillas, G.; Papaporfyriou, A.; Dimakou, K.; Papaioannou, A.I. Pharmacological Treatment of Stable COPD: Need for a Simplified Approach. *Postgrad. Med.* **2020**, *132*, 126–131. [CrossRef]
10. Alshabanat, A.; Zafari, Z.; Albanyan, O.; Dairi, M.; FitzGerald, J.M. Asthma and COPD Overlap Syndrome (ACOS): A Systematic Review and Meta Analysis. *PLoS ONE* **2015**, *10*, e0136065. [CrossRef]
11. Barnes, P.J.; Adcock, I.M. Chronic Obstructive Pulmonary Disease and Lung Cancer: A Lethal Association. *Am. J. Respir. Crit. Care Med.* **2011**, *184*, 866–867. [CrossRef] [PubMed]
12. Durham, A.L.; Adcock, I.M. The Relationship between COPD and Lung Cancer. *Lung Cancer* **2015**, *90*, 121–127. [CrossRef] [PubMed]
13. Wilson, R.; Anzueto, A.; Miravitlles, M.; Arvis, P.; Haverstock, D.; Trajanovic, M.; Sethi, S. Prognostic Factors for Clinical Failure of Exacerbations in Elderly Outpatients with Moderate-to-Severe COPD. *Int. J. Chron. Obstruct. Pulmon. Dis.* **2015**, *10*, 985–993. [CrossRef] [PubMed]
14. Reck, M.; Heigener, D.F.; Mok, T.; Soria, J.-C.; Rabe, K.F. Management of Non-Small-Cell Lung Cancer: Recent Developments. *Lancet* **2013**, *382*, 709–719. [CrossRef] [PubMed]
15. Comer, B.S.; Ba, M.; Singer, C.A.; Gerthoffer, W.T. Epigenetic Targets for Novel Therapies of Lung Diseases. *Pharmacol. Ther.* **2015**, *147*, 91–110. [CrossRef]
16. Tubita, V.; Callejas-Díaz, B.; Roca-Ferrer, J.; Marin, C.; Liu, Z.; Wang, D.Y.; Mullol, J. Role of MicroRNAs in Inflammatory Upper Airway Diseases. *Allergy* **2021**, *76*, 1967–1980. [CrossRef]
17. Zhang, P.; Wu, W.; Chen, Q.; Chen, M. Non-Coding RNAs and Their Integrated Networks. *J. Integr. Bioinform.* **2019**, *16*. [CrossRef]
18. Statello, L.; Guo, C.-J.; Chen, L.-L.; Huarte, M. Gene Regulation by Long Non-Coding RNAs and Its Biological Functions. *Nat. Rev. Mol. Cell Biol.* **2021**, *22*, 96–118. [CrossRef]
19. Kopp, F.; Mendell, J.T. Functional Classification and Experimental Dissection of Long Noncoding RNAs. *Cell* **2018**, *172*, 393–407. [CrossRef]
20. Dong, H.; Zhou, J.; Cheng, Y.; Wang, M.; Wang, S.; Xu, H. Biogenesis, Functions, and Role of CircRNAs in Lung Cancer. *Cancer Manag. Res.* **2021**, *13*, 6651–6671. [CrossRef]
21. Fatica, A.; Bozzoni, I. Long Non-Coding RNAs: New Players in Cell Differentiation and Development. *Nat. Rev. Genet.* **2014**, *15*, 7–21. [CrossRef]
22. Maoz, R.; Garfinkel, B.P.; Soreq, H. Alzheimer's Disease and NcRNAs. *Adv. Exp. Med. Biol.* **2017**, *978*, 337–361. [CrossRef] [PubMed]
23. Zhou, R.; Wu, Y.; Wang, W.; Su, W.; Liu, Y.; Wang, Y.; Fan, C.; Li, X.; Li, G.; Li, Y.; et al. Circular RNAs (CircRNAs) in Cancer. *Cancer Lett.* **2018**, *425*, 134–142. [CrossRef]
24. Zhang, S.-J.; Chen, X.; Li, C.-P.; Li, X.-M.; Liu, C.; Liu, B.-H.; Shan, K.; Jiang, Q.; Zhao, C.; Yan, B. Identification and Characterization of Circular RNAs as a New Class of Putative Biomarkers in Diabetes Retinopathy. *Investig. Ophthalmol. Vis. Sci.* **2017**, *58*, 6500–6509. [CrossRef] [PubMed]
25. Ullah, S.; John, P.; Bhatti, A. MicroRNAs with a Role in Gene Regulation and in Human Diseases. *Mol. Biol. Rep.* **2014**, *41*, 225–232. [CrossRef] [PubMed]
26. Tüfekci, K.U.; Oner, M.G.; Meuwissen, R.L.J.; Genç, S. The Role of MicroRNAs in Human Diseases. *Methods Mol. Biol.* **2014**, *1107*, 33–50. [CrossRef] [PubMed]
27. Shen, Y.; Lu, H.; Song, G. MiR-221-3p and MiR-92a-3p Enhances Smoking-Induced Inflammation in COPD. *J. Clin. Lab. Anal.* **2021**, *35*, e23857. [CrossRef] [PubMed]
28. Li, J.; Chen, R.; Lu, Y.; Zeng, Y. The MicroRNA-1278/SHP-1/STAT3 Pathway Is Involved in Airway Smooth Muscle Cell Proliferation in a Model of Severe Asthma Both Intracellularly and Extracellularly. *Mol. Cell. Biochem.* **2022**, *477*, 1439–1451. [CrossRef] [PubMed]
29. Soni, D.K.; Biswas, R. Role of Non-Coding RNAs in Post-Transcriptional Regulation of Lung Diseases. *Front. Genet.* **2021**, *12*, 767348. [CrossRef]
30. Tanzer, A.; Stadler, P.F. Molecular Evolution of a MicroRNA Cluster. *J. Mol. Biol.* **2004**, *339*, 327–335. [CrossRef]
31. de Rie, D.; Abugessaisa, I.; Alam, T.; Arner, E.; Arner, P.; Ashoor, H.; Åström, G.; Babina, M.; Bertin, N.; Burroughs, A.M.; et al. An Integrated Expression Atlas of MiRNAs and Their Promoters in Human and Mouse. *Nat. Biotechnol.* **2017**, *35*, 872–878. [CrossRef] [PubMed]
32. Alsop, E.; Meechoovet, B.; Kitchen, R.; Sweeney, T.; Beach, T.G.; Serrano, G.E.; Hutchins, E.; Ghiran, I.; Reiman, R.; Syring, M.; et al. A Novel Tissue Atlas and Online Tool for the Interrogation of Small RNA Expression in Human Tissues and Biofluids. *Front. Cell Dev. Biol.* **2022**, *10*, 804164. [CrossRef] [PubMed]

33. Ha, M.; Kim, V.N. Regulation of MicroRNA Biogenesis. *Nat. Rev. Mol. Cell Biol.* **2014**, *15*, 509–524. [CrossRef]
34. Makarova, J.A.; Shkurnikov, M.U.; Wicklein, D.; Lange, T.; Samatov, T.R.; Turchinovich, A.A.; Tonevitsky, A.G. Intracellular and Extracellular MicroRNA: An Update on Localization and Biological Role. *Prog. Histochem. Cytochem.* **2016**, *51*, 33–49. [CrossRef]
35. Munjas, J.; Sopić, M.; Stefanović, A.; Košir, R.; Ninić, A.; Joksić, I.; Antonić, T.; Spasojević-Kalimanovska, V.; Prosenc Zmrzljak, U. Non-Coding RNAs in Preeclampsia-Molecular Mechanisms and Diagnostic Potential. *Int. J. Mol. Sci.* **2021**, *22*, 10652. [CrossRef] [PubMed]
36. O'Brien, J.; Hayder, H.; Zayed, Y.; Peng, C. Overview of MicroRNA Biogenesis, Mechanisms of Actions, and Circulation. *Front. Endocrinol.* **2018**, *9*, 402. [CrossRef] [PubMed]
37. Fan, R.; Xiao, C.; Wan, X.; Cha, W.; Miao, Y.; Zhou, Y.; Qin, C.; Cui, T.; Su, F.; Shan, X. Small Molecules with Big Roles in MicroRNA Chemical Biology and MicroRNA-Targeted Therapeutics. *RNA Biol.* **2019**, *16*, 707–718. [CrossRef] [PubMed]
38. Zhang, T.; Huang, P.; Qiu, C. Progresses in Epigenetic Studies of Asthma from the Perspective of High-Throughput Analysis Technologies: A Narrative Review. *Ann. Transl. Med.* **2022**, *10*, 493. [CrossRef]
39. Gomez, J.L. Epigenetics in Asthma. *Curr. Allergy Asthma Rep.* **2019**, *19*, 56. [CrossRef]
40. Heffler, E.; Allegra, A.; Pioggia, G.; Picardi, G.; Musolino, C.; Gangemi, S. MicroRNA Profiling in Asthma: Potential Biomarkers and Therapeutic Targets. *Am. J. Respir. Cell Mol. Biol.* **2017**, *57*, 642–650. [CrossRef]
41. Farmanzadeh, A.; Qujeq, D.; Yousefi, T. The Interaction Network of MicroRNAs with Cytokines and Signaling Pathways in Allergic Asthma. *MicroRNA* **2022**, *11*, 104–117. [CrossRef]
42. Wang, X.; Chen, H.; Liu, J.; Gai, L.; Yan, X.; Guo, Z.; Liu, F. Emerging Advances of Non-Coding RNAs and Competitive Endogenous RNA Regulatory Networks in Asthma. *Bioengineered* **2021**, *12*, 7820–7836. [CrossRef] [PubMed]
43. ElKashef, S.M.M.A.E.; Ahmad, S.E.-A.; Soliman, Y.M.A.; Mostafa, M.S. Role of MicroRNA-21 and MicroRNA-155 as Biomarkers for Bronchial Asthma. *Innate Immun.* **2021**, *27*, 61–69. [CrossRef] [PubMed]
44. Specjalski, K.; Niedoszytko, M. MicroRNAs: Future Biomarkers and Targets of Therapy in Asthma? *Curr. Opin. Pulm. Med.* **2020**, *26*, 285–292. [CrossRef] [PubMed]
45. Specjalski, K.; Jassem, E. MicroRNAs: Potential Biomarkers and Targets of Therapy in Allergic Diseases? *Arch. Immunol. Ther. Exp. (Warsz).* **2019**, *67*, 213–223. [CrossRef] [PubMed]
46. Polikepahad, S.; Knight, J.M.; Naghavi, A.O.; Oplt, T.; Creighton, C.J.; Shaw, C.; Benham, A.L.; Kim, J.; Soibam, B.; Harris, R.A.; et al. Proinflammatory Role for Let-7 MicroRNAS in Experimental Asthma. *J. Biol. Chem.* **2010**, *285*, 30139–30149. [CrossRef]
47. Lu, T.X.; Hartner, J.; Lim, E.-J.; Fabry, V.; Mingler, M.K.; Cole, E.T.; Orkin, S.H.; Aronow, B.J.; Rothenberg, M.E. MicroRNA-21 Limits in Vivo Immune Response-Mediated Activation of the IL-12/IFN-Gamma Pathway, Th1 Polarization, and the Severity of Delayed-Type Hypersensitivity. *J. Immunol.* **2011**, *187*, 3362–3373. [CrossRef]
48. Dong, J.; Sun, D.; Lu, F. Association of Two Polymorphisms of MiRNA-146a Rs2910164 (G > C) and MiRNA-499 Rs3746444 (T > C) with Asthma: A Meta-Analysis. *J. Asthma Off. J. Assoc. Care Asthma* **2021**, *58*, 995–1002. [CrossRef]
49. Shi, Z.-G.; Sun, Y.; Wang, K.-S.; Jia, J.-D.; Yang, J.; Li, Y.-N. Effects of MiR-26a/MiR-146a/MiR-31 on Airway Inflammation of Asthma Mice and Asthma Children. *Eur. Rev. Med. Pharmacol. Sci.* **2019**, *23*, 5432–5440. [CrossRef]
50. Gagliardo, R.; Ferrante, G.; Fasola, S.; Di Vincenzo, S.; Pace, E.; La Grutta, S. Resolvin D1 and MiR-146a Are Independent Distinctive Parameters in Children with Moderate and Severe Asthma. *Clin. Exp. Allergy J. Br. Soc. Allergy Clin. Immunol.* **2021**, *51*, 350–353. [CrossRef]
51. Marques-Rocha, J.L.; Samblas, M.; Milagro, F.I.; Bressan, J.; Martínez, J.A.; Marti, A. Noncoding RNAs, Cytokines, and Inflammation-Related Diseases. *FASEB J. Off. Publ. Fed. Am. Soc. Exp. Biol.* **2015**, *29*, 3595–3611. [CrossRef] [PubMed]
52. Martinez-Nunez, R.T.; Louafi, F.; Sanchez-Elsner, T. The Interleukin 13 (IL-13) Pathway in Human Macrophages Is Modulated by MicroRNA-155 via Direct Targeting of Interleukin 13 Receptor Alpha1 (IL13Ralpha1). *J. Biol. Chem.* **2011**, *286*, 1786–1794. [CrossRef] [PubMed]
53. Malmhäll, C.; Alawieh, S.; Lu, Y.; Sjöstrand, M.; Bossios, A.; Eldh, M.; Rådinger, M. MicroRNA-155 Is Essential for T(H)2-Mediated Allergen-Induced Eosinophilic Inflammation in the Lung. *J. Allergy Clin. Immunol.* **2014**, *133*, 1429–1438.e7. [CrossRef] [PubMed]
54. Mayoral, R.J.; Deho, L.; Rusca, N.; Bartonicek, N.; Saini, H.K.; Enright, A.J.; Monticelli, S. MiR-221 Influences Effector Functions and Actin Cytoskeleton in Mast Cells. *PLoS ONE* **2011**, *6*, e26133. [CrossRef]
55. Yao, Y.; Chen, C.-L.; Yu, D.; Liu, Z. Roles of Follicular Helper and Regulatory T Cells in Allergic Diseases and Allergen Immunotherapy. *Allergy* **2021**, *76*, 456–470. [CrossRef]
56. Yang, H.-Y.; Barbi, J.; Wu, C.-Y.; Zheng, Y.; Vignali, P.D.A.; Wu, X.; Tao, J.-H.; Park, B.V.; Bandara, S.; Novack, L.; et al. MiR-17 Resulted in Enhanced Suppressive Activity. Ectopic of Genes Encoding Effector Cytokines. Thus, MiR-17 Provides a Potent Layer of Treg Cell Control Expression of MiR-17 Imparted Effector-T-Cell-like Characteristics to Treg Cells via the de-repression. *Immunity* **2016**, *45*, 83–93. [CrossRef]
57. Johansson, K.; Malmhäll, C.; Ramos-Ramírez, P.; Rådinger, M. MicroRNA-155 Is a Critical Regulator of Type 2 Innate Lymphoid Cells and IL-33 Signaling in Experimental Models of Allergic Airway Inflammation. *J. Allergy Clin. Immunol.* **2017**, *139*, 1007–1016.e9. [CrossRef]
58. Cheng, W.; Yan, K.; Xie, L.Y.; Chen, F.; Yu, H.C.; Huang, Y.X.; Dang, C.X. MiR-143-3p Controls TGF-B1-Induced Cell Proliferation and Extracellular Matrix Production in Airway Smooth Muscle via Negative Regulation of the Nuclear Factor of Activated T Cells 1. *Mol. Immunol.* **2016**, *78*, 133–139. [CrossRef]

59. Lou, L.; Tian, M.; Chang, J.; Li, F.; Zhang, G. MiRNA-192-5p Attenuates Airway Remodeling and Autophagy in Asthma by Targeting MMP-16 and ATG7. *Biomed. Pharmacother.* **2020**, *122*, 109692. [CrossRef]
60. Maneechotesuwan, K. Role of MicroRNA in Severe Asthma. *Respir. Investig.* **2019**, *57*, 9–19. [CrossRef]
61. Perry, M.M.; Baker, J.E.; Gibeon, D.S.; Adcock, I.M.; Chung, K.F. Airway Smooth Muscle Hyperproliferation Is Regulated by MicroRNA-221 in Severe Asthma. *Am. J. Respir. Cell Mol. Biol.* **2014**, *50*, 7–17. [CrossRef] [PubMed]
62. Tsitsiou, E.; Williams, A.E.; Moschos, S.A.; Patel, K.; Rossios, C.; Jiang, X.; Adams, O.-D.; Macedo, P.; Booton, R.; Gibeon, D.; et al. Transcriptome Analysis Shows Activation of Circulating CD8+ T Cells in Patients with Severe Asthma. *J. Allergy Clin. Immunol.* **2012**, *129*, 95–103. [CrossRef] [PubMed]
63. Maes, T.; Cobos, F.A.; Schleich, F.; Sorbello, V.; Henket, M.; De Preter, K.; Bracke, K.R.; Conickx, G.; Mesnil, C.; Vandesompele, J.; et al. Asthma Inflammatory Phenotypes Show Differential MicroRNA Expression in Sputum. *J. Allergy Clin. Immunol.* **2016**, *137*, 1433–1446. [CrossRef] [PubMed]
64. Kyyaly, M.A.; Sanchez-Elsner, T.; He, P.; Sones, C.L.; Arshad, S.H.; Kurukulaaratchy, R.J. Circulating MiRNAs-A Potential Tool to Identify Severe Asthma Risk? *Clin. Transl. Allergy* **2021**, *11*, e12040. [CrossRef] [PubMed]
65. Yang, Y.; Sun, Z.; Ren, T.; Lei, W. Differential Expression of LncRNA CASC2 in the Serum of Childhood Asthma and Its Role in Airway Smooth Muscle Cells Proliferation and Migration. *J. Asthma Allergy* **2022**, *15*, 197–207. [CrossRef]
66. Xia, L.; Wang, X.; Liu, L.; Fu, J.; Xiao, W.; Liang, Q.; Han, X.; Huang, S.; Sun, L.; Gao, Y.; et al. Lnc-BAZ2B Promotes M2 Macrophage Activation and Inflammation in Children with Asthma through Stabilizing BAZ2B Pre-MRNA. *J. Allergy Clin. Immunol.* **2021**, *147*, 921–932.e9. [CrossRef] [PubMed]
67. Li, J.; Panganiban, R.; Kho, A.T.; McGeachie, M.J.; Farnam, L.; Chase, R.P.; Weiss, S.T.; Lu, Q.; Tantisira, K.G. Circulating MicroRNAs and Treatment Response in Childhood Asthma. *Am. J. Respir. Crit. Care Med.* **2020**, *202*, 65–72. [CrossRef]
68. Karam, R.A.; Abd Elrahman, D.M. Differential Expression of MiR-155 and Let-7a in the Plasma of Childhood Asthma: Potential Biomarkers for Diagnosis and Severity. *Clin. Biochem.* **2019**, *68*, 30–36. [CrossRef]
69. Kho, A.T.; McGeachie, M.J.; Moore, K.G.; Sylvia, J.M.; Weiss, S.T.; Tantisira, K.G. Circulating MicroRNAs and Prediction of Asthma Exacerbation in Childhood Asthma. *Respir. Res.* **2018**, *19*, 128. [CrossRef]
70. Zhuang, Y.; Hobbs, B.D.; Hersh, C.P.; Kechris, K. Identifying MiRNA-MRNA Networks Associated With COPD Phenotypes. *Front. Genet.* **2021**, *12*, 748356. [CrossRef]
71. Barreiro, E. The Role of MicroRNAs in COPD Muscle Dysfunction and Mass Loss: Implications on the Clinic. *Expert Rev. Respir. Med.* **2016**, *10*, 1011–1022. [CrossRef] [PubMed]
72. Zhu, M.; Ye, M.; Wang, J.; Ye, L.; Jin, M. Construction of Potential MiRNA-MRNA Regulatory Network in COPD Plasma by Bioinformatics Analysis. *Int. J. Chron. Obstruct. Pulmon. Dis.* **2020**, *15*, 2135–2145. [CrossRef] [PubMed]
73. Lacedonia, D.; Palladino, G.P.; Foschino-Barbaro, M.P.; Scioscia, G.; Carpagnano, G.E. Expression Profiling of MiRNA-145 and MiRNA-338 in Serum and Sputum of Patients with COPD, Asthma, and Asthma-COPD Overlap Syndrome Phenotype. *Int. J. Chronic Obstr. Pulm. Dis.* **2017**, *12*, 1811. [CrossRef] [PubMed]
74. Hirai, K.; Shirai, T.; Shimoshikiryo, T.; Ueda, M.; Gon, Y.; Maruoka, S.; Itoh, K. Circulating MicroRNA-15b-5p as a Biomarker for Asthma-COPD Overlap. *Allergy* **2021**, *76*, 766–774. [CrossRef] [PubMed]
75. Barnes, P.J.; Baker, J.; Donnelly, L.E. Cellular Senescence as a Mechanism and Target in Chronic Lung Diseases. *Am. J. Respir. Crit. Care Med.* **2019**, *200*, 556–564. [CrossRef]
76. Wang, L.; Zhao, H.; Raman, I.; Yan, M.; Chen, Q.; Li, Q.-Z. Peripheral Blood Mononuclear Cell Gene Expression in Chronic Obstructive Pulmonary Disease: MiRNA and MRNA Regulation. *J. Inflamm. Res.* **2022**, *15*, 2167–2180. [CrossRef]
77. Kim, R.Y.; Sunkara, K.P.; Bracke, K.R.; Jarnicki, A.G.; Donovan, C.; Hsu, A.C.; Ieni, A.; Beckett, E.L.; Galvão, I.; Wijnant, S.; et al. A MicroRNA-21-Mediated SATB1/S100A9/NF-KB Axis Promotes Chronic Obstructive Pulmonary Disease Pathogenesis. *Sci. Transl. Med.* **2021**, *13*, eaav7223. [CrossRef]
78. Ferraro, M.; Di Vincenzo, S.; Sangiorgi, C.; Leto Barone, S.; Gangemi, S.; Lanata, L.; Pace, E. Carbocysteine Modifies Circulating MiR-21, IL-8, SRAGE, and FAGEs Levels in Mild Acute Exacerbated COPD Patients: A Pilot Study. *Pharmaceuticals* **2022**, *15*, 218. [CrossRef]
79. Cerón-Pisa, N.; Iglesias, A.; Shafiek, H.; Martín-Medina, A.; Esteva-Socias, M.; Muncunill, J.; Fleischer, A.; Verdú, J.; Cosío, B.G.; Sauleda, J. Hsa-Mir-320c, Hsa-Mir-200c-3p, and Hsa-Mir-449c-5p as Potential Specific MiRNA Biomarkers of COPD: A Pilot Study. *Pathophysiol. Off. J. Int. Soc. Pathophysiol.* **2022**, *29*, 143–156. [CrossRef]
80. Liu, P.; Wang, Y.; Zhang, N.; Zhao, X.; Li, R.; Wang, Y.; Chen, C.; Wang, D.; Zhang, X.; Chen, L.; et al. Comprehensive Identification of RNA Transcripts and Construction of RNA Network in Chronic Obstructive Pulmonary Disease. *Respir. Res.* **2022**, *23*, 154. [CrossRef]
81. Qiao, X.; Hou, G.; He, Y.-L.; Song, D.-F.; An, Y.; Altawil, A.; Zhou, X.-M.; Wang, Q.-Y.; Kang, J.; Yin, Y. The Novel Regulatory Role of the LncRNA-MiRNA-MRNA Axis in Chronic Inflammatory Airway Diseases. *Front. Mol. Biosci.* **2022**, *9*, 927549. [CrossRef]
82. Paul, S.; Ruiz-Manriquez, L.M.; Ambriz-Gonzalez, H.; Medina-Gomez, C.D.; Valenzuela-Coronado, E.; Moreno-Gomez, P.; Pathak, S.; Chakraborty, S.; Srivastava, A. Impact of Smoking-Induced Dysregulated Human MiRNAs in Chronic Disease Development and Their Potential Use in Prognostic and Therapeutic Purposes. *J. Biochem. Mol. Toxicol.* **2022**, *36*, e23134. [CrossRef] [PubMed]
83. Mateu-Jimenez, M.; Curull, V.; Rodríguez-Fuster, A.; Aguiló, R.; Sánchez-Font, A.; Pijuan, L.; Gea, J.; Barreiro, E. Profile of Epigenetic Mechanisms in Lung Tumors of Patients with Underlying Chronic Respiratory Conditions. *Clin. Epigenetics* **2018**, *10*, 7. [CrossRef] [PubMed]

84. Rhim, J.; Baek, W.; Seo, Y.; Kim, J.H. From Molecular Mechanisms to Therapeutics: Understanding MicroRNA-21 in Cancer. *Cells* **2022**, *11*, 2791. [CrossRef]
85. Shen, J.; Xia, W.; Khotskaya, Y.B.; Huo, L.; Nakanishi, K.; Lim, S.-O.; Du, Y.; Wang, Y.; Chang, W.-C.; Chen, C.-H.; et al. EGFR Modulates MicroRNA Maturation in Response to Hypoxia through Phosphorylation of AGO2. *Nature* **2013**, *497*, 383–387. [CrossRef] [PubMed]
86. Zhou, Y.; Guo, D.; Zhang, Y. Association of MicroRNA-21 with P53 at Mutant Sites R175H and R248Q, Clinicopathological Features, and Prognosis of NSCLC. *Mol. Ther. Oncolytics* **2020**, *19*, 208–217. [CrossRef] [PubMed]
87. Yan, B.; Zheng, X.; Shi, P. Electrochemical Sensor Propelled by Exonuclease III for Highly Efficient MicroRNA-155 Detection. *Analyst* **2022**, *147*, 4824–4828. [CrossRef]
88. Yadegar, N.; Dadashi, Z.; Shams, K.; Mohammadi, M.; Abyar, M.; Rafat, M. The Prominent Role of MiR-942 in Carcinogenesis of Tumors. *Adv. Biomed. Res.* **2022**, *11*, 63. [CrossRef]
89. Vykoukal, J.; Fahrmann, J.F.; Patel, N.; Shimizu, M.; Ostrin, E.J.; Dennison, J.B.; Ivan, C.; Goodman, G.E.; Thornquist, M.D.; Barnett, M.J.; et al. Contributions of Circulating MicroRNAs for Early Detection of Lung Cancer. *Cancers* **2022**, *14*, 4221. [CrossRef]
90. Guo, C.; Lv, S.; Liu, Y.; Li, Y. Biomarkers for the Adverse Effects on Respiratory System Health Associated with Atmospheric Particulate Matter Exposure. *J. Hazard. Mater.* **2022**, *421*, 126760. [CrossRef]
91. Liu, G.; Li, Y.; Zhou, J.; Xu, J.; Yang, B. PM2.5 Deregulated MicroRNA and Inflammatory Microenvironment in Lung Injury. *Environ. Toxicol. Pharmacol.* **2022**, *91*, 103832. [CrossRef] [PubMed]
92. Hou, T.; Chen, Q.; Ma, Y. Elevated Expression of MiR-146 Involved in Regulating Mice Pulmonary Dysfunction after Exposure to PM2.5. *J. Toxicol. Sci.* **2021**, *46*, 437–443. [CrossRef] [PubMed]
93. Xie, J.; Li, S.; Ma, X.; Li, R.; Zhang, H.; Li, J.; Yan, X. MiR-217-5p Inhibits Smog (PM2.5)-Induced Inflammation and Oxidative Stress Response of Mouse Lung Tissues and Macrophages through Targeting STAT1. *Aging* **2022**, *14*, 6796–6808. [CrossRef] [PubMed]
94. Yang, M.; Ju, L.; Li, C.; Cheng, H.; Li, N.; Zhang, Q.; Sun, S.; Ding, L.; Sui, X.; Zhang, C.; et al. MiR-582-3p Participates in the Regulation of Biological Behaviors of A549 Cells by Ambient PM(2.5) Exposure. *Environ. Sci. Pollut. Res. Int.* **2022**, *29*, 13624–13634. [CrossRef]
95. Wang, C.; Wang, J.; Zheng, X.; Zhang, J.; Zhang, J.; Qiao, G.; Liu, H.; Zhao, H.; Bai, J.; Zhang, H.; et al. Epigenetic Regulation Is Involved in Traffic-Related PM(2.5) Aggravating Allergic Airway Inflammation in Rats. *Clin. Immunol.* **2022**, *234*, 108914. [CrossRef]
96. Weidner, J.; Bartel, S.; Kılıç, A.; Zissler, U.M.; Renz, H.; Schwarze, J.; Schmidt-Weber, C.B.; Maes, T.; Rebane, A.; Krauss-Etschmann, S.; et al. Spotlight on MicroRNAs in Allergy and Asthma. *Allergy* **2021**, *76*, 1661–1678. [CrossRef]
97. Makrinioti, H.; Camargo, C.A.; Zhu, Z.; Freishtat, R.J.; Hasegawa, K. Air Pollution, Bronchiolitis, and Asthma: The Role of Nasal MicroRNAs. *Lancet. Respir. Med.* **2022**, *10*, 733–734. [CrossRef]
98. Rider, C.F.; Yamamoto, M.; Günther, O.P.; Hirota, J.A.; Singh, A.; Tebbutt, S.J.; Carlsten, C. Controlled Diesel Exhaust and Allergen Coexposure Modulates MicroRNA and Gene Expression in Humans: Effects on Inflammatory Lung Markers. *J. Allergy Clin. Immunol.* **2016**, *138*, 1690–1700. [CrossRef]
99. Yamamoto, M.; Singh, A.; Sava, F.; Pui, M.; Tebbutt, S.J.; Carlsten, C. MicroRNA Expression in Response to Controlled Exposure to Diesel Exhaust: Attenuation by the Antioxidant N-Acetylcysteine in a Randomized Crossover Study. *Environ. Health Perspect.* **2013**, *121*, 670–675. [CrossRef]
100. Pan, J.; Xue, Y.; Li, S.; Wang, L.; Mei, J.; Ni, D.; Jiang, J.; Zhang, M.; Yi, S.; Zhang, R.; et al. PM(2.5) Induces the Distant Metastasis of Lung Adenocarcinoma via Promoting the Stem Cell Properties of Cancer Cells. *Environ. Pollut.* **2022**, *296*, 118718. [CrossRef]
101. Szymczak, I.; Wieczfinska, J.; Pawliczak, R. Molecular Background of MiRNA Role in Asthma and COPD: An Updated Insight. *Biomed Res. Int.* **2016**, *2016*, 7802521. [CrossRef]
102. Ramelli, S.C.; Gerthoffer, W.T. MicroRNA Targets for Asthma Therapy. *Adv. Exp. Med. Biol.* **2021**, *1303*, 89–105. [CrossRef]
103. Davis, J.S.; Sun, M.; Kho, A.T.; Moore, K.G.; Sylvia, J.M.; Weiss, S.T.; Lu, Q.; Tantisira, K.G. Circulating MicroRNAs and Association with Methacholine PC20 in the Childhood Asthma Management Program (CAMP) Cohort. *PLoS ONE* **2017**, *12*, e0180329. [CrossRef]
104. Wang, Z.; Song, Y.; Jiang, J.; Piao, Y.; Li, L.; Bai, Q.; Xu, C.; Liu, H.; Li, L.; Piao, H.; et al. MicroRNA-182-5p Attenuates Asthmatic Airway Inflammation by Targeting NOX4. *Front. Immunol.* **2022**, *13*, 853848. [CrossRef]
105. Rodrigo-Muñoz, J.M.; Gil-Martínez, M.; Lorente-Sorolla, C.; García-Latorre, R.; Valverde-Monge, M.; Quirce, S.; Sastre, J.; Del Pozo, V. MiR-144-3p Is a Biomarker Related to Severe Corticosteroid-Dependent Asthma. *Front. Immunol.* **2022**, *13*, 858722. [CrossRef]
106. Palumbo, M.L.; Prochnik, A.; Wald, M.R.; Genaro, A.M. Chronic Stress and Glucocorticoid Receptor Resistance in Asthma. *Clin. Ther.* **2020**, *42*, 993–1006. [CrossRef]
107. Kim, R.Y.; Horvat, J.C.; Pinkerton, J.W.; Starkey, M.R.; Essilfie, A.T.; Mayall, J.R.; Nair, P.M.; Hansbro, N.G.; Jones, B.; Haw, T.J.; et al. MicroRNA-21 Drives Severe, Steroid-Insensitive Experimental Asthma by Amplifying Phosphoinositide 3-Kinase-Mediated Suppression of Histone Deacetylase 2. *J. Allergy Clin. Immunol.* **2017**, *139*, 519–532. [CrossRef]
108. Liang, J.; Liu, X.-H.; Chen, X.-M.; Song, X.-L.; Li, W.; Huang, Y. Emerging Roles of Non-Coding RNAs in Childhood Asthma. *Front. Pharmacol.* **2022**, *13*, 856104. [CrossRef]

109. Mei, D.; Tan, W.S.D.; Tay, Y.; Mukhopadhyay, A.; Wong, W.S.F. Therapeutic RNA Strategies for Chronic Obstructive Pulmonary Disease. *Trends Pharmacol. Sci.* **2020**, *41*, 475–486. [CrossRef]
110. Wang, D.; He, S.; Liu, B.; Liu, C. MiR-27-3p Regulates TLR2/4-Dependent Mouse Alveolar Macrophage Activation by Targetting PPARγ. *Clin. Sci.* **2018**, *132*, 943–958. [CrossRef]
111. Togo, S.; Holz, O.; Liu, X.; Sugiura, H.; Kamio, K.; Wang, X.; Kawasaki, S.; Ahn, Y.; Fredriksson, K.; Skold, C.M.; et al. Lung Fibroblast Repair Functions in Patients with Chronic Obstructive Pulmonary Disease Are Altered by Multiple Mechanisms. *Am. J. Respir. Crit. Care Med.* **2008**, *178*, 248–260. [CrossRef]
112. Ikari, J.; Smith, L.M.; Nelson, A.J.; Iwasawa, S.; Gunji, Y.; Farid, M.; Wang, X.; Basma, H.; Feghali-Bostwick, C.; Liu, X.; et al. Effect of Culture Conditions on MicroRNA Expression in Primary Adult Control and COPD Lung Fibroblasts in Vitro. *In Vitro Cell. Dev. Biol. Anim.* **2015**, *51*, 390–399. [CrossRef]
113. Ikari, J.; Nelson, A.J.; Obaid, J.; Giron-Martinez, A.; Ikari, K.; Makino, F.; Iwasawa, S.; Gunji, Y.; Farid, M.; Wang, X.; et al. Reduced MicroRNA-503 Expression Augments Lung Fibroblast VEGF Production in Chronic Obstructive Pulmonary Disease. *PLoS ONE* **2017**, *12*, e0184039. [CrossRef]
114. Zhang, L.; Valizadeh, H.; Alipourfard, I.; Bidares, R.; Aghebati-Maleki, L.; Ahmadi, M. Epigenetic Modifications and Therapy in Chronic Obstructive Pulmonary Disease (COPD): An Update Review. *COPD* **2020**, *17*, 333–342. [CrossRef]
115. Rüger, J.; Ioannou, S.; Castanotto, D.; Stein, C.A. Oligonucleotides to the (Gene) Rescue: FDA Approvals 2017–2019. *Trends Pharmacol. Sci.* **2020**, *41*, 27–41. [CrossRef]
116. Ma, P.; Han, W.; Meng, C.; Tan, X.; Liu, P.; Dong, L. LINC02389/MiR-7-5p Regulated Cisplatin Resistance of Non-Small-Cell Lung Cancer via Promoting Oxidative Stress. *Anal. Cell. Pathol.* **2022**, *2022*, 6100176. [CrossRef]
117. Fariha, A.; Hami, I.; Tonmoy, M.I.Q.; Akter, S.; Al Reza, H.; Bahadur, N.M.; Rahaman, M.M.; Hossain, M.S. Cell Cycle Associated MiRNAs as Target and Therapeutics in Lung Cancer Treatment. *Heliyon* **2022**, *8*, e11081. [CrossRef]
118. Murugan, D.; Rangasamy, L. A Perspective to Weaponize MicroRNAs against Lung Cancer. *Non-Coding RNA Res.* **2023**, *8*, 18–32. [CrossRef]
119. Mohan, A.; Agarwal, S.; Clauss, M.; Britt, N.S.; Dhillon, N.K. Extracellular Vesicles: Novel Communicators in Lung Diseases. *Respir. Res.* **2020**, *21*, 175. [CrossRef]
120. Li, Y.; Yin, Z.; Fan, J.; Zhang, S.; Yang, W. The Roles of Exosomal MiRNAs and LncRNAs in Lung Diseases. *Signal Transduct. Target. Ther.* **2019**, *4*, 47. [CrossRef]
121. Kaur, G.; Maremanda, K.P.; Campos, M.; Chand, H.S.; Li, F.; Hirani, N.; Haseeb, M.A.; Li, D.; Rahman, I. Distinct Exosomal MiRNA Profiles from BALF and Lung Tissue of COPD and IPF Patients. *Int. J. Mol. Sci.* **2021**, *22*, 11830. [CrossRef]
122. Shan, C.; Liang, Y.; Cai, H.; Wang, F.; Chen, X.; Yin, Q.; Wang, K.; Wang, Y. Emerging Function and Clinical Significance of Extracellular Vesicle Noncoding RNAs in Lung Cancer. *Mol. Ther. Oncolytics* **2022**, *24*, 814–833. [CrossRef]
123. Cao, H.; Zhang, P.; Yu, H.; Xi, J. Extracellular Vesicles-Encapsulated MiR-153-3p Potentiate the Survival and Invasion of Lung Adenocarcinoma. *Mol. Cells* **2022**, *45*, 376–387. [CrossRef]
124. Poroyko, V.; Mirzapoiazova, T.; Nam, A.; Mambetsariev, I.; Mambetsariev, B.; Wu, X.; Husain, A.; Vokes, E.E.; Wheeler, D.L.; Salgia, R. Exosomal MiRNAs Species in the Blood of Small Cell and Non-Small Cell Lung Cancer Patients. *Oncotarget* **2018**, *9*, 19793–19806. [CrossRef]
125. Duréndez-Sáez, E.; Torres-Martinez, S.; Calabuig-Fariñas, S.; Meri-Abad, M.; Ferrero-Gimeno, M.; Camps, C. Exosomal MicroR-NAs in Non-Small Cell Lung Cancer. *Transl. Cancer Res.* **2021**, *10*, 3128–3139. [CrossRef]
126. Zheng, R.; Du, M.; Tian, M.; Zhu, Z.; Wei, C.; Chu, H.; Gan, C.; Liang, J.; Xue, R.; Gao, F.; et al. Fine Particulate Matter Induces Childhood Asthma Attacks via Extracellular Vesicle-Packaged Let-7i-5p-Mediated Modulation of the MAPK Signaling Pathway. *Adv. Sci.* **2022**, *9*, e2102460. [CrossRef]

Disclaimer/Publisher's Note: The statements, opinions and data contained in all publications are solely those of the individual author(s) and contributor(s) and not of MDPI and/or the editor(s). MDPI and/or the editor(s) disclaim responsibility for any injury to people or property resulting from any ideas, methods, instructions or products referred to in the content.

MDPI AG
Grosspeteranlage 5
4052 Basel
Switzerland
Tel.: +41 61 683 77 34

Cancers Editorial Office
E-mail: cancers@mdpi.com
www.mdpi.com/journal/cancers

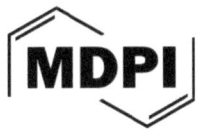

Disclaimer/Publisher's Note: The title and front matter of this reprint are at the discretion of the Guest Editors. The publisher is not responsible for their content or any associated concerns. The statements, opinions and data contained in all individual articles are solely those of the individual Editors and contributors and not of MDPI. MDPI disclaims responsibility for any injury to people or property resulting from any ideas, methods, instructions or products referred to in the content.

www.ingramcontent.com/pod-product-compliance
Lightning Source LLC
LaVergne TN
LVHW072355090526
838202LV00019B/2552